The laboratory, or school of arts: in which are faithfully exhibited and fully explain'd, A variety of curious and valuable experiments in refining, A dissertation on the nature and growth of saltpetre. The second edition

Godfrey Smith

The laboratory, or school of arts: in which are faithfully exhibited and fully explain'd, I. A variety of curious and valuable experiments in refining, ... VI. A dissertation on the nature and growth of saltpetre : ... The second edition. Illustrated with

Smith, Godfrey
ESTCID: T072112
Reproduction from British Library
Compiled and translated by Godfrey Smith, who signs the dedication. A reissue of the 1738 edition, with a cancel title page, and with the addition of a separately paginated appendix with separate titlepage and register. The appendix is priced and was pr
London : printed for J. Hodges; J. James; and T. Cooper, 1740.
[8],242;[2],lxxx;[6]p.,plates ; 8°

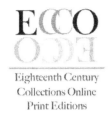

Eighteenth Century
Collections Online
Print Editions

Gale ECCO Print Editions

Relive history with *Eighteenth Century Collections Online*, now available in print for the independent historian and collector. This series includes the most significant English-language and foreign-language works printed in Great Britain during the eighteenth century, and is organized in seven different subject areas including literature and language; medicine, science, and technology; and religion and philosophy. The collection also includes thousands of important works from the Americas.

The eighteenth century has been called "The Age of Enlightenment." It was a period of rapid advance in print culture and publishing, in world exploration, and in the rapid growth of science and technology – all of which had a profound impact on the political and cultural landscape. At the end of the century the American Revolution, French Revolution and Industrial Revolution, perhaps three of the most significant events in modern history, set in motion developments that eventually dominated world political, economic, and social life.

In a groundbreaking effort, Gale initiated a revolution of its own: digitization of epic proportions to preserve these invaluable works in the largest online archive of its kind. Contributions from major world libraries constitute over 175,000 original printed works. Scanned images of the actual pages, rather than transcriptions, recreate the works *as they first appeared.*

Now for the first time, these high-quality digital scans of original works are available via print-on-demand, making them readily accessible to libraries, students, independent scholars, and readers of all ages.

For our initial release we have created seven robust collections to form one the world's most comprehensive catalogs of 18th century works.

Initial Gale ECCO Print Editions collections include:

History and Geography
Rich in titles on English life and social history, this collection spans the world as it was known to eighteenth-century historians and explorers. Titles include a wealth of travel accounts and diaries, histories of nations from throughout the world, and maps and charts of a world that was still being discovered. Students of the War of American Independence will find fascinating accounts from the British side of conflict.

Social Science

Delve into what it was like to live during the eighteenth century by reading the first-hand accounts of everyday people, including city dwellers and farmers, businessmen and bankers, artisans and merchants, artists and their patrons, politicians and their constituents. Original texts make the American, French, and Industrial revolutions vividly contemporary.

Medicine, Science and Technology

Medical theory and practice of the 1700s developed rapidly, as is evidenced by the extensive collection, which includes descriptions of diseases, their conditions, and treatments. Books on science and technology, agriculture, military technology, natural philosophy, even cookbooks, are all contained here.

Literature and Language

Western literary study flows out of eighteenth-century works by Alexander Pope, Daniel Defoe, Henry Fielding, Frances Burney, Denis Diderot, Johann Gottfried Herder, Johann Wolfgang von Goethe, and others. Experience the birth of the modern novel, or compare the development of language using dictionaries and grammar discourses.

Religion and Philosophy

The Age of Enlightenment profoundly enriched religious and philosophical understanding and continues to influence present-day thinking. Works collected here include masterpieces by David Hume, Immanuel Kant, and Jean-Jacques Rousseau, as well as religious sermons and moral debates on the issues of the day, such as the slave trade. The Age of Reason saw conflict between Protestantism and Catholicism transformed into one between faith and logic -- a debate that continues in the twenty-first century.

Law and Reference

This collection reveals the history of English common law and Empire law in a vastly changing world of British expansion. Dominating the legal field is the *Commentaries of the Law of England* by Sir William Blackstone, which first appeared in 1765. Reference works such as almanacs and catalogues continue to educate us by revealing the day-to-day workings of society.

Fine Arts

The eighteenth-century fascination with Greek and Roman antiquity followed the systematic excavation of the ruins at Pompeii and Herculaneum in southern Italy; and after 1750 a neoclassical style dominated all artistic fields. The titles here trace developments in mostly English-language works on painting, sculpture, architecture, music, theater, and other disciplines. Instructional works on musical instruments, catalogs of art objects, comic operas, and more are also included.

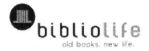

The BiblioLife Network

This project was made possible in part by the BiblioLife Network (BLN), a project aimed at addressing some of the huge challenges facing book preservationists around the world. The BLN includes libraries, library networks, archives, subject matter experts, online communities and library service providers. We believe every book ever published should be available as a high-quality print reproduction; printed on-demand anywhere in the world. This insures the ongoing accessibility of the content and helps generate sustainable revenue for the libraries and organizations that work to preserve these important materials.

The following book is in the "public domain" and represents an authentic reproduction of the text as printed by the original publisher. While we have attempted to accurately maintain the integrity of the original work, there are sometimes problems with the original work or the micro-film from which the books were digitized. This can result in minor errors in reproduction. Possible imperfections include missing and blurred pages, poor pictures, markings and other reproduction issues beyond our control. Because this work is culturally important, we have made it available as part of our commitment to protecting, preserving, and promoting the world's literature.

GUIDE TO FOLD-OUTS MAPS and OVERSIZED IMAGES

The book you are reading was digitized from microfilm captured over the past thirty to forty years. Years after the creation of the original microfilm, the book was converted to digital files and made available in an online database.

In an online database, page images do not need to conform to the size restrictions found in a printed book. When converting these images back into a printed bound book, the page sizes are standardized in ways that maintain the detail of the original. For large images, such as fold-out maps, the original page image is split into two or more pages

Guidelines used to determine how to split the page image follows:

• Some images are split vertically; large images require vertical and horizontal splits.
• For horizontal splits, the content is split left to right.
• For vertical splits, the content is split from top to bottom.
• For both vertical and horizontal splits, the image is processed from top left to bottom right.

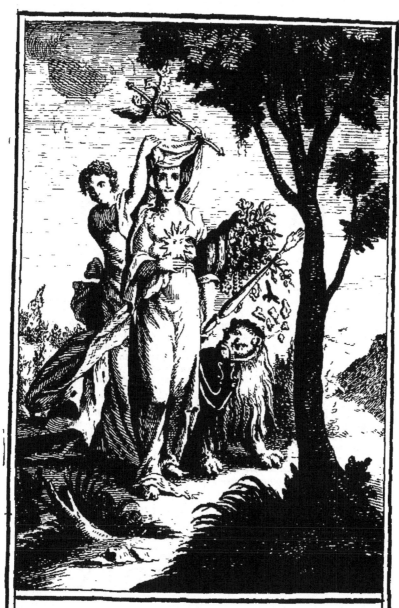

No vulgar Eye enjoys a fond Delight
In Nature Beauty and Productions bright,
This nursing Mother, is ye Second Cause
Of Plenty, Life, and uncontroling Laws,
When Art doth Court her, She unveils her Face,
And shews her Charms to her adopted Race

THE
LABORATORY,
OR
SCHOOL *of* ARTS:

In which

Are faithfully exhibited and fully explain'd,

I A Variety of curious and valuable Experiments in Refining, Calcining, Melting, Assaying, Casting, Allaying, and Toughening of *Gold* With several other Curiosities relating to *Gold* and *Silver*

II Choice Secrets for *Jewellers* in the Management of *Gold* in *Enameling*, and the Preparation of *Enamel* Colours, with the Art of copying Precious Stones of preparing Colours for *Doublets*; of colouring *Foyles* for *Jewels*, together with other rare Secrets

III Several uncommon Experiments for Casting in *Silver, Copper, Brass, Tin, Steel*, and other Metals, likewise in *Wax, Plaifter of Paris,*

Wood, Horn, &c With the Management of the respective Moulds

IV The *Art* of making *Glass* Exhibiting withal the Art of Painting and making Impressions upon *Glass* and of laying thereon Gold or Silver, together with the Method of preparing the Colours for *Potters-work*, or *Delft ware*

V A Collection of very valuable Secrets for the Use of *Cutlers, Pewterers, Brasiers, Joiners, Turners, Japanners, Book binders, Distillers, Lapidaries, Limners,* &c

VI A Dissertation on the Nature and Growth of *Saltpetre* Also, several other choice and uncommon *Experiments*

The SECOND EDITION.

Illuftrated with COPPER-PLATES

To which is added

An APPENDIX:

TEACHING

I The Art and Management of Dying *Silks, Worfteds, Cottons,* &c. in various Colours

II The Art of preparing *Rockets, Crackers, Fire globes, Stars, Sparks,* &c. for Recreative *Fire works.*

Translated from the HIGH DUTCH.

LONDON

Printed for J HODGES, at the *Looking glass* on *London Bridge*, J JAMES, at *Horace's Head* under the *Royal Exchange*, and T. COOPER, at the *Globe* in *Pater-nofter Row*

M,D,CC,XL.

1740

JAMES THEOBALD, *Esq.*
F. R. S.

A Dedication fill'd with Flattery and Compliments, would, I know, be as unacceptable and diſpleaſing for you to read, as it would be improper and diſagreeable for me to write.

YOUR Affability, Candour, Openeſs of Heart, and the many Civilities you have for ſeveral Years paſt, condeſcended to honour me with on the one Hand; and the Delight and Pleaſure you take in the Search and Knowledge of the various Productions and Curioſities of

A 2   Art

DEDICATION.

Art and Nature, on the other Hand, are,
I hope, sufficient to excuse the Freedom
I take in offering and inscribing these
my mean Endeavours to your Patro-
nage and Protection; and in laying hold
of this Opportunity to assure you of
my Gratitude, and of the Value and
Esteem I have, and will always enter-
tain for your Person, Merit and Friend-
ship.

BE pleased, Sir, to accept of this
with the sincere Wishes for your long
Life and Prosperity, from,

S I R,

Y O U R most obedient

and most humble

Servant,

G. SMITH

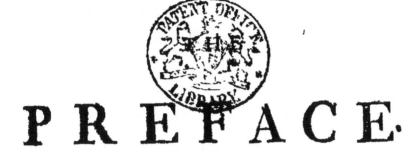

PREFACE.

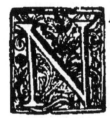ATURE, the Mother of all visible Beings, or, to speak more Christian-like, the Wisdom and Power of God has shewn itself throughout the Universe, in the most admirable and surprising Productions The Wonders and innumerable Curiosities of our particular System ravish the Eyes of every Beholder, who is thereby prompted to acknowledge and adore the Supreme Being, and first intelligent Cause of so glorious a Frame

But the Manifestation of Gods Perfections, was not the only Design of such a Profuseness and Variety of Wonders, it was also design'd for the present Use and Benefit of Mankind. In them we find a Plenty of every thing to supply our Wants, and all Manner of Helps to bring to Perfection the most useful Arts. For though Nature has hid the best, and even the richest Part of her Productions, either in the Deep, or in the Bowels of the Earth; yet is she willing and ready to lay her Treasures open to our diligent Enquiries,

to

to our Contemplation and Use. The more a Man applies himself to such Researches, the better he answers the End of his Creation. But the less he is indued with that Spirit of Enquiry, the nearer he resembles the Brutes, who enjoy the present Objects, without reflecting on their Beauty, Variety, and Usefulness, without minding any thing else but what makes an actual Impression upon their Senses. Such are the People who tread under-foot Arts and Ingenuity, and despise those who apply to Mechanicks, and do their Endeavours to be as useful in that Respect to their Fellow Creatures, as in them lies.

I don't doubt but there will be many of that Kind (for of such the World abounds) who will set their Wits at work to find fault with this Performance, either as to the intrinsick Merit of it, the Truth of some Experiments, or the Translator's Stile. But to be beforehand with those Gentlemen, and to save them some Trouble, I freely own my self to be a Foreigner, that has had no great Share of School, much less of University Learning. Nevertheless, I can say without Pride, that I am not destitute of Common Sense and Reading.

I have endeavour'd to translate this Work in as plain, easy and intelligible a Manner as I am Master of, and if there is any Fault, in Point of Grammar or Orthography, I hope Gentlemen of good Sense and good Nature will easily excuse such Trifles, in Consideration of the Goodness of the Work itself. It was not design'd for profess'd Scholars, but for People of Ingenuity and Lovers of Arts.

As to the Truth of the Experiments mentioned in it, I must own, that had my Fortune answer'd my Inclination, I would have carefully try'd them all before-hand. But I leave that to those Gentlemen whose Ingenuity and Purse may go together, to satisfy their Curiosity. I have however try'd some of them, and they

they have anfwered my Expectation, which gives me room to believe that the reſt are as true. Befides, I have confulted about it People whoſe Province it was to be better acquainted with thoſe Particulars. Or, when I could not have ſuch an Opportunity, I have weigh'd them the beſt I was able, and duly examined their Probability, and the Credit of the Authors thereof. So I dare ſay, that moſt (if not all) of thoſe Experiments will ſtand the Teſt.

WHILE this Book was in the Preſs, I have had ſome Hints given me, that the Publication thereof would give Offence to thoſe Tradeſmen or Artificers, whoſe Myſteries in their reſpective Profeſſions would be by that means lay'd open to every Body. But as this Argument ſeem'd to me to be of little Weight, I did not think proper to deſiſt from my Undertaking. Thoſe that are in a good Way of Bufineſs, will hardly negleſt it or leave it off, in Hopes of making a better Fortune by trying the Experiments mentioned in this Work: And thoſe that get only their Livelihood by their Trade, will find ſo many Difficulti′ ſand Obſtruſtions in ſuch Trials, that they will never be able to go thro' them. But ſuppoſing ſome ingenious Perſon ſhould by following theſe Experiments, better his Fortune, and diftinguiſh himſelf in his Profeſſion (as no doubt it may happen ſo) where ſhould be the Harm? Muſt a Man for fear of difpleaſing a few private Perſons, hide Things whoſe Knowledge not only would prove entertaining but alſo advantageous to the Publick, and hinder Thouſands of People of their Satisfaſtion in curious Inquiries.

My Aim, in the Publication of this Book, is not to hurt Any Body or any Set of Men in their Profeſſions, God forbid! But it is (to ſpeak ingenuouſly) firſt to get Money in an honeſt Way, which is no doubt the main View of moſt Authors, though they dare not own it publickly, as I do here, and ſecondly to oblige the World, eſpecially the Curious who are

Lovers

The PREFACE.

Lovers of Art and Ingenuity, and take a Pleasure in try-ing Experiments of one Sort or other, Amusements much more delightful and satisfactory to some Gentle-men than Gaming, Hunting, or Reading of Novels, Ballads, and such like The Artists and Crafts-Men will also, I hope, find it a very useful Performance They will perhaps make some new and advantageous Discoveries in it, relating to their Trade, which they never knew before The Selfishness and Ill-nature of some Masters is such, that they will keep their Apprentices ignorant of the most essential Parts of their Business, employ them during seven Years on particular Branches, and conceal from them what they themselves do in a private Room It concerns those who have labour'd, or do labour under such an unjust or ungenerous Proceeding, to strive to be better inform'd in all the Branches of their Trade: And to many of such this Book, I venture to affirm, will not be a needless Purchase, if they peruse it with Attention, and will try the Experiments, as far as it lies in their Power

I hope these my Endeavours will meet with a fa-vourable Reception from the Publick, as they are the Fruits of a good Intention, presented to the Curious with Sincerity

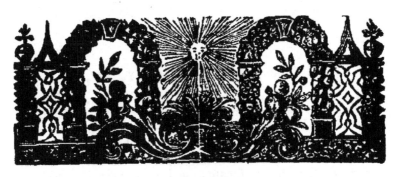

LABORATORY,

SCHOOL of ARTS, &c.

6 7c 08

PART I.

A Variety of Curious and Valuable Experiments in *Refining, Calcining, Melting, Affaying, Cafting, Allaying* and *Toughening* of GOLD, with feveral other Curiofities relating to GOLD and SILVER

S *Gold*, of all other Metals is the moft noble and moft valuable, it is juftly diftinguifh'd from all the reft by the Name of the *King of Metals* *Europe*, as well as the other Parts of the World, affords feveral Gold Mines, but *Peru* in the *Spanifh Weft Indies* particularly abounds in them, and as they contain the richeft Oar, almoft every Nation endeavours to be furnifh'd and fupply'd therewith

Of all Metals, Gold is the moft folid It confifts of Particles fo fine and clofely interwoven, that it is a difficult Matter to feparate them from one another It will refift the Fire, and not fuffer any Diminution by the Heat thereof, though never fo fierce and violent. It is not fubject to ruft, but retains its natural Colour Its Weight is ten times heavier then Earth, and a Piece of Gold contains feven times the Matter what a Piece of

B

Glafs

Glaſs doth of the ſame Magnitude It is of a Malleable Temper, and ſpreads under a Hammer more than any other Metal, and by the Hand of a ſkilful Artiſt, may be wrought into any Form or Shape There is no ſolid Body that can be extended ſo much than Gold, one Ounce of it being capable to furniſh 750 Leaves, each of four Inches ſquare , and it is affirm'd, that one Ounce, thus beaten out, would cover 10 Acres of Ground. Wire-Drawers extend out of an Ounce of Gold a Thread of 230800 Foot long

THE fineſt Metal, next to Gold, is Silver, which is of a more ſmooth and poliſhed Nature than Gold, and is as malleable, but will not ſo eaſily yield or extend under the Hammer, neither is it ſo weighty as Gold

SILVER is ſeldom found in Mines by itſelf, but commonly accompanied or mixed with *Copper*, *Lead*, or *Gold* That mixed among *Lead* lies in a Kind of black Oar, but what is found in *Copper*, is for the generality in a hard white Oar, reſembling Cryſtal Sometimes Pieces of pure Silver are found in Mines, ſo hard that it cannot be melted without the Addition of a Quantity of other Silver

Of REFINING

REFINING or purifying of Gold or Silver, is an Art by which the Impurities that are mix'd with theſe Metals, are ſeparated, and this is generally done, when in large Quantities, by the * *Teſt*, and in ſmall Quantities, by the † *Coppel*, in the following Manner.   TAKE

---

* The *Teſt* is a round Iron Ring, ſome are made Oval, about two or three, or more Inches deep , according to their largeneſs, and the Quantity of the Silver to be refin d This Ring is fill d with Wood-Aſhes well cleanſed and preſſed very cloſe At the Top there is a Cavity, commonly ſunk with an Iron Canon-Ball, for to contain the Silver Before the Aſhes are quite dry, you put a Cloth over it with fine Aſhes of Trotter-Bones, which you ſift upon, through a fine Hair Sive, then place it on a Tile, in a Wind Furnace, cover it with a Muffel, and make it red Hot, when ſo, then put in the Silver to be refined Vid Plate I Fig 1

† The *Coppel* is made like an earthen Cup, not glas'd, but able to withſtand the Fire, this is lin d throughout with a Paſte, made either of Wood-Aſhes, or the Aſhes of Bones, mixed up to a Maſs with either ſtrong Beer, Siſs, or the Whites of Eggs. The Wood-Aſhes are waſh d in ſeveral Waters, till they have loſt all their Filt and Salt, and the Water comes off clear and ſweet, as when firſt put on The Bone-Aſhes looſe their Salt in the Fire, and are commonly burnt of Trotter-Bones, or thoſe of Calfs-Head,

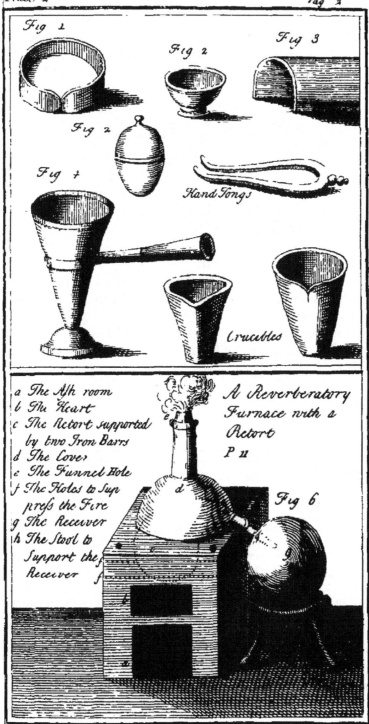

Fig 1

Fig 2

Fig 3

Fig 2

Fig 4

Hand Tongs

Crucibles

a The Ash room
b The Heart
c The Retort supported
by two Iron Barrs
d The Cover
e The Funnel Hole
f The Holes to Sup
press the Fire
g The Receiver
h The Stool to
Support the
Receiver

A Reverberatory
Furnace with a
Retort
P 11

Fig 6

Hulett Sculp

TAKE your Coppel, and put it under a † Muffel, which cover all over with live Coals, adding dead ones to them, and by Degrees augmenting the Heat, till both the *Muffel* and *Coppel* are red hot   Then put, according to your Quantity of Silver, a proportionable Quantity of Lead into the *Coppel*, which is commonly four parts of Lead to one part of Gold or Silver   When the Lead is melted, and of a sparkling and fine Quickfilver Colour, then put your Gold or Silver upon it, and it will melt presently   Give it a brisk Fire, and the baser Metals will mix and unite with the Lead, but the Gold or Silver remain in the middle, clean and purified from all Drofs, which fixes itself to the Sides like a Scum, this you take off, preventing its entering into the Pores of the Coppel, and this is what is commonly known by the Name of *Litharge*, and according to the Degree of Calcination becomes of diverse Colours, fome is call'd *Litharge of Gold*, and fome *Litharge of Silver*   Continue the Fire till you obferve no rifing of Fumes.

By thefe Means Gold and Silver is feparated or purified from other Metals, except the Silver from Gold, or the Gold from Silver, the Separation of thefe two Metals being accomplifh'd after another manner, commonly call'd *Departing*, and is perform'd in the following Manner

To feparate Silver from Gold.

PUT three Parts, or more, of Silver, to one part of Gold, into a Crucible, give it a brisk Fire, and when in Fusion, granulate it, then, after you have dry'd the Grains, put them into *Aqua Fortis*, wherein the Silver will diffolve, and the Gold will precipitate and fettle to the Bottom, in a Powder   After the Gold is fettled, pour off the Diffolution of Silver, wafh the Gold Powder with clean Water, and fweeten it from all the fharpnefs of the *Aqua Fortis*   Then dry and melt it

---

Heads, fome prefer Fifh Bones before any other   The Afhes, which foever are ufed muft be fifted through a fine Hair Sive   After having prepared this Pafte or Mafs, the Cup is lined all over the Infide very finoo h and neat leaving only a Cavity or a hollow in the middle, to hold the Matter that is to be *Coppel'd*, and then it is fet to dry   The Size of thefe *Coppels* are made to the Quantity of the Metal to be purifed See Plate I Fig 2

† A Muffel is made of one Part of Clay mix'd with one Part of Sand, and two Parts of Horfe Dung   Work up this, frit in a fquare Flat, with a Rowling Pin, to the Thicknefs of a Crown Piece and then bend it in to an Arch, and Let it dry Some only ufe Pipe Clay by itfelf See Plate I Fig 3

in a fmall Crucible, with a little *Borax* or *Saltpetre*; and when in Fufion, and looks of a bright Colour, caft it into an Ingot or Mould you have for that purpofe.

To bring the Solution of the Silver into a Body, pour it in a thick-bottom'd Copper Bowl, that is thorough clean; add to it ten times the Quantity of clean Water, and the whole will turn of a Sky Colour, fling a little Salt into it, ftir it about with a clean wooden Stick, and the Silver will precipitate to the Bottom, of the Confiftence of a thin Pafte After it has fettled for three Hours, or longer, pour off the Water into another clean Copper Bowl, and add fome warm Water to the Settlement, this will alfo turn of a Sky Colour, but paler than the firft Repeat this till the Water comes off clear, and the Silver remains free from all Sharpnefs or Salt Warm the firft blue Water in the Bowl, fling a little Salt into it, and the Silver that remaind, will fettle at the bottom Pour off the Water, dry the Settlements, and then, after you have greas'd or wax'd your Crucible, melt them therein with a little Borax.

How to granulate Silver in the beft Manner.

TAKE a Twig or two of a Birch Broom, with thefe ftir the Water, in which you defign to granulate, in a circular Motion, at the fame time pour your Silver with difcretion into it, between the Branches of the Twigs, and the Procefs will anfwer to your Satisfaction

To feparate Gold from Silver

TAKE Silver, which contains Gold, as it comes from the Coppel or Teft, granulate it, or elfe caft it into an Ingot, then hammer it into thin Plates, and cut them in little Pieces, fo as to be eafily convey'd through the Neck of the Matrafs Then pour to one Ounce of Silver, two Ounces of *Aqua Fortis*, ftop your Matrafs, yet fo as to give it a little Vent, place it over a gentle Coal Fire, and let it leifurely advance to working and boiling, continuing it thus till the Silver is wholly diffolv'd, and the *Aqua Fortis* looks of a clear Colour If the Silver contained any Gold, you will fee it fettled at the Bottom of the Matrafs, in a blackifh Powder, but if there appears little or no black Settlement, it is a Sign the Silver contain'd no Gold   Iou a

POUR off the Silver Water very gently and carefully into a Glafs or Pan, for in every Drop thereof is a Mixture of Silver, but take particular Care of the black Settlement, for that is the Gold Calx

To this Silver Water put ten times as much of Rain or River Water, which is better than that of Springs, and at the Bottom of the Pan, put a Plate of Copper red hot, this will caufe the Silver to precipitate to the Bottom, and by Degrees hang itfelf to the Plate, and cover it

ON the black Settlement pour about an Inch heigh of clear Water, which will for the firft and fecond time turn whitifh, becaufe of the Silver that remains therein, this Water put to that in the Glafs, and keep on pouring of Water on the Gold Calx, till it comes off clear Then put the Gold Calx in a fmall Crucible, drain off the Water, and let it dry, mett it in the fame Crucible with a little Borax, and you will have the pureft Gold

To try whether there is any Silver remaining in the Water, fling a little Salt in it, and let it ftand all Night to fettle, if there is any, the water will turn turbulent and cloudy, but if there is no Silver remaining, the Salt will fettle at the bottom of the Glafs, and the Water remain clear After it has fettled 24 Hours, or more, pour off the clear Water from the Top, and the Settlement, which is the Silver Calx, put into a Crucible, which has been warmed, and the Infide wax'd all over, in this let the Calx fettle, then pour off the clear Water When the Calx is dry, melt it as has been directed, and you will have the pureft Silver for Ufe This is the fhorteft Manner of feparating thefe Metals.

To refine Gold when coarfe, by cafting it through Antimony.

TAKE to one ounce of Gold four ounces of *Antimony*, melt the Gold in a proportionable Crucible, at the fame time put the *Antimony* in another larger Crucible, and let that alfo be melted, when both are melted, caft the Gold into the melted *Antimony*, then make it red hot, when it is fo, caft it into a Brafs * *Cone*, but let the Infide be a little warmed and greafed with Tallow before you ufe it; then with a Piece of Wood, or with the Handle of a Hammer knock pretty hard and quick upon the

---

* See the Figure of a *Cone*, Plate I. Fig 4.

Rim,

Rim, which helps the Gold's sinking to the Bottom, when cold, turn it out of the *Cone,* and you will see the *Regulus;* beat it gently off with a Hammer, and lay it by   Then take the *Antimory,* put it in the same Crucible, melt it as before, and separate it from the   *Gold*   When turned out, you will find a little *Regulus,* and if you think you have not all your Gold, you may repeat it a third time When this is done, in order to separate the remaining *Antimony* from the Gold, do it thus. Take a pretty large Crucible, put the *Regulus,* and a Handful of *Saltpeter* into it, then take another Crucible that fits in the former, make a Vent-Hole in the Bottom of it, and turn it upside down, that the Hole may come uppermost. When the wide Ends of the Crucibles fit well, take a Lutum, mix it with some pounded Glass, and lute it well, let it dry very well before a Fire, then take a Brick-bat, put it in your melting Place, and lute your Crucible upon it Then lay a little Fire around it, upon that lay dead Charcoal, up to the Top of the upper Crucible, but take care the Hole be not covered As the Heat of the Fire augments, so the *Saltpeter* goes off in strong Fumes through the Hole. When the Fumes cease, give it a strong Heat for an Hour long, or less, according to your Quantity, then take your Crucible out of the Fire, and let it cool, or else when you see the Crucible turn black, you may quench it in a Pail of Water; knock off the Bottom of the Crucible, and you will find your Gold, fine in a Cake, then take a clean proportionable Crucible, put a little *Borax* and the Gold into it, and melt and cast it into an Ingot   This is the finest Gold that can be

A Method of purifying Gold, by way of Cementation.

CEMENTATION is a singular and useful Art, by which Gold may be purified from the Allay it may have of any other Metals, and this is done by Virtue of a moistened Powder, which eats and consumes the impurer Metals from it: But it is to be observ'd, that this Cementation is only to be made use of where the Gold has the Predominancy, otherwise if there should be more Silver or other Metal than Gold, it is better to perform the Separation with *Aqua Fortis,* as has been directed

THE Cementing Powders are prepared of such Salts and Ingredients as attack, and with their Sharpness devour the Silver or Copper.

To thefe are alfo added, * *Æs uftum*, which gives the Gold a fine Colour, *Blood-ftone*, *Tutia*, *Crocus Martis*, calcin'd *Vitriol*, and feveral other Things, as are inducive to advance the Beauty of that Metal

BRICK Duft is ufed in this Cement, in order to receive the Allay, let it be Silver or Copper, or what it will, from the Ingredients that draw and feparate them from the Gold, which otherwife would ftick and hang to the Gold I fhall here fet down a few Receipts of fuch Cements as have been experienc'd, and are approv'd off

TAKE fine Brick Duft, one part, and fine beaten Salt, one part, moiften and mix it with Vinegar, and with it fill a Crucible half full, then ftratify Plates of Gold, or Gold Coin, and the forefaid Mixture or Pafte, and prefs it clofe down, repeat this as you have Occafion, and give it a thick Lay at Top, then cover and lute the Crucible clofe, that nothing may evaporate When this is done, fix your Crucible upon a high Brick, in the Middle of the Furnace, give it a violent Heat for 12 Hours, and the Salt will eat and confume the Impurities of the Gold, and draw it into the Brick-Duft

Another

TAKE in Weight one part of Saltpeter, one part of Allum, one part of Sal-armoniack, two parts of Vitriol, four parts of Salt, eight parts of Brick-duft, and mix it with Vinegar, ftratify this and the Gold, as before directed, in the Crucible, cover and lute it well, and give it a violent Fire for an Hour or two and let it cool of itfelf, but before it is quite cold, take out the Gold, fling it into White-Wine Vinegar, and boil it therein, then brufh it, and after you have done this, heat it red hot upon an Iron Plate

Another

TAKE Blood-ftone two Ounces, Ruft of Iron one Ounce, calcined Vitriol one Ounce, Sal-armoniack one Ounce, Verdegreafe one Ounce, Boli-armeniæ $\frac{1}{4}$ of an ounce, Tutia $\frac{1}{4}$

---

* *Æs uftum* is prepared thus Stratify Plates of Copper with powdered Sulphur in a large Crucible, cover and lute it with a Cover that has a Hole in the Middle, to give vent for the Fumitation, give it a ftrong Fire in a Wind-Furnace, fo long till you fee no exhalation of Vapours; then take off your Plates whilft hot, feparate them, and when cold, beat them to a Powder Which is the *Æs uftum*.

of

of an ounce, Salt-petre ⅛ of an ounce, Allum ¼ of an ounce, moisten this three or four times with Vinegar, let it dry between while, grind it fine, and proceed as directed, give it a strong Fire for three Hours, which repeat three times

To bring the Silver out of the Cementing Powder or Brick-dust, mix it with Glass and granulated Lead, let it melt together, put it to the Test, and you will have the Silver again which was in the Gold

To separate Gold and Silver, out of the Sweepings

TAKE Sweepings, put them into a Pan well glazed, add Mercury to them, in Quantity as you think proper, mix and mingle the Dust and Mercury with your Hands well together, so long till you think the Mercury has contracted all the Gold and Silver from the Dust, then put the Mass into a Piece of Wash-leather, and wring out the Mercury, what remains in the Leather will be like a Paste, put that into a Alembick, and drive the Mercury from it into a Dish with Water, which you put under the Head to receive it, what remains, put to the Test, refine it with Lead, and separate it with *Aqua Fortis*

To separate the Gold from gilded Copper

TAKE four ounces of yellow Brimstone, two ounces of Sal armoniack, one ounce of Saltpetre, half an ounce of Borax, take these and grind them fine and clear with strong Vinegar, to a Paste, this wipe thin over the gilded Copper, give it a gentle Heat, till the Paste is burned away, and the Copper looks black, then take it out, and with a Knife or other such Instrument scrape off the Gold in a clean Dish, and it will come off very easy.

Another Method.

TAKE the Root of *Bertram*, cut it fine, pour one Quart of strong White wine Vinegar upon it, put it into a boiling-Pot, cover it with a Lid, lute it well, and let it boil a little, then take it from the Fire, and let it cool. After this take your Copper Cup or other Thing that is gilded, real it well, quench it in that Liquid, and the Gold will peel off the Copper and fall to the Bottom, which wash, and then melt together in a Crucible

Another

Another Way

TAKE fine Sal armoniack two parts, Sulphur one part, grind it well together, anoint your Work with Linfeed Oil, ftrew the Powder upon it, hold the Utenfil of Copper to the Fire, over an earthen Difh with Water, beat againft it with an Iron, and the Gold will fall off into the Difh

Another Way

TAKE Saltpetre and Borax, one ounce of each, diffolve it in a little Quantity of Water, then neal your Copper, and quench it in this Water, repeat this feveral Times, and the Gold will fall to the Bottom

Another Way to feparate the Gold from any gilded Metal, Silver or Copper

TAKE one part of Borax, and three parts of live Sulphur, grind this together with very ftrong Whitewine Vinegar, as thick as Oil Colour, with this wipe the gilded Side of the Metal, let it dry gently before a Fire, and when dry, wipe this Compofition with a Feather, into a Bafon with Water, wafh and melt it, as has been taught before.

To fepaiate Copper fiom Silver, let it be Money or any Thing elfe

TAKE half an ounce of Verditer or Spanifh Green, White Vitriol one ounce, Sulphur one ounce, Allum half an ounce, feeth all together in Vinegar, in a Glafs, put in your mixt Silver, this will diffolve and extract the Copper, and the Silver remain whole

To extract the Silver out of a Ring that is ftrong gilded, fo as to keep the Gold intire, a curious Secret.

TAKE a Silver Ring that is ftrong gilded, pierce a little Hole through the Gold into the Silver, then lay the Ring into Spirit of Nitre, and put it in a warm Place, it will hollow out the Silver, and the Gold remain whole

To

To make Brittle Gold malleable

PUT Gold into a Crucible, and give it a brisk Fire in a Wind-Furnace, or before the Bellows, when the Gold is nigh melting, then fling gently upon it some good, dry and clear *Saltpetre*, which will presently turn into Flames, and occasion the Fusion of the Gold the sooner, and the *Saltpetre* will spread and cover the Gold, then cast it into an Ingot, which before has been warm'd and anointed over with Wax.

Another Method

THE best way of all to make Gold malleable, is this Take human Excrements, which dry, and calcine in a Crucible to a black Powder, when the Gold is in Fusion, then fling some of this Powder upon it, and give it a brisk Fire, when the Powder is consumed, cast the Gold into an Ingot, and it will be fine and malleable If you extract the Salt from the black Powder before you use it, it will still have a better Effect, and that with a less Quantity

To make Silver that is brittle, pliable

TAKE one Mark of Silver, half an Ounce of Glass, one Ounce of Saltpetre, a quarter of an Ounce of *Borax*, half an Ounce of *Sal Gemmæ*, put all this into a Crucible, and cover it with a lesser one that has a Vent-hole at Bottom, and lute it well, Then give it a brisk Fire, and continue it so long 'till you think the Silver is dissolv'd, then cover the Crucibles all over with live Coals, except the Vent-hole, and leave it till cold Take off the Upper Crucible, and you will find therein hanging all the Filthiness and Impurities the Silver contain'd, and was the Occasion of its hardness. Then melt the Silver again in a Crucible, and fling into it half an Ounce of *Tartar* finely ground, and when in Fusion, cast it into an Ingot, and you will have fine and malleable Silver

To give Gold, Silver or other Metals a good and quick Fusion.

TAKE calcined *Venetian* Soap, Borax, Glass gall, or *Venice* Glass, of one as much as the other, grind it well and mix it together, it will cause a quick Fusion

Another

Another.

TAKE yellow Amber, Borax, Glafs-gall and Soap, even Quantities, grind them together to a Powder, and what you defign to caft, let it be melted with that Compofition

To try whether granulated Silver contains any Gold.

TAKE fome of thofe Silver Grains, and rub them on a Touch-ftone, then with the End of a Feather drop one or two Drops of *Aqua Fortis* upon the Strokes, let it ftand upon it for a little while, if it contains Gold, you will fee fome remains of the Strokes, but if not, the Strokes will be vanifh'd.

To Amalgamate Gold, or to mix it with Mercury, ufeful for Gilders

TAKE a penny weight of fine Gold, beat it in very thin little Plates, heat them in a Crucible red hot, then pour upon it 8 penny-weight of Quickfilver, † revived from Cinnaber; ftir the Matter with a little Iron Rod, and when you fee it begin to rife in Fumes, which quickly happens, caft your Mixture into an earthen Pan, fill'd with Water, it will coagulate, and become tractable, wafh it feveral times to take away its Blacknefs; Thus you have an *Amalgama*; from which feparate the Mercury which you find is not united, by preffing it between your Fingers, after you have wrapt it in a Linnen Cloth.

Gilding upon Silver, Brafs, Copper, and Iron

IF you will gild Silver, take of the forefaid *Amalgama*, and with it rub that which you defign to gild, clofe

---

† Reviving of Quickfilver from Cinnaber is thus perform'd Take a pound of Artificial Cinnaber powder it, and mix it exactly with three Pound of Quick lime, alfo powdered, put the Mixture into an Earthen Pot, or Glafs Retort, whofe third part at leaft remains empty, place it into a Reverberatory Furnace, and after having fitted to it a Receiver filled with Water, let it reft 24 Hours at leaft, give your Fire by Degrees and at laft encreafe it to the Height, and the Mercury will run in Drops, into the Receiver, continue the Fire untill no more will come, the Operation is commonly at an End in fix or feven Hours Pour the Water out of the Receiver, and having wafh d the Mercury to cleanfe it from the little portion of Earth it might carry along with it, dry it with Linnen or the Crums of Bread, and keep it for Ufe *Lemery*

every

every where, that the Gold may be received all over, then hold it over a Charcoal Fire, or lay it upon it, and it will cause the Quickfilver to fly away, after which you heighten the Colour with Gilding Wax, as fhall be directed

A particular Secret, to Gild Silver to the greatest Perfection.

TAKE * *Crocus Veneris* and Vinegar, put into it Quick-filver, let it boil together, till it comes to the Confiftence of a Pafte, with this quicken (anoint or wipe over) the Silver you intend to gild, and where-ever you quicken, it will turn of a reddifh Gold Colour, which doth not happen when done with *Quickfilver* only, for then it looks white   This is a curious Secret, you may gild upon this Pafte with Leaf Gold, when otherwife it requires to be ground, it makes the Gilding look rich and of a high Colour

Another Advantageous Gilding on Silver

TAKE Tartar one part, Salt two parts, pour Water upon it, add to it fome Steel Filings, boil the Silver therein, till it becomes reddifh, and this will require only the third Part of what Gold you would ufe otherwife

A particular Method of Gilding, which may be done in a Moment, and better than with Quickfilver

TAKE the fineft Gold, diffolve it in † *Aqua Regis,* which has been prepar'd with Salt, let the *Aqua Regis* be evaporated to half the quantity, then put the Glafs into a damp Cellar, on Sand, and the Gold will over Night fhoot into Cryftals, which take out, and let them diffolve again in

---

* Take the Slips of Copper, and fquench them in Urine   repeat this till it eafily pulverizes   The Powder you will find at the Bottom of the Urine, which preferve for Ufe
† The Preparation of this *Aqua Regis* only differs from the following Receipt, in ufing of Salt inftead of *Sal armoniack*, the ufual Way of making *Aqua Regis* according to *Lemery* is thus
Powder four Ounces of *Sal armoniack* and put it into a Matrafs or other Glafs Veffel of a good Bignefs pour upon it 16 Ounces of *Spirit of Nitre*, place the Veffel in Sand a little warm, until the *Sal-armoniack* is all diffolv'd, then pour the Diffolution into a Bottle, and ftop it with Wax This is the right *Aqua Regis*

ftill'd

ftill'd Vinegar, put it again upon the Fire, and let the half thereof evaporate, then put the Glass again in the Cellar, as before, in moist Sand, and over Night the Gold will shoot in Cryftals These diffolve in Rain Water, let that evaporate to half the Quantity, and again shoot into Cryftals, when this is done, take the Cryftalline Gold, break it to a Powder with a Knife, put that Powder into the White of an hard boil'd Egg, after the Yolk has been taken out, set it in a cool and damp Place, and over Night it will diffolve to an Oil, and what Silver you anoint with ever so thin, drying it gently, you will find the Gilding of a high and fine Colour, to the greatest Perfection

A Gilding after the Grecian *Manner*

TAKE * *Mercur. Sublimat* and clear Sal armoniac, of each one Ounce, make a Solution thereof in *Aqua Fortis*, then diffolve in it fine Gold which is beaten very thin, let this Solution evaporate over a Coal Fire, till it becomes an Oil, then dip in it a Silver Wire, if it comes out black, and by nealing it in the Fire, turns out gilded, it is right, and fit to be ufed for gilding any Sort of Silver

A right Italian *Gilding*

TAKE common Vitriol four Ounces, Allum two Ounces, White Vitriol one Ounce, *Plum Alb* one Ounce, Salt two Handfuls, River-Water one Quart, let it boil to half, then let it ftand till it fettles and looks clear, and it is fit for Ufe

---

* Mercury fublimate or fublimate Corrofive, is a Mercury that s impregnated with Acids, and by Fire is raifed to the Top of the Matrafs or other Veffel

Put one pound of Mercury, reviv'd from Cinnaber, into a Matrafs, pour on it 18 Ounces *of Spirit of Nitre*, fet it on a warm Sand, and let it ftand till all is diffolv d, this Diffolution put into a Glafs Veffel or Earthen Pan, fet it on warm Sand to evaporate all the Moifture, the remains will be a white Mafs, which beat to Powder in a Glafs Mortar, and mix with one Pound of white calcin d Vitriol and as much decripitated Salt, put this Mixture into a Matrafs, fo as to leave two thirds empty, place it in Sand, give it firft a gentle warmth for three Hours then augment the heat with laying on more Coals, and a Sublimate will rife to the Top of the Matrafs The Operation will require fix Hours Time, when the Matrafs is cold, break it, but take care to avoid a Kind of light Powder that flies in the Air, when the Matter is ftirred You will have one Pound and above of very good Sublimate Corrofive.

To deaden Quickfilver for Gilding.

TAKE clear Quickfilver which is free from the Mixture of Lead, put it into a Matrafs, and fling into it a handful of fine white Salt, fhake it well together, and let it ftand for two days, then pour upon it ftrong Vinegar, let it reft a Day, and you will find a good Quickfilver for gilding, and come cheap

A Gold Powder.

TAKE Leaf Gold or other thin beaten Gold, to the Quantity of a Penny-Weight, or as much as you pleafe, diffolve it in twice the Weight of *Aqua Regis* Let half the Solution evaporate on warm Sand, then take dry'd Linnen Rags, foak them in the remaining Liquid, dry them by a gentle Heat, and burn them on a flow Fire in a Crucible, the Powder whereof will remain at the Bottom, and be of a yellowifh Colour, wherewith the gilding is performed

Another for cold Gilding

TAKE half a Pound of *Aqua Fortis*, put in it two Ounces of Sal-armoniac finely pulverized and white, let it diffolve over a Fire, and then filter it through a Paper, put it into a Matrafs, with as much fine beaten Gold as will make two Penny Weights; fet it on a flow Fire, in order to diffolve the Gold in the *Aqua Regis*. When this is done, add to it two Ounces of *Sal-gemmæ*, fine and clear, powdered. and let it diffolve upon the Fire, then take fine clean linnen Rags, each about ¼ of an ounce in Weight, dip them into that Liquid, till all the Solution is foaked in, and having dryed them, burn them to a Powder, which preferve for Ufe When you gild any Thing with this Powder, let the Metal you defign to gild be boiled and fcraped, to have it clean and frefh, wet a Piece of Cork with Spittle or Water, and with it take up fome of the Powder, rubbing the Places of the Metal you are about to gild, till it is yellow, after which brufh and polifh it. You may ufe inftead of Cork, a foft Leather fowed or tied to a round End of a little Stick.

Another

Another Method

TAKE of the fineſt Gold the Quantity of two Penny-weight, and diſſolve it in *Aqua Regis*, add to this Solution the Weight of the Gold refined *Saltpetre*, let that alſo diſſolve, this done, dip a fine little linnen Rag, till it is all ſoak'd up, dry it gently, and burn it to Powder. With this Powder and freſh Water gild your Silver, by rubbing it with your Cork, or a Leather, faſtened to the Knob End of a Stick.

Another Powder to Gild withal

TAKE refined Gold, beat it very thin, roll it in little Rolls, fling it in *Aqua Regis*, hold it in a Matraſs over a ſlow Fire, till all the Gold is diſſolv'd, and the Solution is turned of a yellow Colour, then fling into it ſome pulverized Cryſtalline *Saltpetre*, by little and little, as much as it will conſume, then take ſome long narrow Slips of old fine Linnen, draw them through that Liquid, and when they are thorough wet, hang them into the Air to dry, in a Glaſs Bowl, or a Piece of a broken Bottle, and when thoroughly dry, light them with a Coal, and let them thus, without Flame, conſume to Aſhes. With theſe Aſhes you may gild, rubbing it on the Silver a Piece of Cork

Another

TAKE a Penny-Weight of Gold, put the ſame Weight of *Saltpetre*, alſo the ſame Weight of *Sal-armoniack* into a Matraſs, to three Quarts of *Aqua Fortis*, then put the Gold nealing hot into it, and as ſoon as the Gold is diſſolved, take ſome dry Linnen Rags, dip them therein, dry and burn them at a Candle to Tinder, which preſerve for Uſe, as has been mentioned

A Quickening Water.

TAKE one Ounce of Quickſilver, one Ounce of *Aqua Fortis*, let it be put together into a Glaſs, and after the Quickſilver is diſſolv'd, put to it five Ounces of freſh Water; warm it, and it will be fit to gild withall

Another

Another.

TAKE one Ounce of *Aqua Fortis*, put it into a Matrass add to it ¼ of an ounce of Mercury, let this diffolve, then take frefh River Water, and mix it with that in the Glafs, to that Degree that you may put your Hands in without hurting them; then let it ftand clofed up, and you will have a good Quick-Water for gilding

Another Water-Gilding upon Silver.

TAKE Copper-flakes, pour ftrong Vinegar thereon, add to it Allum and Salt, of one as much as the other, fet it on a Fire, and when the Vinegar is boiled the fourth part away, fling into it what Metal you defign to gild and it will attract a Copper Colour. If you let it boil on further, it will change into a fine Gold Colour. This is a fine Secret for Goldfmiths, to gild Silver all over, for the boiling it in that Liquid, gives the Gold a high and rich Colour

A Method to Work a Cup, One Side Gold and the other Silver.

TAKE a Piece of fine Silver, form it into a flat Square, and with a rough File, rough it all over one Side, raife alfo with a Graver little Points upon it   Then take a Piece of Gold in Proportion to what Thicknefs you would have it, form it exactly to the Dimenfion of the Silver, in a flat Square, neal both the Gold and the Silver red Hot, then lay them quick on one another, and with a wooden Hammer beat it gently together   When thus you have united thefe two Metals, you may form thereof what you pleafe, one Side will be Silver and the other Gold.

To embellish Gold, Silver, or Brafs, with Ornaments of Glafs

TAKE fine pulverifed Venice Glafs of what Colour you pleafe, grind it upon a Stone, temper it with Oil, then put it in Circle of a clear Charcoal Fire to melt, it will look fine and beautiful, especially if the Ornaments and Things are well defign'd

OF

Of feveral Sorts of Gold-Colours, Gilding-Wax, and other Embellifhments of Gold or Gilded Work.

THE Gold, as well as gilded Silver, wants confiderably of that Luftre and Brightnefs it appears in, after it is placed in Goldfmiths Shops, for before this, it undergoes feveral Operations, and is raifed to its Beauty by *Gilding Wax, Colouring*, and *Helling*, each of which fhall be feparately explain'd under the following Heads.

Gilding Wax ufed for Gold, or gilded Work.

TAKE four ounces of clear Wax, one ounce and a half of Verditer, one ounce of Copper Flakes, one ounce of Red Chalk, one ounce of Alom, melt the Wax, and put the other Things, finely powdered, into it, and ftir it well together let it cool and form thereof round Sticks like Sealing Wax. When you have Occafion to make ufe of it, then firft heat your Gold, and then rub it over with this Wax, Then neal it, and draw it nimbly through boiling hot Water and Tarter, and it will give the Gold a deep Colour

Another

TAKE two pound of Wax, one 'pound of Red Chalk one pound of White Vitriol, and four ounces of *Æs uftum*.

Another.

TAKE 12 ounces of fine yellow Wax, eight ounces of Red Chalk, four ounces of Verditer, two ources of *Æs uftum*, one ounce of Vitriol, half an ounce of Borax, melt the Wax floly in a glazed Pipkin, on a gentle Fire, not too hot, then put the fore-mentioned Things one Spoon ful after another, into it, ftirring it, till you have mixt it well, and when cool, form it into Sticks for your Ufe Let every Matter be ground by itfelf, the finer the better.

C

Another

Another

TAKE 16 ounces of Wax, one Grain of Copper Flakes, three ounces of Vitriol, four ounces of Verditer, and nine ounces of Red Lead.

Another.

TAKE eight Ounces of clear Wax, one Ounce and a half of *Terra Vert* one Ounce of *Æs uftum*, one Ounce of red Chalk, and half an Ounce of Alom, diffolve the Wax, and put thefe Ingredients in, let it cool, then form it into Sticks like fealing Wax, with this, after you have heated your gilded Metal, rub it over, then burn it off, and it will give the Geld a deep Colour

Nurimberg Gilding Wax.

TAKE two Pound of Wax, two Pound and one ounce of Red Chalk, one ounce of Vitriol, half an ounce of *Æs uftum*, three ounces of Verdegreafe, half an ounce of Borax.

Another.

TAKE two Pound of Wax, one Pound of Red Chalk, one ounce of Verditer, three Grains of *Æs uftum*, three ounces of Verdegreafe, and two ounces of Borax

Another

ONE Pound of Wax, one Pound of Red Chalk, one ounce of Verditer, three Grains of *Æs uftum*, two ounces of Venice Borax, two ounces of Vitriol

Another

TAKE four pound of clear Wax, one pound eight ounces of Red Chalk, one pound eight ounces White Vitriol, 15 ounces of Verdegreafe, three ounces of Venice Borax, 15 ounces of *Æs uftum*, be it it fine, mix it together, and when the Wax is melted, ftir it, till you perceive it to cool, then put in the Ingredients, and ftir them well together, and when cold, form them into Sticks like Scaling-Wax

Of several Gold Colours, whereby the Gold or gilded Work, after it has been heightned with Gilding-Wax, receives its proper Colour

A Silver Gold Colour, or a Colour for gilded Silver.

TAKE one ounce of Verdegrease, one ounce *Salt petre*, one ounce Vitriol, half an ounce *Sal Armoniac*, half an ounce of Borax, grind them fine, boil it in half a Pint of Urin to half the Quantity, then with a Brush dipt in this Liquid, brush over your gilded Work, put it upon a clear Charcoal Fire, and when you see it turn black, take it off the Fire, and quench it in Urin.

A Green Gold Colour.

TAKE two ounces of Salt-petre, two ounces of Vitriol, two ounces of Verdegrease, and one ounce of Sal-armoniac, mix and grind them with Vinegar.

Another

TAKE four ounces of Verdegrease, four ounces of Sal-armoniack, two ounces of Vitriol, two ounces of *s uftum*, one ounce of Salt petre, grind them with Vinegar, and colour your Gold therewith.

A French Gold Colour.

TAKE four ounces of Salt, two ounces of Alum, two ounces of Sal armoniac, two ounces of *Æs uftum*, one ounce of Saltpetre, and grind them with Vinegar.

Another

TAKE four ounces of Sal-armoniac, four ounce of Verdegrease, two ounces of Salt petre, one ounce and a half of clean Copper Flakes, grind it with Vinegar.

A fine

A fine Gold Colour

TAKE melted Salt-petre, and black Vitriol, of one as much as the other, let it boil half away in a clean Pipkin

Another Gold Colour

TAKE one ounce of Verdegreafe, one ounce of Sal-armoniac, one ounce of Red Chalk, one ounce of fine Salt, grind all together, and boil it with Vinegar.

Another.

TAKE one ounce of Salt petre, one ounce of Verde-greafe, one ounce of Vitriol, one ounce of Sal-armoniac, grind each Piece feparately in a clean Morter, then mix and put it in a clean Pan, with Water, and boil it for almoft half an Hour

A Green Gold Colour

TAKE four ounces of Sal-armoniac, four ounces of Verdegreafe, one Grain of Salt-petre, and grind it in Vinegar.

A White Colour for Gold.

TAKE two ounces of Salt-petre, one ounce of Alum, one ounce of Salt, pulverize and mix this well toge-ther ; then take a piece of a broken Muffle or Crucible, put it in the Fire, and let it be red hot, wet the Work you defign to colour, and roll it in the Powder, then put it on the red hot Piece of the Muffle, and the Colour will ebullate, when it melts, turn the Work with your Tongs about, when the Colour is quite fluid and yellow, take the Work out, and lay it upon a clean Brick or Anvil till it is cold   Then take an unglaz'd Pot, or elfe a large Crucible, fill it almoft up with clean Water, put into it a Handful of Salt, the Bignefs of a Filbeard of Tartar, ground, and fix or eight Drops of *Aqua Fortis*, let that boil, then put your Work into it, and boil it fo long, till the Drofs of the white Colour is clean off, then Scratch brufh it

To colour an old Gold Chain, as new.

TAKE Urin, diffolve therein Sal-armoniac, boil in this the Gold Chain, and it will have a fine Colour.

A Green Colour for Gold Chains

TAKE four ounces of Sal armoniac, four ounces of Verdegreafe, one ounce and a half of Salt-petre, half an ounce of white Vitriol, make a Powder thereof, mix it with Vinegar, and boil your Chain in it.

To give Gold a high and fire Colour.

TAKE red calcin'd Vitriol three ounces, Sal armoniac two ounces, and Verdegreafe one ounce, grind them together, and keep it dry When you will colour your Gold, moiften it, and ftrew this Powder over it, let it often neal, and quench it in Pump Water.

Another fine Colour for Gold

TAKE Verdegreafe, Sal-armoniac, Salt petre, and Vitriol, of one as much as the other, grind it well together, pour Vinegar upon it, grind it again, as the Painters do their Colours, and let it dry, then moiften, grind, and dry it again, repeat this for feveral Times· Then lay up your Powder carefully, and when you will colour Gold, wet it with Urin, rub it with a Brufh, then fling the Powder upon it, lay it on red hot Coals, and it will turn black, then quench it in Urine, and rub it with a Wire-Brufh, in this Manner you proceed with the other Colours.

To bring Pale Gold to a high Colour.

TAKE Verdegreafe, pour Vinegar upon it, ftir it well, anoint your Gold therewith, heat it in the Fire, and quench it in Urin.

To make Silver throughout Yellow, and to tincture it the Colour of Gold

TAKE common Aqua fortis, diffolve therein as much Silver as you pleafe; if you have eight Ounces, take

four

four Ounces of *Hepatic Aloes,* six Ounces of *Gurgian,*, two Ounces prepared *Tutty,* that has been several Times quench'd in Urin, put these to the Solution of the Silver, and they will dissolve, and raise up in the Glass like a Spunge, the Glass must be large, to prevent the running over, then draw it off, and you will have ten Ounces of Silver, which is yellow as Gold. *N B* These two Ounces, increased in the Weight of the Silver, will not stand the Test, but be lost when melted down with Lead

A Water to Tincture any Metal of a Gold Colour.

TAKE fine Sulpher, and pulverize it, then boil some stale Spring or Rain Water, pour it hot upon the Powder, and stir it well together, boil it and put into it one Ounce or more of Dragon's Blood, and after it is well boil'd, take it off and filter it through a fine Cloath. Put this Water into a Matrass, after you have put in what you design to Tincture; close it well and boil it, and the Things will be of a fine Gold Colour.

Another Water wherewith one may tinge any Metal a Gold Colour, a curious Secret

TAKE *Hepatic Aloes,* Salt-petre, and Roman Vitriol, of one as much as the other, distil it with Water in an Alembeck, give it fire so long till all the Spirits are extracted, it will at last yield a yellowish Water, which will tinge any Sort of Metal a Gold Colour.

To colour Gold.

TAKE a Lock of human Hair, of about a Fingers thick, lay it on live Coals, and hold the Gold with a pair of Tongs over it, to receive the Fumes thereof.

To give Gold a high and fine Colour.

TAKE one Ounce of *Sal-armoniac,* two Ounces of Copper Flakes, one Ounce of distill'd Verdegrease, grind all well together, put it into a Matrass, pour upon it one Quart of good distill'd White-Wine Vinegar. Let it thus dry and boil away, then grind it fine, strew it on a Glass Plate, and let it in a Cellar, where it will turn into an Oil, this is again to be gently coagulated, then ground and mix'd with Mercury Sublimate; put half an Ounce of it, wrapt up in Bees-Wax, into the Quantity of a Pound of Gold that's in Fusion, and it will give it a high and fine Colour.

To give the Guilded Work a fine Colour.

TAKE clean Salt and Brimstone, boil it together with Water in an Egg-shell, after you have pealed the inside Film, take care you don't give it too much Fire to burn the Egg-shell With this Liquid wipe over your Gilding, and it will make it of a much brighter Colour than it was before

Another.

TAKE Powder of Sulpher, and bruised Garlick, boil these in Urin, neal your Gold, quench it therein, and it will give it a fine Colour

To brighten Spots in Gilding.

TAKE Alom, boil it in clean Water, put your Work into it, this will fetch the Colour again, and dispel the Spots.

To give old Silver Lace or Trimmings their Beauty and Colour, as if new.

TAKE Powder of Alablaster, put it dry into a Pipkin, and let it boil as long as it can; then take it off the Fire, and when cold, lay your Lace upon a Cloth, and with a Comb Brush, take up some of that Powder, and rub therewith both Sides, till it is as bright as you would have it, afterwards polish it with a smooth Stone.

Another Method.

TAKE Ox Gall, and the Gall of a large Jack, and some Water, mix it together, and with it rub your Gold or Silver, and you will see the Colour change to your liking.

✿✿✿✿✿✿✿✿✿✿✿✿✿✿✿✿✿✿✿✿✿

Of the HELL, or HELLING of Gold.

This is the finifhing Stroke of either Gold or gilded Work, and is perform'd after it has undergone the Operations with the Gilding-Wax and Gold Colours as has been fhewn in the preceeding Articles The following are the different Receipts of different Mafters The ingenious and judicious will by experimental Enquiry foon difcover which of them is beft, and make his Choice of fuch as he approves.

The Hell of Gold, or gilded Work.

TAKE two ounces of Tartar, two ounces of Sulphur, and four ounces of Salt, boil this in half Water, and half Urin, dip your Gold or gilded Work into it, and it will give it a fine Luftre.

Another

TAKE eight ounces of Salt, two ounces of Tartar, two ounces of Sulphur, two ounces of *Cap Mort* half an ounce of Alom; if you boil this in Water and Urin, and draw your Work through, it will anfwer your Expectation.

Another

TAKE eight ounces of Sulphur, eight ounces of Alom, eight ounces yellow Arfenick, 16 ounces of Tartar, 16 ounces of Salt, boil it in Water and Urin.

Another.

TAKE three ounces of Sulphur, one ounce of Alum, one ounce of Arfenick, half an ounce of *Gurgums*, and half a Grain of Antimony, grind them very fine together, then boil them in Urin and Water, and ftir the Ingredients by little and little well together, give it a little boiling, put the gilded Plate into it, and boil it till the Colour is bright.

Another

Another.

TAKE eight ounces of yellow Arfenick, 16 ounces of Sulphur, 16 ounces of Tartar, 16 ounces of burnt Alom, three ounces and a half of Salt; boil it in Urin and Water.

Another.

TAKE fifted Afhes and Antimony, finely pulveriz'd, with thefe make a Lee, and with a Brufh rub over the gilded Silver.

Another.

TAKE one ounce of white Tartar, one ounce of green Sulphur, nine ounces of Salt, grind it together like Flower; then take a Copper Sauce Pan with frefh Water, and let the Water boil, put into it one Grain crude yellow Arfenick; take of the grounded Ingredients three Spoonfuls, and let it boil, after that, you may draw your Work through, and make it as high as you will, it will come out clear and with a fine Luftre.

How to take off the Gold from gilded Silver Tankards or Cups.

TO take off the Gold from fuch Plate, take *Sal Armoniack* one part, *Sal-petre* one half part, grind them both to a Powder, wipe over the gilded Part with Oil, ftrew the Powder upon it, and lay your Plate into the Fire to heat it well; then take it out, hold your Plate over an earthen Difh, in one Hand, and with the other beat it with an Iron, and the Powder will fall into the Difh, together with the Gold, which you may feparate in the Manner as has been directed.

Another Method.

PUT Quickfilver in an earthen Difh, heat it fo much as juft to fuffer your Finger in, in this turn your
Silver

Silver Cup or other Utenſil, and the Gold will ſeparate from the Silver, and join the Quickſilver, when you ſee the Gold all off the Plate, take it out, pour the Quick-ſilver with the Gold, after it is cool, into another Diſh, and if any Place ſtill retains ſome Gold, repeat it, till you perceive no more upon it, then ſtrain the Quickſilver through a Leather, what remains put into a * Retort, and on hott Sand or Aſhes force the reſt of the Mercury from it into a Receiver with Water, and what is left, melt together, and refine the Gold as has been taught before.

An approved Method to take off the Gilding from Silver.

FIRST take a Glaſs, or a glazed Utenſil, with *Aqua Fortis,* the Quantity whereof muſt be according to the Bigneſs of your Work, take no more than half ¼ of an ounce of *Sal Armoniack* to one Ounce of *Aqua Fortis,* beat your *Sal Armoniack* fine, put it into the *Aqua Fortis,* and ſett it over the Fire, till it grows warm, and when you perceive the *Sal Armoniack* to work, then lay in the gilded Silver, and when you obſerve your work to change to a black Colour, then the Gold is off on it, if there is a pretty large Quantity of Work, let it lay for half an Hour or an Hour before you take it out, which you do with a Pair of wooden Plyers, when it is taken out, put it into clean Water then neal it, and afterwards boil it with Tartar; repeat this three times running, and your Silver will look freſh and new

How to get the Gold out of Aqua Fortis

TAKE a Copper Bowl or Cup, put into it a Glaſs full of Water, then pour in the *Aqua Fortis* which contains Gold, in Order to ſweeten it a little, then put to it ¼ of an ounce of Venice Borax, and boil it up, let it ſtand over Night, in the Morning pour it off gently, and the Gold will be ſettled at the Bottom, dry it by Degrees, and when dry, put a little Borax to it, and melt it.

---

* Vid Plate I Fig 6 The Neck, through which the Mercury is conveyed, muſt be half Way in the Water, thatʼs in the Receiver

To separate Gold from gilded Silver, by Cementation.

TAKE red calcined * Vitriol or *Colcothar* one part, Salt one part, also red Lead half a part, pulverise and mix it all well together, with this mixed Powder cover your gilded Silver all over in an earthen Pan, put it into a Furnace, and give it a slow Fire, to prevent the Melting of the Silver, the Powder will contract the Gold, which you reduce by Melting it with Lead, and by Separating it in the Coppel.

❀❀❀❀❀❀❀❀❀❀❀❀❀❀❀❀❀❀❀❀❀

Of several Sorts of SOLDER, used for GOLD and SILVER.

Filings Solder for Silver Chain-Work.

MELT three parts of fine Silver and one part of Brass; when in fusion, fling into it a little quantity of yellow Arsenick Or,

Take one part yellow Arsenick, and one part of Copper, melt and granulise it, Of this take one part, and of fine Silver four parts; melt it together, cast it into an Ingot, and when cold file it to a fine Dust.

A Solder for Silver

MELT two parts of Silver, then put to it one part of thin beaten Brass or Tincal, but don't keep it too long in Fusion, least the Brass should fly away in a Fume.

Another, for coarse Silver.

FOUR ounces of Silver, three ounces of Brass, ¼ of an ounce of Arsenick, melt this together, and pour it out quick.

---

* The Calcination of Vitriol is perform'd thus Put what Quantity you please of green Vitriol into an earthen Pot unglazed, set the Pot over the Fire and the Vitriol will dissolve into Water boil it till the Moisture is consumed, or the Matter turns into a grayish Mass, drawing towards white, this is called White calcined Vitriol If you calcine this white Vitriol a good while over a strong Fire, it will turn as red as Blood. This is call'd *Colcothar*.

Another,

A good Silver Solder.

MELT two ounces of Silver, one ounce of Tincal, add to it half an ounce of white Arfenick, pour it out quick, and it is a very good Solder.

Another.

MELT one ounce of fine Silver, one ounce of thin Brafs, when both are well melted together, then fling one ounce of white Arfenick upon it, let it liquidate, ftir it well together, and pour it out quickly.

A good Solder for Gold.

MELT Copper and fine Silver, of each one part, fine Gold two parts. *Or,*

TAKE one penny-weight of the fame Gold your Work is of, and allay it with three grains of Copper and three grains of Silver.

___

The Manner and Way of Soldering GOLD or SILVER.

BEAT the Solder thin, and cut it in little Bits or Pallions, then take the Work which is to be foldered, join it together with fine Wire, wet the Joinings with a Pencil with Water, mix'd up with Borax; then lay the Bits or Pallions of Solder upon it, and ftrew fome powdered Borax over it, lay the Work, if it be a Button or fome other fmall Thing, upon a large Coal, and blow with your Blowing Inftrument through a large Lamp Flame upon it, for to melt it

AFTER this, you boil the Work either in Alom-Water, or elfe, in Aqua Fortis, to clear it from the Borax, and then dry it on a Charcoal Fire, then file or turn it; If it is Silver, boil it white in the following Manner.

TAKE the Work, lay it on a clear Fire, and when red hot, take it out, and put it by to cool; in the mean while
fett

fett a Copper Sauce-Pan with Water upon the Fire, into which put one part of fine Salt, and one part of Tartar; this boil together, yet not too fierce, to prevent its boiling over, after it is well boiled, lay the Work when it is a little cold, into it, and let it boil about six Minutes, then take it off the Fire, take out the Work, and put it immediately into clean Water, take it out and fcratch it well with a Wire Brufh, to clear it of the Coat, then repeat this Work over again, neal it once more, boil it in Tartar and Salt, and proceed as before, then take black burnt Tartar, mix it with a little Water into a Pafte, with which rub over the Work, then neal it on a clear Coal Fire, take it out, and brufh the Work well of the burnt Tartar in clean Water; put it once more in the Tartar Water in which it was boiled, and let it boil four Minutes, then wafh it in cold Water, and dry it with a clean Rag, it will be of a white and beautiful Pearl Colour

To folder a Ring fet with Stones.

TAKE a large Charcoal, put two or three Penny Weights of Silver upon it, melt it with your Blowing Inftrument and the Lamp, then, after you have clap't a thin Pallion of Silver Solder betwixt the opening of the Ring, dip it into it; but as foon you fee the Pallion run, take off your Ring, or elfe the Silver will devour it.

For Soldering.

TAKE the beft hard Venice Soap, fcrape it as thin as poffible, let it dry between two Papers in the Air; then rub it to a Powder, put it in an unglaz'd Pipkin, fet it on a gentle Coal Fire, and let it by Degrees fumigate, till it has no moifture at all, then is it right, this Borax you may ufe for all Manner of Work, and it will do better than the Venice Borax.

To melt in a Moment feveral Sorts of Metals, over a Table.

TAKE two ounces of Salt-petre, Tartar one ounce, Sulphur half an ounce, beat it in a Morter to a Powder, then take one ounce of filed Metal, or fine pulverized Oar, mix it well together, put it in a fmall Crucible, or a hollowed Charcoal, light it with a little Splinter, and it will melt immediately. *Another*

Another Manner of doing it.

TAKE one ounce of Saltpetre, half an ounce of Sulphur, ¼ of an ounce of Gun-Powder, grind it well together, and put half of this Powder into a small Crucible, or if you will, into an Egg shell, then put a Farthing or Sixpence, or any other Metal upon it, and upon that, put the other half of the Powder, press it down with your Finger, then let it on a Stone, light it, and it will melt immediately.

N B. A gilded Cup, or other Plate, if anointed with Sallet Oil, and this Powder flung upon and lighted, takes off the Gold, and melts it to a Mass

To prepare Aurum Fulminans.

TAKE Gold that's refin'd with Antimony, beat it in thin Plates, put it into a Phial or Matrass, pour Aqua Regis upon it, then set the Phial or Matrass upon warm Sand, till the Aqua Regis has dissolv'd as much of the Gold as it is able to contain, which you will know when you see the Ebullitions cease, pour your Solution by Inclination into another Glass, and if you see there remains any Gold in the Matrass, dissolve it as before with a little fresh Aqua Regis, mix your Dissolution, and pour to it six times as much common Water, afterwards drop into this Mixture, by Degrees, the volatile Spirit of *Sal Armoniack*, or Oil of Tartar, and you will see the Gold precipitate to the Bottom of the Glass, let it rest a good while for the Gold to settle, then pour off the Water by Inclination, wash your Powder with warm Water, till it grows insipid, dry it to the Substance of a Paste, then form it in little round Corns, the *Bigness* of Hempseed, dry them by the Sun; if you put one of them into the Fire, it will fly and disperse with a terrible Noise, and beat about with great Violence.

To make Aurum Sophisticum, or mimick Gold.

TAKE fine distill'd Verdegrease eight Ounces, Crude Alexandrian Tutty four Ounces, Borax 12 Ounces, Salt-peter one Ounce and a half, pulverize and mix them all together, temper them with Oil, with a wooden Spattle, to the Consistence of a Paste, then put a *German* Crucible in a Wind-Furnace, heat it red hot, and convey your Mass into it
with

with a wooden Spattle, by little and little, when all is in, cover it, fill your Furnace with Coals all over the Crucible; let it stand in a fierce Fire and melt, let it cool of itself, then break the Crucible, and you will find at the Bottom a fine *Regulus* like Gold, weighing about four Ounces, out of which you may form and make what you please, it will work as malleable as real Gold

Another.

TAKE fine and clear Wire Copper four ounces, melt it; then fling into it one ounce of *Speltar*, stir it well together with an Iron Spattle, blow the Fire brisk, to bring it in Fusion, but before you pour it out, put in some Borax and it will give it a peculiar Beauty Then cast it into an Ingot, out of this Ingot you may draw Wire for Chains, and work it in what Form or Shape you please, and after you have filed it, and rubb'd your Work well with Tripoly, then give it the Finishing with a Mixture of one Grain of Tripoly, and six Grains of Flower of Sulphur, which put upon a Piece of Leather, and rub your Work as usual, and it will have a fine Gold Colour

Another.

TAKE *Speltar* one ounce, of the finest and softest Copper two ounces; melt the Copper in a Crucible; when melted, fling into it Venice Borax one Grain, and Salarmoniac one Grain, and lastly fling in the *Speltar* Pour it into an Ingot, and you will have a fine Gold colour'd Metal

To make a curious yellow mix'd Metal, which resembles Gold, and may be drawn into fine Wire.

TAKE eight Ounces of Tartar, put it into a Crucible, and let it neal by Degrees, then take pulverized dry *Salt-petre*, and fling it on the red hot Tartar, and it will melt into a yellow Matter, take it from the Fire, let it cool, then take clean Copper, put it in Fusion till it is like fair Water, and fling to eight Ounces of Copper the above Matter, give the Crucible a strong reverberatory Heat, till in Fusion, then take the best *Speltar* or *Gosslar Zink* half an Ounce, Tutty and Venice *Sublacani* half an Ounce, put it to the melted

Copper,

Copper, and presently you will hear a crackling Noise, and see a yellow Fume and Flame ascend, stir this Copper and the other Ingredients well together with an Iron Wire till it is burnt away, let it stand a little in the Flux, and then after you wiped your Ingot with Wax, pour it in, and it will be playable as to be drawn into Wire, and of a high Gold Colour, you may work, form, finish, and colour it as you do other Gold.

Another Method to make a Metal resembling Gold.

TAKE fine Copper Filings one Pound, fine *Salt-petre* eight Ounces, prepared *Tutty* six Ounces, *Borax* six Ounces, *Hepatic Aloes* four Ounces, mix all well together, and incorporate it with Linseed Oil into a Mass, put it in a clean Crucible, and cover it a-top, a Finger's Height, with subtil pulverized Venice Glass, lute it well, put it into a Wind-Furnace; fill the same with dead Coals, then put live Coals upon them, and light the Fire from the Top to go downwards, blow it for an Hour long, and give it a fierce Fire, then let it cool of itself, take out the Crucible, break the same, and you will find at the Bottom thereof a very fine *Regulus* like Gold, this you melt again, and add to one Pound two Ounces of *Mercury Sublimate*, and two Ounces of prepared *Tutty*, both clap'd up in red Sealing-Wax, stir it well with a dry Stick, then cast it into a Mould, and make of it what you please.

Another

TAKE six ounces of distill'd Verdegrease, grind it fine in a Marble Mortar, eight ounces of prepar'd Tutty, four ounces of Saltpetre, four ounces of Borax, beat it to a coarse Powder, moisten it with Oil of Turneps, and stir it in an earthen Dish all together, till all is well mix'd. Then put a Crucible into a Wind-Furnace, and when red hot, convey the said Mixture into it with a wooden Spattle, cover it, add more Coals, and give a brisk and strong Fire, all over the Crucible. In about half an Hour put a little Stick into it, and search whether the Matter is dissolved, and in Fusion like Water, if so, then it is time to pour it out, but if you find still some Matter remain, you stir it about with your Stick; cover it, and repeat giving it a brisk Fire, till you find it is all dissolv'd. Then pour it out, into a Morter, or Brass Cone, and you will have a fine Gold-colour'd Regulus

To

To silver Copper or Brass.

TAKE fine Silver one ounce, *Sal gemmæ* and *Sal-armoniac* of each six ounces, Glass-Gall six ounces; beat the Silver thin, and then lay it in one ounce of *Aqua Fortis*, let it dissolve, when dissolved, fling a little Salt into it, and the Silver will settle like a white Calx at the Bottom; then pour off that Water, and put on fresh; repeat it, till the Silver Calx has lost all the Flavour of the *Aqua Fortis*, dry this Silver Calx, then take the above Ingredients and grind them well on a clean Stone, when you have well grounded them, mix and grind them and the Silver Calx together, with a little Water, till it is like a thick Paste, put this up in a clean Glass, and when you will silver, take Care that your Metal be filed and brush'd clean, strike it over with the above Matter, and lay it on live Coals, when it has done smoaking then scratch it well, and strike it over again with the Silver Matter, do this three Times successively, and you will have a fine Silvering.

To silver Copper or Brass.

TAKE fine Silver, dissolve it in *Aqua Fortis*, then add to it the same Quantity of warm Water, as you had *Aqua Fortis* Take common Salt, fling it in the mixt Waters, and the Silver will precipitate to the Bottom like a Powder; when settled, pour off the mixt Water, and sweeten the Silver Calx, by pouring fresh Water to it, shifting it, till all the Sharpness is gone from it. Then drain off the Water, and let the Silver dry, whereof take a $\frac{1}{4}$ of an ounce, white calcin'd Tartar one ounce, common Salt half an ounce; beat and mix this well together, and with *Aqua Fortis* grind it upon a Stone; then let it dry, and you have the Powder to silver withal ready. If you will silver, either poor Silver, Copper, or Brass, then rub the Powder after you have moistened it with Water, with a Piece of Cork well in, so long till you see the Execution thereof to your Mind, then lay it on a Coal Fire, till it is red hot, let it cool; then boil it in Water with Tartar and Salt, and after it is boiled, wash it in clean Water.

To silver Brass in Fire

TAKE Calx of fine Silver half an ounce, one ounce of Sal-armoniac, three ounces of Salt, mix and grind these well together. When you use it, grind and temper it together with Water, and rub your Brass therewith, neal it brown, then quench it in Water wherein Tartar has been dissolv'd; scratch it, and finish your Work by polishing it, as you see requisite.

A Powder to silver Copper or Brass withal, by rubbing it with one's Finger

DISSOLVE a little Silver in *Aqua Fortis,* add to it as much Tartar and Sal armoniac as to make it like a Salve, whereof make little Balls, dry and pulverize them. If you take some of this Powder with your wetted Thumb, and rub it upon Copper or Brass, it will give it the Colour of Silver.

A Silvering on Copper.

DISSOLVE fine Silver in *Aqua Fortis,* pour it upon pulverized Tartar, and then draw your *Aqua Fortis* clear off, and there remains a black Matter, with this rub your Copper, then neal it well and boil it in Tartar and Salt.

To silver Copper or Brass, with boiling it.

TAKE three ounces of Salt, 26 Leaves of Silver, ¼ of an ounce of Tartar, half an ounce of Alom, this boil in an earthen Panniken, and stir it well together, put what you design to silver, into it; pour Water upon it, and let it boil; after it is well boil'd, scratch-brush it, put it in again and boil it; then scratch it again, and repeat this so often, till it is to your Satisfaction

To boil Brass like Silver.

TAKE one part of the Filings of good Pewter, add to it one part of white Tartar, and mix it together: Then take an unglaz'd Pipkin, put these two Ingredients, and the Brass (which before must be well scratch'd and clean'd) into it, and let it boil.

To

To silver Copper, Brass, Steel, or Iron, so as not to come off,
except it is made red hot.

TAKE Urine which is made in the Morning, cover it, and let it stand a whole Month, and it will foment, put it into a Kettle or earthen Pot, and let it boil, skim it, and when the third Part is evaporated, take to two Pints of Urine one ounce of Tartar, and one ounce of Galiz-stone; put it in, and let it boil once up This Liquid keep clean, and if you will silver any Metal, take Brick-Duft on a damp woolen Rag, and rub therewith your Iron or other Metal, till it is clear and fine and put it 24 Hours in the prepared Urine; afterwards dry it, and where you defign to silver it, rub it over with Quickfilver, you muft lay it on thin with an Iron Spatula that has alfo lain 2 Hours in the Urine, then rub it on with a foft woolen Rag, and it is a fine bright Silvering

To silver all Sorts of Metals.

TAKE as much *Aqua Fortis* as you think there is Oc-cafion for in a Glafs, and fet it on hot Afhes; then put in your Quantity of Silver, which firft has been beaten very thin, and cut in little Shreads When your Silver is diffolv'd, take it from the Afhes, and mix that Liquid with as much White Tartar as to make it like a Dough. If you rub Brafs, Copper, or any other Metal over with this, it will be like Silver itfelf

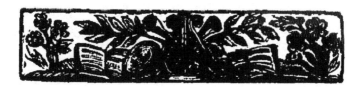

PART II.

Choice Secrets for JEWELLERS, in ENAMELLING, and the Preparing of ENAMEL-Colours, the Art of Painting Portraiture on Enamel'd Plates Several curious Inftructions how to make Artificial Pearls, of DOUBLETS and FOYLES, how to prepare and colour them The Art of copying Precious Stones, together with other rare Secrets.

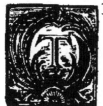HE foregoing Part will, no doubt, give a fufficient Idea, and direct the ingenious Reader in the Management of *Gold* and *Silver,* in all the different Branches fpecified We fhall in this Second Part prefent him with feveral choice Secrets, peculiarly relating to JEWELLERS, and firft fhew that admirable Branch

Of ENAMELLING

To prepare the Flux for Enamel Colours.

TAKE four ounces of Red Lead, one ounce of well wafh'd and clean'd Sea Sand, melt it together, and pour it into a cold Ingot   Or,

TAKE Pebble one part, prepared as fhall be directed; mix one part thereof with five parts of Red Lead.

Another Sort of Flux, which is very foft.

TAKE one ounce of White Lead, ¼ of an ounce of Red Lead, fix Grains of Pebble, heat the Pebbles red hot, and quench them in Urin, repeat this, till you can
rub

rub them to an inpalpable Powder between your Fingers, then beat them fine, put them with the Ingredients into a clean Crucible, lute it well, and when dry, give it a fierce Fire for half an Hour, or longer, then take it off the Fire, and let it cool of itself, break the Crucible afterwards, and you will find a *Regulus*, which melt again in another clean Crucible, and pour it into a clean Ingot, or a bright Brass Weight Scale, and then it will be fit for Use, beating and grinding it in an Agat Mortar to an impalpable Powder When you mix your Colours therewith, temper as much as you have occasion for, with Oil of Spike.

A Green Colour.

TAKE Copperas, and neal it, take of it one part, and four parts of Flux. *Or*,

TAKE Brass, diffolve it in *Aqua Fortis*, then neal it well, take of this one part, and three parts of Flux.

Another.

TAKE Copper Plates, and with a Piece of Pumice-Stone rub it over with Water, receive the Water in a Bason or Dish, so long till you have wore it off pretty thin, then let it settle; pour off the Water, and neal the settling; then take thereof one part, and three parts of Flux, which makes a good and fine Green

Dark Green.

TAKE green Enamel two parts, yellow Smalt one eighth part, and fix parts of Verditer.

Yellow Colour.

TAKE fine King's Yellow, neal it in a Crucible, one part Yellow, and three parts Flux.

A High Yellow.

TAKE Gold-Yellow Enamel, Vitriol and Flux, grind and temper it as you would have it with Oil of Spike.

Brimstone

Brimstone Colour

TAKE calcin'd Naples Yellow one part, three parts of burn'd Lead Yellow, and three parts of Flux

A Black Colour

TAKE six eight parts of black Enamel, and one eighth part of Scales of Iron of a clean enamelling Plate This grind together with Water in an Agat Mortar very fine, draw the Water from it, and dry it upon hot Plates, then grind it with Oil of Spike.

Another.

TAKE Hungarian Vitriol, boil it over a little Fire, like Borax, and melt it in a new Crucible, three different Times, one part Vitriol, three parts Flux, grind this with Oil of Spike as quick as possible.

Another

TAKE Magnesia, neal it upon a Tile, the blacker it comes off the Fire, the better, one part thereof with three parts of Flux, ground with Oil of Spike

Several other FIRE COLOURS for *Enamelling.*

A Good Red

TAKE Hungarian Vitriol, grind it fine, and dry it in the Sun, then neal it between two Crucibles, well luted, so as to prevent the Air coming to it. Take thereof one part, and two parts and a half of Flux, melt it together, and when you use it, grind it with Oil of Spike.

Another.

TAKE Roman Vitriol, about the Quantity of a Walnut; grind it in a Stone Mortar very fine, dry it, and

then

then neal it to a brown Colour, take the heavy Lumps, put them in a new glaz'd Pipkin, and pour *Aqua Fortis* upon it, then wash the *Aqua Fortis* from it again, and let it evaporate, take afterwards one part thereof, and three parts of Flux, grind it with Oil of Spike

Another.

TAKE Brown Red, or *Caput Mortis* of *Aqua Fortis*, or Paris Red, and a little Flux, grind it fine with Oil of Spike.

Another.

TAKE Vitriol, let it boil up in a clean Crucible, and when dry, pour a little *Aqua Fortis* and Vinegar to it, neal it well, after that wash it with clean Water, till it has no Taste, dry it over a Fire, and when dry, neal it again, then take of this one part, and three parts of Flux

Blew Colours

TAKE fine Smalt, wash it well with clear Water, as fine as possible, put a little Flux to it, and grind it with Oil of Spike.

Another.

TAKE Ultramarine one part, Flux four parts; grind it with Oil of Spike.

Another

SIX ounces of Lead, four ounces of Sand, two ounces of Saffera, two Quarts of Pot-Ashes, and two Quarts of Lead Salt

SMALT may also be used without the principal Powder, only ground with Oil of Spike.

Green.

TAKE Verditer, and a little grounded Flux, grind it with Oil of Spike.

Grass

Grass Green

TAKE Verditer; neal it in a Crucible, one part of this, and three and a half of Flux

Brown Colours

TAKE *Crocus Martis* one part, Flux two parts, grind it with Oil of Spike.

Purple Colour.

TAKE one part *Crocus Martis*, one part Smalt, and three parts Flux.

Another

TAKE Bloodstone, grind it with Vinegar; when it is fine, wash it clean, and burn it over a Candle on a thin Plate.

A Hair Colour.

TAKE Umber, neal it in a Crucible, then take one part thereof, and three parts of Flux, grind it with Oil of Spike.

Fawn Colour.

TAKE Vitriol, glow it as hot as you possibly can, then take of it one part, and three parts Flux.

Carnation Colour.

TAKE yellow Oaker, glow it in a Crucible very hot, and after that let it cool, and beat it in an Iron Mortar, and if it is not of a fine Colour, neal it again, of this one part, and three and a half of Flux

A Steel Red for Enamel

TAKE fine thin beaten Plates of Steel, cut them into small Shreads, put them into a Viol with *Aqua Fortis*, and when reduced to a Calx over a slow Fire, then neal it; of this one part, and three parts of Flux

Of

❀❀❀❀❀❀❀❀❀❀❀❀❀❀❀❀❀❀❀❀❀❀❀❀❀❀❀❀❀❀

Of the ART of PAINTING on ENAMEL.

THE Ancients that laboured in this noble Art, were unacquainted with the Beauties the Moderns have discovered, particularly in the Art of compounding Colours for representing Portraitures and History; the fine Performances in those Particulars are the Admiration of every curious Beholder· Besides their peculiar Beauty and Lustre, they have the Pre-eminence before all other Paintings, in that they are not subject to the Injury of the Air or Weather, as most all other Paintings, either in Oil or Water-Colours are, and unless being rubb'd or scratch'd with any Thing harder then itself, the Colours will retain their Beauty for Ages, and be as fine and bright as when first done

THIS curious Art cannot be effected without Fire, which always must be Reverberatory, or in a Furnace, so artfully contriv'd that the Fire may play all over the Muffle that covers your Work, but to explain this more fully Take the half of a large Crucible, namely one that is split down lengthways, but as thin as possible you can get When your Reverberatory is building, let the Mouth Part of the Crucible, the split Side downwards, be placed fronting the Mouth of the Furnace, and be fixt in such a Manner, that the Furnace-Fire may not play into it, nor the Ashes drop upon your Work

YOUR Furnace may be either round or square, let it be of Iron or Earth, it is no Matter which, only let there be so much room in the Inside as will contain the split Crucible or Muffle with a good Charcoal Fire round about, to cover it. You must have a Slice or Iron Plate to put your Work upon, which, with a pair of Tongs, you convey into the Furnace, and bring it out again

THE Metals fittest to enamel upon are Gold, Silver, and Copper, but the best Work is perform'd on Gold, for Silver makes the white Enamel appear of a yellowish Hue, and Copper is apt to scale, whereby the Enamel is subject to break in Pieces, besides, the Colours loose a great Deal of their Charms and Lustre to what they appear upon Gold And the Gold, used for this Purpose, should be the finest,

else

elfe the Impurities of a bad Allay will have the fame Effect in the Enamel Colours as the Silver or Copper

YOUR Plate, of whatever Metal it be, muſt be very thin, raiſed in the Nature of a Convex, both that and the Concave Side are laid over with white Enamel, that on the Convex Side whereon you Paint muſt be lay'd on a ſmall Matter thicker than the other. You muſt obſerve that the white Enamel which you lay on the Convex, muſt be ground with fair Water in an Agat Mortar, and with an Agat Peſtle till it be fit for Uſe · The Enamel for the other Side muſt be tempered with Water wherein you have before ſteep'd ſome Quince Kernels

As to the Enamel Colours which you paint with, you muſt take great care that they be equally tempered or your Work will be ſpoil'd, if one be ſofter than the other, when your Work comes into the Furnace and to be hot, the ſoft Colour will intermix with the hard, ſo as to deface your Work intirely This may ſerve to caution you to make tryal upon a white enamel'd Plate for that Purpoſe, of all your Enamels, before you begin your work, Experience will direct you further

TAKE particular Care that not the leaſt Dirt imaginable may come to your Colours while you are either painting or grinding them, for the leaſt Speck thereof, when it is workt up with it, and when the Work comes to be put into the Reverberatory to be red hot, wherever the Dirt is, will leave a Hole, and ſo deface your Work

AFTER you have prepared your Plate with a white Enamel, and ready to paint upon, apply your Colours on an Ivory Pallat or a Piece of Glaſs in a juſt Order, as in Limning, and firſt delineate your Deſign with a dark Red, made out of *Caput Mortus* or *Crocus Martis*, ground with Oil of Spike, put the Piece in the Muffle, and with a reverberatory Fire, as before directed, fix that Colour; and then proceed to Painting, remembring to delute the thick and opaque Enamel Colours with Oil of Spike, and the tranſparent ones with fair Water By mixing blew and yellow Enamel Colour you have a fair green, blew and red, a Violet, red and white, a Roſe Colour, and ſo of other Colours.

WE ſhall here ſet down ſeveral other Receipts for preparing Enamel Colours to the greateſt Perfection, which will not only be fit in beautifying and adorning of Gold; but alſo for Portraiture or Painting on Enamel.

To

To prepare the principal Matter for Enamel Colours

TAKE Lead 15 pound, Plate-Tin Afhes 16 pound, mix and calcine thefe as directed in the Firft Part. After you have calcined your Lead and Tin, fearce the Calx, and put them into an earthen Pot fill'd with Water, fet it over a Fire, and let it boil a little, after which take it off, pour the Water into another Veffel, which will carry the more fubtil Calx along with it, repeat this fo long till you can fubtilize no more of the Calx, and the Water comes off clear without any Mixture What grofs Part remains in the Pot, calcine as before, and this repeat fo often till you can draw off no more of the fubtil Matter Then pour the Waters out of all your Receivers into one that is larger, and evaporate it on a flow Fire, leaft by a fierce one the Calx fhould founder or fettle to the Bottom, but continue more fine and fubtil then when firft calcined

Of this Calx take 12 pound, Frit of white Sand beaten and fearced 12 pound, Saltpetre purified 12 Pound, Salt of Tartar purified * and fearced two ounces. Put thefe Powders all together in a Pot, place it into a Glafs-Houfe Furnace for 10 or 12 Hours to digeft and purify Then take and reduce it to an impalpable Powder, keep it in a clofe dry Place for Ufe. Thus is your firft or principal Matter for Enamel-Colours prepared.

---

* To purify Salt of Tartar, Calcine Tartar of red Wine in an Earthen Pot, till it comes black, continue the Fire till it changes to a White Then put it into an Earthen Pan, glaz'd, fill the Pan with clear Water, and boil it over a gentle Fire, fo that in four Hours the Water may evaporate the fourth Part, then take it off the Fire, and after the Water is fettled and cold, pour it off by Inclination, into a clean glaz'd Pan, and you will have a ftrong Lee Then pour clean Water on the Feces, and let them boil as before This repeat, till the Water becomes infipid Then filter the Lees, put them in Glafs Bodies upon the Afhes in a gentle Heat to evaporate, and at the Bottom there will remain a very white Salt Diffolve this Salt again in fair Water, and let it ftand two Days, for the Feces to fettle, then filter it, and evaporate it at a gentle Fire as before, and you will have a Salt whiter then the former, repeat this three or four times, and your Salt will be whiter than Snow itfelf

To make Enamel of a Milk white Colour

TAKE three pound of the fore mentioned principal Powder, and 24 Grains of *Magnesi* prepared *, Arsenick two pound, put this together into a melting Pot to melt and to purify over a fierce Fire When the Matter is thus melted, throw it out of the Pot into fair Water, and having afterwards dry'd it, melt it again as before, do this for the third Time, changing the Water. When you have thus purified it, and find the White answer your Intent, it is well, but in Case it has still a Tincture of a greenish Hue, add a little more *Magnesi,* and in melting it over again it will become as white as Milk, and be fit to enamel with upon Gold or other Metals Take it off the Fire, make it in Cakes, and preserve it for Use

A Turcoise blue Enamel.

TAKE of the principal Matter or Powder three pound, in a white glaz'd Pot, melt and purify it; then cast it into Water, when dry, put it again into a Pot, and being melted over again, add to it at four times this Composition Scales of Copper thrice calcined † two ounces and a half, prepared Zaffer 43 Grains, of prepared *Magnesi* 24 Grains, Some blew two ounces, mix and reduce these to a very fine Powder, stir the Matter very well with an Iron Rod, for the Powders to incorporate When your Matter is thus ting'd, observe well whether your Colour answers your Intent before you empty the Pot If you perceive the Tinging-powders are too predominant, add more of the principal Powders, and if too faint, add more of the Tinging powder Your own Judgment must direct you in the Management of this Preparation

---

* The Preparation of the *Magnesi* is thus Put some Pieces in an Iron Ladle into a Reverberatory Fire, and when it begins to whiten, sprinkle it with good Vinegar, after which beat it, and wash it whilst hot, then dry it, and reduce it into a Powder

† To calcine Copper Scales, such as come from the Hammer of Braziers or Copper Smiths Wash them from their foulness, put them into a Crucible place it in the Mouth of a reverboratory Furnace for four Days after which let them cool, then pound, grind, and searce them This Powder put a second time into the Furnace, to reverberate four Days longer, proceed as before, and after it has stood again the third time for four Days, reduce it into Powder, and it will be fit for the Use design'd for

A fine

A fine Blew Enamel

TAKE two pound of the principal Powder, purified, 1 Ounce of prepared Zaffer, or of Indigo Blew, 22 Grains of Copper thrice calcin'd, mix and reduce these to a fine Powder, put it into a white glaz'd Pot When the Metal is melted, cast it into Water, then dry it, and put it into the Pot again, let it stand upon the Fire, till it is well incorporated Take it off, make it into Cakes, and keep it for Use

A Green Enamel

TAKE two pound of the principal Powder, purified; one ounce of Copper Scales thrice refin'd, 24 Grains of Scales of Iron, Copperas two ounces, yellow Arsenick one ounce, mix and reduce these to an impalpable Powder, and at three several times or Portions, fling it into the principal Matter, stirring the Metal so as to tinge it equally. When the Colour is to your liking, let it stand for a while in the Fire, to incorporate thoroughly, then take it off, and you will have a delicate Green.

Another

TAKE * Feretto of Spain two ounces, 48 Grains of Crocus Martis prepar'd with Vinegar, yellow Arsenick two ounces, pulverize and mix this well, and put it into a white glaz'd Pot, set it in the Furnace to melt, and refine the Matter, after which cast it into Water, and when dry'd, again into the Pot When melted, observe whether the Colour is to your liking· If so. let it stand for some time longer to refine If you find the Colour too faint, add more of the tinging Powder.

---

* *Feretto of Spain* is thus prepared Stratify thin Plates of Copper with Vitriol, in a Crucible put it in the Mouth of a Glass Furnace, for three Days then take it out and add to the Copper new Rows or Layers of Vitriol, stratifying them as before, Then put the Crucible again in the same Place of the Furnace This repeat six Times successively, and you will have an excellent *Ferretto*, which beat to Powder, and it will tinge Glass of an extraordinary beautiful Colour.

A Black

A Black Enamel.

TAKE of the principal Powder two pound, prepar'd Zaffer one ounce, and prepared *Magnefi* one ounce, pulverize and mix this, and proceed as directed in the preceeding Colours.

Another

OF the principal Powder three pound, Zaffer one ounce, *Crocus Martis* one ounce, *Feretto of Spain* one ounce; pound and mix it, and proceed as directed before.

A Velvet Black Enamel.

OF the principal Powder two pound, Red Tartar two ounces, prepar'd *Magnefi* one ounce, pulverize this; and put it into a glaz'd Pot, bigger than ordinary, because the Metal will raile; for the reft, proceed as directed before.

A Purple Colour Enamel.

OF the principal Powder two pound, prepar'd *Magnefi* one ounce, Indigo Llew halt an ounce, proceed as above.

Another.

PRINCIPAL Powder three pound, prepar'd *Magnefi* one ounce and a half, of twice calcin'd Scales of Copper three ounces, Stone Blew one ounce, pulverize, and proceed as directed.

A Violet Enamel

OF the principal Powder three pound, prepar'd *Magnefi* one ounce, thrice calcin'd Copper Scales 24 Grains, Terra Vert one ounce, pulverize and mix this all together, and proceed as before directed

A Yellow Enamel.

OF the principal Powder three pound, Tartar one ounce and a half, prepar'd *Magnefi* 36 Grains, yellow Orpiment two ounces, Arfenick one ounce, pulverize it, and proceed as before directed.

An

An excellent Red Enamel, of a very Splendid Ruby Colour.

THIS Enamel is of a surprizing Beauty, and its Lustre equals that of a real Ruby. To prepare this, take equal Quantities of *Magness* of *Piedmont*, and *Saltpetre*; let them reverberate and calcine in an Earthen Pot in a Furnace for 24 Hours, take it then off, and wash it well in warm Water, to separate the Saltpetre, dry it well, and the Mass will be of a red Colour. To this add an equal Quantity of Sal armoniac, grind this on a Marble with distill'd Vinegar, as Painters do their Colours; dry it, and pulverize it. Then put it into a strong Matrass, let it sublimate for 12 Hours; break off the Neck of your Matrass, and mix all the volatile and fixed Parts together, adding the same Quantity of Sal armoniac as there are Flowers, and take care to weigh them before the Composition, grind, pulverize and sublimate as before, repeating this until your *Magness* remains fusible at the Bottom of the Matrass. This preserve to tinge your Crystal with, and according to your liking, add either a greater or lesser Quantity of the *Magness*, or else of the Crystal, till you have brought it to its Degree of Perfection

A Rose Colour'd Enamel.

TAKE five Pound of Crystal ground, melt it in a glaz'd Pot, add at four different times two ounces and a half of thrice calcin'd Copper, stir the Metal every time, then pour into it *Crocus Martis* and *Magness*, prepared as directed, let it stand for six Hours to cleanse, and if the Colour is too light, add a little more *Crocus Martis*, till it be of a fine Rose Colour

OBSERVE that all the Colours, which are not pure Enamel, must be incorporated with the Crystalline Matter, to the End they may vitrify the better, which else they would not easily do. Most Workmen make use of Rocailli, but that does not answer the Purpose so well as Crystal ground.

A fine Purple.

TAKE half an ounce of fine Gold; neal it, and beat it in very thin Plates, dissolve this in four ounces of *Aqua Fortis*, regulated with Sal-armoniac, or old strong Salt; put it into a Glass Cucurbit, which set on warm Ashes or Sand,

to

to diffolve, put to it a fmall Matter of Saltpetre, when all is diffolved, drop two or three Drops of Oil of Tartar into it, and ftop the Cucurbit clofe, to prevent its boiling over. Then put in fome more Drops of Oil, and repeat this fo long, till it ebullates or boils no more. After this, put fome lukewarm Rain-Water to it, and let it ftand for fome Time, and a Powder will fettle at the Bottom of the Cucurbit, then pour off the Water leifurely into an earthen or glazed Receiver, put more frefh Water to the Settlement, and repeat this till the Water comes off clear, and free from the Sharpnefs of the *Aqua Fortis* When the Powder is fettled, and all the Water pour'd from it, then put it upon a Piece of whited brown Paper, to feparate it from the reft of the Water, and dry it on a warm Tile, or in the Sun. To one part of this Powder, add fix parts of the principal Powder, grind it with Oil of Spike, and it will make a good Purple.

A good Red Enamel Colour

TAKE clean Hungarian Vitriol, put it into a Copper Cup, hold it over a Fire, and ftir it with a Silver or Copper Wire, till it is reduc'd to a white Powder, this burn upon a hot Tile, on which let it cool of itfelf, then wafh it with Rain-Water, and when fettled, pour off that, and put frefh Water on, and thus repeat it feveral Times

But fome Artifts, inftead of wafhing this Powder, boil it in fair Water, and think this Method better then that of wafhing. With this Powder you tinge the principal Matter to what Height you would have your Colour

Another good Red Enamel

DISSOLVE Vitriol in an Earthen Pan, and it will fix and fhoot at the Sides therof into Cryftals, which take and burn over a gentle Fire between two Crucibles well luted. When thus you have burnt it to a Powder, take and boil it in clean Water, and when done, dry it, of this take one part, of the principal Powder three parts, and of tranfparent yellow one and one eighth part

Another.

PUT Vitriol into a Crucible, pour a little *Aqua Fortis* upon it, and neal it gently, then put it in a clean Earthen Pipkin, pour clean Water upon it, and boil it one Hour; then

then pour off that, and put fresh Water upon it, wash it, and when settled, dry it; neal it once more, and it is fit for Use. Of this Powder take two parts, and of the principal Powder or Flux, three parts.

A Flux for Red Enamel.

TAKE of Red Lead four ounces, white scouring Sand one ounce, melt it, and pour it into an Iron Mortar.

Some General Observations.

BEFORE we proceed to another Subject, we will conclude this Article with a few Observations and general Rules, for the more easy apprehending of what has been said already.

You may observe, That Gold is the most proper Metal to enamel upon · That every Colour, except a Violet or Purple, receives an additional Beauty from it, to what it does from Silver or Copper That it is most agreeable to enrich Gold with such beautiful Colours, since they raise an agreeable Admiration in the Beholder, when a skilful Artist places them in due Order

THE Ancients only painted in black and white, with something of a Carnation or Flesh Colour, in Success of Time they indeed made some few Improvements, but all their Enamel Colours were equally alike on Gold, Silver, or Copper; every one transparent, and every Colour wrought by itself. But since the Modern Artists have found out to Enamel with opaque Colours, and to compound them in such a Manner as to shade or heighten the Painting therewith, in the same Manner as is done in Miniature or Oil Painting, this Art has gain'd the Præeminence in small Pourtraitures, it having the Advantage of a natural and lasting Lustre, which is never tarnish'd nor subject to decay.

THE purple colour'd Enamel agrees best upon Silver, from which it receives an agreeable Beauty, so doth the Egmarine, Azure and Green. All other Colours, as well clear as opaque, disagree therewith Copper suits with all thick Enamels, but is unfit for that which is clear

You must observe to make choice of good, hard, and lasting Enamel The soft is commonly full of Lead, which is apt to change the Colours, and makes them look sullied and foul,

E

but

but if you follow our Prefcriptions, you will meet with no fuch Inconveniences.

REMEMBER when you lay on your white Enamel on either Gold, Silver, or Copper, to dilute it with Water of Quince Kernels, as has been directed, your clear Enamel Colours mix only with fair Water, and the opaque, when mix'd with Flux or the principal Powder, dilute with Oil of Spike.

BE careful not to keep your Work too long in the Fire, but take it often out, to fee when it has the proper Glazing, and then it is finish'd

BEFORE you ufe your Enamels, give it a little Preparation The beft approv'd by Goldfmiths is, to take the Enamel, and after you have ground it to a fine Powder, pour on it a little *Aqua Fortis,* and afterwards purify and refine it in a fmall Glafs Cucurbit, then wafh it feveral times in fair Water, dry it, and lay it up carefully to keep it from Duft When you ufe it, grind as much as you have occafion for, with fair Water, in an Agat Mortar, thus you do with all your clear and tranfparent Enamels, and by this Means you will have all Things in Readinefs to go on in your Work with Pleafure

ALL opaque Colours that will ftand the Fire, are fit to be ufed in painting Enamel, and the ingenious Artift will not be at a great Lofs, but in fearching after them will meet with feveral Colours not yet difcover'd, as it frequently happens to thofe who try Experiments, and are in Purfuit of new Difcoveries, in this as in any other Art.

Of

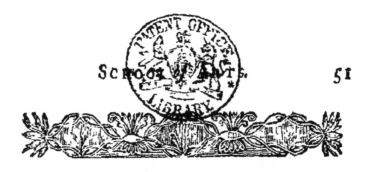

Of Artificial PEARLS.

IT will not be improper to treat in this Place on this Subject, as it is a Branch relating to Jewellers.

THE Ancients, who did write about the several Sorts of
Precious Stones, did range Pearls among the Jewels of the first
Class, they having at all Times been in high Esteem, and have
been eagerly fought for, particularly for the Ornament of
Ladies

THE Oriental Pearls are the finest, on Account of their
Largeness, Colour, and Beauty, being of a Silver White,
whereas the Occidental or Western Pearls seldom exceed the
Colour of Milk The best Pearls are brought from the *Per-
sian* Gulf, above the Isle of *Ormus, Bassora* They are found
in *Europe* both in salt and fresh Waters, *Scotland, Silesia,
Bohemia* and *Frisia*, produce very fine ones, tho' those of
the latter Country are but very small.

ART, which is always busy to mimick Nature, has not
been idle to bring counterfeit Pearls to the greatest Perfection;
they are imitated so near, that a naked Eye cannot distinguish
them from the Pearls of the first Class, or the real ones,
and by this Means the wearing of Pearls is become a uni-
versal Fashion

WE shall here present the Curious with several Receipts
how to counterfeit Pearls in the best Manner, and after a Method both easy and satisfactory, so as to render his Labour pleasant and delightful, and to answer his Expectation

To imitate fine ORIENTAL PEARLS.

TAKE of thrice distill'd Vinegar two pound, Venice
Turpentine one pound, mix it together into a Mass and
put it into a Cucurbit, fit a Head and Receiver to it, and
after you have luted the Joints, set it, when dry, on a Sand
Furnace, to still the Vinegar from it, don't give it too much
Heat, least the Stuff should swell up.

AFTER this, put the Vinegar into another Glaſs Cucurbit, in which there is a Quantity of Seed Pearl, wrapt in a Piece of thin Silk, but ſo as not to touch the Vinegar, put a Cover or Head upon the Cucurbit, lute it well, and put it in *Bal Maine,* where you may let it remain a Fortnight. The Heat of the Balneum will raiſe the Fumes of the Vinegar, and they will ſoften the Pearls in the Silk, and bring them to the Conſiſtence of a Paſte, which being done, take them out, and mould them in what bigneſs, Shape and Form you pleaſe. Your Mould muſt be of fine Silver, gilded the Inſide, you muſt alſo refrain from touching the Paſte with your Fingers, but uſe Silver gilded Utenſils, with which fill your Moulds. When you have moulded them, bore them through with a Hog's Briſtle, or Gold Wire, and let them dry a little, then thread them again on a Gold Wire, and put them in a Glaſs, cloſe it up, and ſet them in the Sun to dry, after they are thorough dry, put them into a Glaſs Matraſs, in a Stream of running Water and leave 'em there 20 Days, by that Time they will contract the natural Hardneſs and Solidity. Then take them out of the Matraſs, and hang them in * Mercury-Water, where they will moiſten, ſwell, and aſſume their Oriental Beauty, after which ſhift them into a Matraſs, Hermetically cloſed up, to prevent any Water coming to them, and let it down into a Well, to continue there about eight Days, then draw the Matraſs up, and in opening it, you will find Pearls exactly reſembling Oriental ones. This Method is very excellent, and well worth the Trouble, ſince by experimenting ſo fine a Secret one will have the Satisfaction of ſeeing the Performance anſwer the Direction above Expectation.

---

* Mercury-Water is thus prepar'd. Take Plate Tin of *Cornwall* calcine it, and let the Calx be pure and fine; then with one ounce of the Calx, and two ounces of prepared Mercury, make an Amalgamate waſh it with fair Water, till the Water remains inſipid and clear, then dry the Amalgamate thoroughly, put it into a Matraſs over a Furnace, giving it ſuch a Heat as is requiſite for Sublimation. When the Matter is well ſublimated, take off the Matraſs, and let it cool. Take out that Sublimate, add one ounce of Venice Sublimate to it, and grind it together on a Marble, put this into another Matraſs, cloſe it well, and ſet it upſide-down in a Pail of Water, and the whole Maſs will reſolve itſelf in a little Time into Mercury Water. This done, filter it into a Glaſs Receiver, ſet it on a gentle Aſh Fire to coagulate, and it will turn into a Cryſtalline Subſtance. This beat in a Glaſs Mortar with a Glaſs Peſtle to a fine Powder, ſearce it through a fine Sieve and put it into a Matraſs ſtop it cloſe up, and place it in *Bain Marie* there let it remain, till it reſolves again into Water, which is the Mercury Water, fit for the above mentioned Uſe.

Anoth-

Another Way to make Artificial Pearls

TAKE Oriental Seed Pearl, reduce them into a fine Powder on a Marble, then diffolve them in Mercury Water, or clarified Juice of Lemons To make the more difpatch, fet them in a Cucurbit on warm Afhes, and you will fee prefently a Cream arife at the Top, which take off immediately: Take the Diffolution off the Fire, and when fettled, pour off the Liquid in another Glafs, and fave it You will have the Pearl-Pafte at the Bottom, with which fill your Silver gilded Moulds, and fo put them by for 24 Hours Then bear them through with a Briftle, clofe up the Moulds in Barley Dough, and put it in an Oven to bake, and when about half bak'd, draw it out, take out your Pearls, and fteep them in the Liquid you fav'd before, putting them in and out feveral times, then clofe them up in their Moulds, and bake them again with the like Dough, but let it remain in the Oven till it is almoft burnt, before you draw it out After you have taken your Pearls out of their Moulds, ftring them on one or more Gold or Silver Threads, and fteep them in Mercury-Water for about a Fortnight, after which Time take and dry them by the Sun, in a well clofed Glafs, and you will have very fine and bright Pearls

Another Way

DISSOLVE very fine pulverized Oriental Pearls in Alom-Water; when the Diffolution is fettled, pour off the Water, and wafh the Pafte that's fettled, firft in diftill'd Waters, then in Bean-Water, and afterwards fet it in *Bal Marie* or Horfe Dung, to digeft for a Fortnight, this done, take out your Glafs, and the Matter being come to the Confiftence of a Pafte, mould it as you have been directed before, bear and ftring the Pearls on a Silver Thread, and hang them in a wellclofed-up Glafs Limbeck, to prevent the Air coming to them. Thus dried, wrap every one up in Leaves of Silver, then fplit a Barbel, and clofe them up in the Belly thereof, make a Dough of Barley Meal, and bake the Fifh, as you do a Batch of Bread, then draw him, take out your Pearls, and dry them in a clofed-up Glafs in the Sun

To give them a Tranfparency and Splendour, dip them in Mercury-Water, or inftead thereof, take the Herb *Gratuli* fqueez'd in Water, put therein fix ounces of Seed Pearl, one

ounce

ounce of Saltpetre, one ounce of Roch-Alom, one ounce of
Litharge of Silver, the whole being diſſolv'd, heat firſt the
Pearls, and then dip them in this Diſſolution to cool, repeat
this about ſix times running

IF your Pearls ſhould not have their natural Hardneſs, then
take two ounces of *Calamy*, or *Lapis Calaminaris* in impalpable Powder; add to this two ounces of Oil of Vitriol, and
two ounces of the Water of the Whites of Eggs, put it together
into a Retort, lute a Receiver to it, and you will ſtill a fair
Water, with which, and ſome fine Barley Flower, make a
Paſte, in which coffin your Pearls, and bake them as before,
thus they will become exceeding hard.

Another Method.

TAKE Chalk, well purified and cleanſed from all groſ-
neſs and Sand, of this make a Paſte, and form thereof Pearls, in a Mould for that Purpoſe, pierce them through
with a Briſtle, and let them dry in the Sun, or in an Oven;
then ſtring them on a Silver Thread, colour them lightly over
with Boli-Armoniac deluted in the Water of the White of
Eggs, and drench them with a Pencil and fair Water, lay
them over with Leaf Silver, and put them under a Glaſs in
the Sun to dry, when dry, poliſh them with a Wolf's
Tooth

To give them the true Colour, make a Glue of Vellum
Shavings thus After you have waſh'd them in warm Water, boil
them in fair Water, in a new earthen Pot or Pipkin, to ſome
thickneſs, and then ſtrain it through a Cloath When you
will uſe it, warm it firſt, and dip your String of Pearls into it, but
let there be an Interval between each Pearl, not to touch one
another, this will give your Pearls a natural Luſtre.

To form large Pearls out of ſmall ones, as directed by Korndorffer.

TAKE of Mercurial Water 14 Ounces, put two ounces
of Sulph Solis into a low Matrais, pour the Mercurial Water upon it, and let it diſſolve and extract. Then take of
the whiteſt ſmall Pearls 20 ounces, put them into a proper
Matrais, and pour the ſaid Water upon it. The Pearls will by
Degrees reſolve, and at laſt turn to a clear Calx, much like
reſolved Silver Calx; Pour off the Mercurial Water, boil
the

the Calx well out, and dry it, then put it into a clean Crucible by itself, and melt and cast it into what form you please. When cold, polish it in the same Manner as you do Gems or Crystals, and you will have your Work of the Consistence and Beauty of the finest and clearest Oriental Pearl.

To make out of small Pearls a fine Necklace of large ones,

TAKE small Oriental Pearls, as many as you will, put them into Mercurial Water 15 Days and Nights together, and they will turn soft, like a Paste; then have a Pearl Mould, made of Silver; into this convey the Paste by a Silver Spatel or such like Implement, but you must not touch the Paste with your Fingers, and be very careful to have every Thing nice and clean about this Work. When it is in the Mould, let it dry therein, boar a Hole with a Silver Wire thro' it, and let it stick thereon till you have more, but take care they don't touch one another; then have a Glass wherein you may fix, as upon a Pair of Stands, your Wires with Pearls, put them well closed up in the Sun to harden, and when you find them hard enough, put them into a Matrass, lute the Neck thereof very close, and sink it in running Spring Water for 20 Days, in which time they contract their natural Colour.

To clean Pearls, when of a foul Colour.

TAKE Pigeons Dung, moisten it with Alom-Water, to the Consistence of a Paste, this put into a Glass, big enough to hold four times the Quantity, put into this your yellow-colour'd or foul Pearls, so that they may be cover'd all over, and set them in a warm Place, behind an Oven; let them stand for a Month: then take them out, fling them into fresh cold Alom-Water, and dry them carefully, and your Pearls will become fine and white: If you repeat the Operation once or twice, they will be done to a greater Perfection.

To Blanch and Cleanse Pearls.

FIRST soak and cleanse them in Bran-Water, then in Milk warm Water, and last of all steep them in Mercury-Water Then string and hang them in a Glass, close it well, and set them in the Sun to dry.

THE Bran-Water is made thus Boil two good handfuls of Wheaten Bran in a Quart of Water, till all the Strength of the

Bran

Bran is drawn out, which ufe thus: Take a new glaz'd earthen Pan, in which put your Pearls on a String, and pour the third part of the Bran-Water upon it, when they have foak'd, and the Water juft warm, rub your Pearls gently with your Hands, to cleanfe them the better and continue this till the Water is cold; then throw off that, and pour on another third part of the Bran-Water that's boiling, proceed with this as you did before, and when cool, throw it away, and pour on the Remainder of the Water ftill proceeding as before, after this, heat fair Water, and pour it on your Pearls, to refrefh them, and to wafh away the Remains of the Bran, by fhifting them, and pouring on frefh warm Water. This do thrice, without handling your Pearls, then lay them on a Sheet of clean white Paper, and dry them in a Shade, then dip them into Mercury-Water, to bring them to Perfection.

Other Methods us'd in Blanching of Pearls

POUND Alablafter to an impalpable Powder, rub the Pearls therewith very gently, this will not only cleanfe them, but if you let them remain in this Powder 24 Hours afterwards, they will ftill be the better for it White Coral has the fame Effect, ufed in the like Manner

TARTAR calcin'd white, and divefted of all its Moifture, is very good for the fame Purpofe

SALT diffolv'd, filter'd, coagulated, well dried and ground, is as effectual as any of the former Things, for cleanfing of Pearl, by rubbing them therewith, and if afterwards you will lay them up in fome coarfe ground Millet, it will contribute to their natural Brightnefs

Of DOUBLETS.

DOUBLETS being much in Vogue, and the Lapidaries arrived to such a Perfection in the making of them, that they often deceive even tolerable Judges: I shall, for the Sake of such as are unacquainted with the Secrets thereof, set down some Instructions, how they are made; and also how they may be known and distinguish'd from real Gems.

TAKE two Drams of clear Mastick, and of the finest and clearest *Venetian* or *Cyprian* Turpentine 16 Drams; dissolve this together in a Silver or Brass Spoon. If you find there is too much Turpentine, then add a little more Mastick to it, to bring it to a right Temper. Then take what Colour you please, as *Florentine* Lake, Dragon's Blood, distill'd Verdegrease, or what Colour else you design, for representing a particular Stone; grind each by itself, in the nicest Manner you possibly can, and mix each apart with the Mixture of Mastick and Turpentine, which you ought to have ready by you, and you will find the *Florentine* Lake to imitate the Colour of a Ruby, the Dragon's Blood that of a Hyacinth, and the Verdegrease the Colour of an Emerald But in case you would have your Colours, as it were, distilled, then get a little Box, made of Lime-Tree, in the Shape of an Egg or Acorn, as represented in Plate II. Fig. 2

THIS Box must be turned at the Bottom as thin as possible, so that the Light may be seen through it. Then make a Quantity of any one of the abovesaid Colours, mix'd with the Mixture of Mastick and Turpentine, and put it into that little Box, hung over a gentle glowing coal Fire, or in Summer-time in the Heat of the Sun, where the Colour will distil through very fine · Scrape and put this in little Boxes of Ivory, to preserve it from Dust, for your use, It is necessary to have to every different Colour such a different wooden Box

WHEN the Colours are ready, take your Crystals (first ground exactly to fit upon one another) and make your Colours and Stone of an equal Warmth, lay your Colour with a fine Hair Pencil on the Sides of the Crystals that are to be join'd together,

ther; then clap them again each other as nimble as poffible; prefs them with your Fingers clofe together; let them cool; and it is done.

How to know a Doublet from a natural Stone.

TAKE a Stone, in Cafe you are dubious about it, and look upon it edge-ways againft the Light, and if it is a Doublet, you will prefently fee the clear Cryftal, or the Glafs, and fo find out the Impofter.

The Cryftal Glue of Milan.

IS Nothing elfe but Grains of Maftick, fqueezed out by Degrees over a Charcoal Fire, and like a clear Turpentine. The Pieces which are to be glued together, are firft warm'd over a Coal Fire, then the Maftick is put on a Point of a Bodkin and warm'd, when both are of an equal warmth, wipe your Cryftal or Stone over with it, clap them upon one another, and prefs them together, what comes out about the Sides, fcrape as foon as it is dry, with a Knife This withftands as well cold as hot Water, except a fierce Fire.

Some Remarks on DOUBLETS.

WE muft know that all falfified Jewels are made, either of a Saphir, or two Cryftals, by putting a Foyl between them, and cementing 'em together, as has been mentioned before, with Maftick Thefe mimick'd Stones may eafily be difcern'd, by taking one of them between the two Nails of your Thumbs, and holding 'em againft the Light, directing your Eye towards the Middle of the Stone, if the two outer Parts appear white, and the Middle of a different Colour, you may conclude the Stone to be falfe and made thus by Art.

A Peremptory Instruction concerning the Foyles or Leaves which are laid under Precious Stones.

IT is customary to place thin Leaves of Metal under Precious Stones, in order to make them look transparent, and to give them an agreable different Colour, either deep or pale. Thus if you want a Stone to be of a pale Colour, put a Foyl of that Colour under it; again, if you would have it deep, then lay a dark one under it. Besides, as the Transparency of Gems discovers the Bottom of the Ring they are set in, Artificers have found out these Means, to give the Stone an additional Beauty, which without these Helps it would be depriv'd of.

These Foyles are made, either of Copper, Gold, or Gold and Silver together. We shall first speak of such as are made of Copper only, and are generally known by the Name of *Noremberg* or *German* Foyles.

Buy the thinnest Copper Plates you can get, because the thinner they are, the less Trouble they will give you in reducing them to a finer Substance. Beat these Plates gently upon a well polish'd Anvil, with a polish'd Hammer, as thin as possible: But before you go about this Work, take two Iron Plates, about six Inches long, and as wide, and no thicker then Writing-Paper, bend them so as to fit one in the other; between these neal the Copper you design to hammer for the Foyles, to prevent the Ashes or other Filthiness coming to them. Put your Copper Foyles between these bended Irons, lay them in the Fire, and let them neal. Then, taking them out, shake the Ashes from them, and hammer them, till cool. Take than your Foyles to the Anvil, and beat them till they are very thin, and whilst you beat one Number, put in another between the Irons to neal. This you may repeat eight times, till they are as thin as the Work requires. You must have a Pipkin with Water at hand, in which put Tartar and Salt, of one as much as the other. This boil, put the Foyles in, and stir them continually, till by boiling they become white. Then take them from the Fire, wash them in clean Water, dry them
with

with a clean fine Rag, and give them another hammering on the Anvil, till they are fit for your Purpose

N B CARE muſt be taken in the Management of this Work, not to give the Foyles too much Heat, to prevent their melting, neither muſt they be too long boil'd, for fear of attracting too much Salt

How to poliſh the FOYLES

TAKE a Plate of the beſt Copper, one Foot long, and about five or ſix Inches wide, poliſh'd to the greateſt Perfection This bend to a long Convex, faſten it upon a half Roll, and fix it to a Bench or Table, then take ſome Chalk, waſh'd as clean as poſſible, and filter'd through a fine linnen Cloath ſo often till you think it cannot be finer, and having laid ſome thereof on the Roll, and wetted the Copper all over, lay your Foyles upon it, and with a Poliſh-Stone and the Chalk, poliſh your Foyles till they are as bright as a looking Glaſs; and when ſo, dry them between a fine Rag, and lay them up, ſecure from Duſt. I ſhall now ſhew how theſe Foyles are colour'd, but firſt give a ſhort Deſcription of the Oven or Furnace that's requiſite for that Purpoſe

THE Furnace muſt be but ſmall and round, about a Foot high, and as wide, cover the ſame with a round Blade, in which muſt be a round Hole, about four Inches wide, upon this Furnace put another without a Bottom, of the ſame Dimenſion as the former, and let the Crevices of the Sides round about be well cloſed and luted This Furnace muſt alſo have a Hole at Top. The lower Furnace muſt have a little Door at Bottom, about five Inches big Before this fix a Sort of a Funnel, like a Smoak-Funnel to an Oven, and lute it cloſe to the Furnace, then light ſome Charcoal on your Hearth, and when they burn clear, and are free from Smoak, convey them through the Funnel into the Furnace, till they come up ſo high as to fill half the Funnel. When every Thing is ready, and you have a clear Fire, then begin to colour your Foyles in the following Manner

LAY the Foyles upon a Pair of Iron Tongs, hold them over the Hole that is a-Top the Furnace, ſo that the Fumes of the Coals may reverberate over 'em, and move them ſo long about, till they are of a browniſh Violet Colour, and this is done without any other Vapour or Smoak When you have done with this Colour, put it by, and if you will colour others,

of

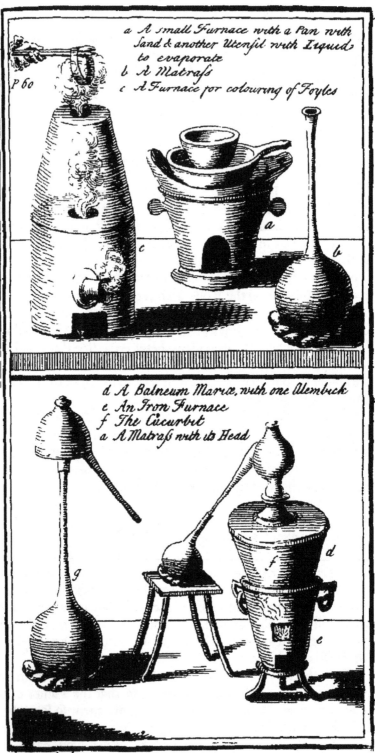

a A small Furnace with a Pan with Sand & another Utensil with Liquid to evaporate
b A Matrass
c A Furnace for colouring of Foyles

P 60

d A Balneum Mariæ, with one Alembick
e An Iron Furnace
f The Cucurbit
a A Matrass with its Head

Hulett Sculp

of a Saphir or Sky Blew, then put the Foyles upon the Tongs as before, and whilft you with one Hand are holding the Foyles over the Holes, fling with the other fome Down Feathers of a Goofe, upon the live Coals in the Funnel, and with a red hod Poker prefs them down, to drive the Smoak of the Feathers up through the Holes of the Oven, which by fettling upon the Foyles, gives 'em a fine Sky Colour. But you muft have your Eyes very quick upon them, and as foon you fee that they have attracted the Colour you defign, take them away from the Oven, to prevent their changing into fome other Colour: But if you will have your Foyles of a Saphir Blew, then firft filver them over, which is done in this Manner.

TAKE a little Silver, and diffolve it in *Aqua Fortis*, when diffolv'd, put Spring-Water to it, fling thin Bits of Copper into it, and the Water will look troubled, and the Silver precipitate and hang to the Copper, pour off that, fweeten the Silver with fair Water, and let it dry in the Sun, when dry, grind it on a Porphyr-Stone. Then take one ounce of Tartar, and as much of common Salt, mix and grind 'em all together, till they are well mixed. This Powder fling upon the thin Foyles, and rub them with your Finger backwards and forwards, and it will filver 'em, then lay them upon the Polifher, pour Water over them, and fome of the Powder, rub with your Thumb, till they are as white as you would have 'em. Polifh them with the Polifher of Blood-Stone, and holding them over the Goofe Feather Smoak, they will take a fine dark Blue.

To colour Foyles of a green Colour for an EMERALD.

YOU muft firft colour your Foyles of a Sky Blew, as directed before, then hold them over the Smoak-Hole, and below in the Funnel lay upon a red hot Iron Plate, Leaves of Box, from which afcends a Smoak that gives the Foyles a green Colour, but before they attract that Colour, they undergo feveral Changes, as Blew, then red, and again yellow, wherefore you muft hold them fo long, till you have the green Colour to your Mind.

To colour the Foyles of a RUBY Colour.

PUT the Shearings of Scarlet Cloath upon the Coals, and holding the Foyles over the Smoak-Hole, they will attract a fine red Colour.

The

The Colour of an Amethist

MAY be had in proceeding with your Foyles, as for the blew or Saphir Colour; for before that blew Colour comes, it first changes to an Amethist, as soon as you perceive this, take them off, and polish them.

How the Foyles are mix'd with Copper, and other Metals.

THESE are more difficult to make, but more lasting in their Colour Take one pound and a half of Copper, and melt it in a Crucible, fling into this two ounces and 11 Penny-Weight of Gold, when in Fusion, pour it out into a flat Ingot, and let it cool. This beat and work, as has been taught, into thin Foyles, then boil them in Tartar and Salt These Sorts of Foyles will take a fine Ruby Colour; nor can that Colour be well done without this Mixture.

Another Way to make the Foyles.

TAKE Small-Coal Dust, put it in a little Iron Oven, and in the midst thereof a live Charcoal, blow it till all the small-Coal Dust is lighted, and let this glow for two Hours: When it is most all glown out, add such another Quantity to it, and let it glow for an Hour. At the Top of your Oven must be a round or square Hole, with a close Cover to it, in which hang the Foyles to some Copper or Iron Wire When your Small-Coal has glow'd for about an Hour, take a little Iron Bowl, and warm it well, put in it a little Quantity of Fox Hair, and then set it upon the Small-Coal Dust, shut the Oven Door, and open the Top. This will draw the Smoke through, and give the Foyles first the Colour of a Ruby, then of an Amethist, and at last of a Saphir. You may take out such Colours as will serve your Purpose; and if you want a Green, let those Foyles hang, and burn Sage Leaves, so long till the Foyles turn to a green Colour. Take care to put but a few Sage Leaves in at a Time.

To the Ruby and Hiacynth Colour you use pure Copper, but to an Emerald and Saphir you must take one part of Gold and two parts of Silver, and eight Parts of Copper, melted and work'd together.

Choice

Choice Secrets to imitate Precious Stones, or to make Artificial Gems.

THIS curious Art is arrived to that Perfection that it is capable of imitating Precious Stones in their Lustre, Colour, and Beauty, and even to surpass the natural ones, except in Hardness, which to obtain, has been, and no doubt are still the Endeavours of several ingenious Men.

The Art of making artificial Gems, consists chiefly in rightly imitating the Tinctures of those that are real These must be extracted from such Things as resist the Fire, and don't change their Colour, though of a Volatile Nature: Thus Verdegrease being put into the Fire, changes to another Colour, but when put in Fusion with Crystal, it retains its natural Colour.

You must therefore take such Colours as change not, when you have occasion to mix them together As Blew and Yellow makes a Green, you must take such Blew that may not hurt the Yellow you mix with, and such a Yellow, that cannot be detrimental to the Blew, and so for the rest of the Colours. We shall give most plain and certain Instructions, to carry the ingenious Artist with Ease and Pleasure through this Labour, and first shew him,

The Way of preparing Natural Crystal.

TAKE natural Crystal, the clearest you can get, let the Pieces be bigger or less, it is no Matter, fill a large Crucible with them, and cover it with a Cover broader than the Mouth of the Crucible, to prevent the Ashes or Coals falling into it Then put it into a small Furnace, on burning Coals, and when the Crystal is thorough hot, cast it into a pretty large Vessel of cold Water Then take it out of the Water, dry it on an Earthen Plate, and put it into the same Crucible again: Cover it, and proceed as before, repeating it 12 times running, and changing each time the Water When the Crystal easily breaks and crumbles, and is thorough white, it is a Sign that it is calcin'd enough. If there appears any black in the Veins, break off the white, and put the black again into the Furnace,

and

and proceed therewith as before, till only the white remains behind.

AFTER you have dried this Calcination thoroughly, grind it to an impalpable Powder, on a Marble or Porphir Stone, after you have fearced it through a filken Sieve. Of this Powder of Cryftal, as it is ufed for all artificial Gems, of which we fhall treat, it will be beft to have a fufficient Quantity by you, to have recourfe to, when at Work; and if you will fucceed in this Art, you muft not ufe ordinary Frit of Cryftal, let it be ever fo good; for that will not anfwer or come up to the Refplendency or Fairnefs of natural Cryftal

To make a fair Emerald.

TAKE of natural Cryftal four ounces, of Red Lead four ounces, Verdegreafe 48 Grains, *Crocus Martis* prepared with Vinegar eight Grains, the whole finely pulverized and fifted   This put together in a Crucible, leaving one Inch empty, lute it well, and put it in a Potter's Furnace, where they make their Earthen Ware, and let it there ftand as long as they do their Pots. When cold, break the Crucible, and you will find a Matter of a fine Emerald Colour, which, after it is cut and fet in Gold, will furpafs in Beauty the Oriental Emerald   If you find that your Matter is not refined or purified enough, put it again the fecond time in the fame Furnace, and in lifting off the Cover you will fee the Matter fhining, you may then break the Crucible, but not before, for if you fhould put the Matter into another Crucible, the Pafte would be cloudy, and full of Blifters   If you cannot come to a Potter's Furnace, you may build one yourfelf with a fmall Expence, in which you may put 20 Crucibles at once, each with a different Colour, and one baking will produce a great Variety of artificial Gems. Heat your Furnace with hard and dry Wood, and keep your Matter in fufion 24 Hours, which Time it will require to be thoroughly purified, and if you let it ftand four or fix Hours longer, it will not be the worfe for it.

A Deeper Emerald.

TAKE one ounce of natural Cryftal, fix ounces and a half of Red Lead, 75 Grains of Verdegreafe, 10 Grains of *Crocus Martis*, made with Vinegar, proceed as directed before.   *Another*

Another Emerald Colour.

TAKE prepar'd Cryſtal two ounces, Red Lead ſeven ounces, Verdegreaſe 18 Grains, *Crocus Martis* 10 Grains, and proceed as before directed

To make a Paſte for imitating an Oriental Topaze.

THE Colour of this Stone is like Water tinged with Saffron or Rhubarb. To imitate it, Take of prepared natural Cryſtal one ounce, of Red Lead ſeven ounces, finely pounded and ſearched, mix the whole well together, and put it into a Crucible, not quite full by an Inch, leaſt the Matter ſhould run over, or ſtick to the Cover of the Crucible in riſing, then proceed as directed above

Another.

TAKE prepar'd Cryſtal two ounces, native Cinnaber two ounces, *Æs uſtum* two ounces, all fine pulveriz d and ſearced, four times as much calcined Tin, put it all together into a Crucible well covered and proceed as before.

To make an Artificial Chryſolite

THIS Stone is of a green Colour, and ſome have the Caſt of Gold, To imitate it, take natural Cryſtal prepar'd, two ounces, Red Lead eight ounces, *Crocus Martis* 12 Grains, mix the whole finely together, and proceed as above, only leaving it a little longer than ordinary in the Furnace.

To Counterfeit a Beryl.

THIS Stone is of a Blueiſh Sea-Green To imitate it, take two ounces of natural Cryſtal prepared, five ounces Red Lead, 21 Grains of * Zaffer prepared, the whole finely pulverized, put it in a Crucible, and cover and lute it, then proceed as directed above, and you will have a beautiful Colour.

---

* Preparing of Zaffer may be done, by putting ſome Pieces into an Iron Ladle, heating it red hot, and then ſprinkling it with ſtrong Vinegar, when cold grind it on a Stone, then waſh t n clean Water

F A Sa-

A Saphire Colour

A Saphir is generally of a very clear Sky C⸻ ⸻, ⸺ highly esteemed for its Beauty. There a ⸻ ⸻ of ⸻, Whitish Colour, like Diamonds, others a full Blue ⸺ ⸺ ⸺ are of a Violet

To make this Paste, take of prepar'd Rock Cryst⸻ ⸻ ounces, Red Lead four ounces and a half, Sm⸻ ⸻ ⸺; pulverize and proceed as directed This C⸻ ⸻ ⸺ ne near to a Violet

Another more beautiful, and nearer t ⸻

TAKE two ounces of Natural Crystal prepar'd, six ounces of Red Lead, two Scruples of prepared Zaffer, and six Grains of prepared Manganese; all reduced to a fine Powder, mix and proceed as before.

Another deeper colour'd Saphire.

OF prepared Natural Crystal take two Ounces, Red Lead five Ounces, prepar'd Zaffer 42 grains, prepar'd Manganese eight Grains, the whole reduc'd to an impalpable Powder, and mixed together, proceed as you have been directed, and you will have a Colour deeper than the former, tending to a Violet.

To make a Paste for an Oriental Granat.

A Granat is much like the Carbuncle; both, if exposed to the Sun, exhibit a Colour like burning Coals, between red and yellow; and this is the true Colour of Fire. To imitate this Stone, take two Ounces of Natural Crystal prepared, and six Ounces of Red Lead, also 16 Grains of prepared Manganese, and two Grains of prepar'd Zaffer; pulverize and mix the whole, put it together into a Crucible, and proceed as directed

Another deeper Granat.

OF Natural Crystal prepared two ounces, Red Lead five ounces and a half, prepared Manganese 15 grains, pulverize all, and proceed as before directed

Another

Another Proce∫s for counterfeiting of PRECIOUS STONES.

TAKE of black Flint Stones what Quantity you plea∫e, and put them into a Pail of hot Water, and being wet, put them into a hot Furnace, this will prevent their flying into ∫mall Pieces; or el∫e warm them thoroughly by degrees, before you put them into the Furnace. When you ∫ee that they are thorough red hot, then quench them in fair Water, and they will look of a fine White Colour, dry and pulverize them very fine: This you may do in an Iron Mortar; but as it may contract ∫ome of the Iron, it will be proper after you have taken it out, to pour on it ∫ome *Aqua-Fortis*, which will clear it of the Iron, and to di∫engage it from all the Filth and Impurities, wa∫h it in ∫everal clean hot Waters.

THIS Powder thus prepared is fit to be u∫ed for making the fine∫t Gla∫s, and for imitating the mo∫t cleare∫t and tran∫parent Gems, e∫pecially tho∫e as require the Lu∫tre of a Diamond or Ruby, as for a Saphir, Emerald, Topaze, Chry∫olite, Spirel, Amethi∫t, *&c.* your Labour with *Aqua-Fortis* may be ∫aved, if your Mortar is bright and free from Ru∫t Such as have a Mortar of *Porphire*, or ∫uch like Stone, have no occa∫ion to u∫e an Iron one, but will ∫ave them∫elves a good deal of Trouble.

IN ca∫e you cannot have black Flint Stones, you may content your ∫elf with Pebble, but Flint is far preferable, and makes the Gla∫s of a harder Sub∫tance than that made of Pebble.

An Approved Compo∫ition.

OF the above Powder three parts, Fine refined Salt-petre two, Borax and Ar∫enick one part.

Another.

OF the Flint Powder three parts, Salt-petre two, and Borax four parts.

Another

Another.

OF the forefaid Powder two parts, of refined Cryftalline Pot-Afhes, or Salt of Tartar and Borax, of each one Part.

Another.

TAKE of the above Powder feven Parts and a half, purified Pot-Afhes five Parts· Or,

Powder, fix Parts and a half, Salt-petre two and a half; Borax one half, Arfenic one half, and Tartar one Part.

How to melt thefe Compofitions, and how to tinge and finifh your Work

TAKE any one of the above fpecified Compofitions, and weigh what quantity you pleafe, one or two ounces, then mix it with fuch a Colour as you defign to have it of, as for Inftance

To make a Saphir.

TAKE to one Ounce of the Compofition four grains of *Zaffer*, mix it well together, and melt it in a Crucible ; if you fee the Colour to your liking, you proceed to finifh it· you may make a Saphir either deeper or paler, according to what Quantity you take of each Ingredient, and 'tis the fame with refpect to other Colours A new Practitioner in this Art may make Experiments in fmall Crucibles, in order to acquaint himfelf with the Nature thereof

I have already given Receipts of moft Colours for imitating of Precious Stones, but neverthelefs I fhall here lay down fome experimental Rules, neceffary to be obferv'd

You muft know, that the *Crocus Martis* may be prepared different Ways, and each will have a particular Effect in Colouring of Cryftals, the one is prepared with Vinegar, another with Sulpher, a third with Aqua-Fortis, and a fourth by only a reverberatory Fire.

To prepare Crocus Martis with Vinegar.

TAKE Iron; or, which is better, Steel-filings, moiften and mix them up with good Strong Vinegar in an
Earthen

Earthen Diſh or Pan, after which ſpread them and let them dry in the Sun, when dry, beat them fine in a Mortar. This Powder you moiſten again with freſh Vinegar, and dry and beat it again as before, this you repeat eight times running, afterwards you dry and fift it through a fine Hair Sieve, and it will be the Colour of Brick duſt. but when mixt with Glaſs, of a fine Crimſon Colour Put this Powder up carefully to preſerve it from Duſt

To prepare *Crocus Martis with Sulphur, or Brimſtone*

TAKE Iron or Steel Filings, one Part, Sulphur three parts, mix it together and put it into a Crucible, cover and lute it well; then ſet it into a Wind Furnace, and give it a ſtrong Fire with Charcoal, for four Hours together, then ſhake it out, and when cold, pulveriſe and ſift it through a fine Sieve This Powder you put into a Crucible, lute it, and place the ſame in the Eye or Hole of the Glaſs Furnace, let it ſtand there for 14 Days or more, and it will turn to a red Powder inclining to Purple, this is a very uſeful Ingredient for Tinging of Glaſs.

To prepare *Crocus Martis with Aqua Fortis.*

MOISTEN ſome Iron or Steel Filings in a glaz'd earthen Plate or Diſh with *Aqua Fortis*, ſet it to dry in the Sun or Air; when dry, ground it to a fine Powder: Moiſten it again with freſh *Aqua Fortis*, dry it, and proceed as before, repeating it ſeveral Times, till you ſee it of a high red Colour, then grind and ſift it through a fine Hair Sieve, and put it ſafe from Duſt for Uſe

To prepare *Crocus Martis by a reverberatory Fire.*

TAKE clean Iron or Steel File-duſt, put thereof into a large Pot or Pan about the quantity of an Inch high, cover it well, and put it in a Reverberatory Furnace, or any other place where it may be ſurrounded with a ſtrong Heat and Flame. The Iron will ſwell and riſe in a fine red Powder, ſo as to fill the Pot, and will even force up to the Cover Lid, this Powder you take off, and you will find a good part of Iron cak'd together at the Bottom, which you put again in the Furnace, where it will ſwell, and raiſe in a Powder, as before, this continue ſo long till you have a ſuf-

ficient

ficient Quantity. This is the moſt valuable *Crocus,* and of great uſe in the Art of Colouring or Tinging of Glaſs for counterfeiting of precious Stones.

To make a fine Hyacinth,

YOU take of *Crocus Martis,* or of that by Reverberation prepared Iron Powder, 8 or 10 Grains, to one Ounce of the Compoſition.

The Opal

IS made of Silver diſſolved in *Aqua Fortis,* precipitated with Salt, add to it ſome Load Stone, and mix it up with the above Compoſition, it gives divers Colours, ſo as to repreſent a natural Opal.

A reddiſh Stone

MAY be made of the Fragments or Waſt of Calcedon, mix'd with Borax and melted ; with which you may make as many Changes as you pleaſe.

Such as will ſave themſelves the Trouble of preparing the Compoſition for counterfeiting precious Stones, may uſe fine Cryſtal or Venice Glaſs, beat in a clean Mortar to a fine Powder, of this take eight Ounces, Borax two Ounces, refin'd Salt-petre one Ounce. Out of this Mixture you may melt and colour all Manner of Stones, with little Trouble.

Bartholomew Korndorffer's *Secret, to make a Diamond out of natural Cryſtal.*

TAKE the beſt poliſh'd Cryſtal, no matter whether large or ſmall, ſo it is but clear and tranſparent, put it in a Crucible, with three Times as much of my fix'd Sulphur of Gold, ſo that the Cryſtal may be cover'd all over with it. Then, after you have put a Lid over it and luted the Crucible well, let it for three Days and Nights neal in a ſtrong Fire, then take it out and quench it in Spring-Water, in which a red hot Steel has been quenched 46 Times running, and you will have a Diamond which reſembles a natural one in every Reſpect, and is right and good.

Thus

Thus far *Korndorffer*, but how to come at his Sulpher he has left us in the dark.

How to make a Diamond out of a Saphir, according to Porta's Description.

WE ufed to make it (the Diamond) the moſt fureſt Way in this Manner: We fill'd an Earthen Pipkin or Crucible, with Quick-Lime, and lay'd the Saphir in the midſt thereof, covering it firſt with a Tile, and then with Coals, all over, blowing them gentle till we had a clear Fire, for if it is blown too much, it may occaſion the breaking of the Stone

When we thought that the Saphir had chang'd its Colour, we let the Fire go out of it ſelf; and took it out to ſee whether it was turned white, if ſo, then we laid it again in the Crucible, in order to let it cool with the Fire, but if it had not the right Colour, then we augmented the Heat again as before, and looked often to ſee, whether the force of Fire had taken away all the Colour, which was done in about five or ſix Hours; if then the blue Colour was not quite gone, we began our Operation from the firſt over again, till it was white and clear. It is to be obſerv'd, that the Heat of the Fire in the beginning of your Operation, muſt increaſe by ſlow Degrees, and alſo when done, it muſt in the ſame manner decreaſe; for if the Stone, comes either too quick in the Heat, or from the Heat in the Cold, he is apt to turn dark, or fly to Pieces

In like Manner all other Precious Stones looſe their Colour, the one ſooner than the other, according as they are either harder or ſofter. The Amethiſt is very light, and requires but a ſlow Fire, for if he hás too much Heat, he becomes dark, or turns into Chalk.

This is the Art whereby inferior Precious Stones are changed into Diamonds, they are afterwards cut in the middle, and a colour given them; and from hence comes the ſecond Sort of falſe Diamonds, or Doublets.

To make a fine Amethiſt.

TAKE calcin'd Flint-Stone, and ſift it thro' a Cambrick, whereof take one ounce and a half, of fix'd Salt-petre half an ounce; of Borax one ounce and a half; of *Tinct. Ven* and *Mart* 108 grains; Manganeſe, 100 grains; put
F 4   both

both these Tinctures together, and then mix them with the Ingredients. Then add fix'd *Nitre* * and *Borax* well mixt to it, put it into a Crucible in a Wind Furnace, give it at first a gentle Heat, till it is red hot, and thus keep it for a quarter of an Hour, then give it for two or three Hours a strong Fire, at last you pour it into a Mould, and let it cool by Degrees, to prevent its flying afunder

To make a Ruby, or a fine Hyacinth.

TAKE Vitriol one Ounce, and the same Weight of Water, mix it well together, in this diffolve Filings or very thin beaten Steel, fet the Glafs on a warm Sand, filtrate the Solution before it is cold, then let it into a Cellar, and it will shoot Cryftals, which pulverife, put it under a Muffel, and ftir it fo long, till you fee it of a crimfon Colour. Then take it off the Fire, put it in a Vial, pour on it good ftill'd Vinegar, and after it has ftood four Days in a gentle Warmth, pour off that Vinegar, pour fresh to it, and let it ftand four Days more, this you repeat till the Vinegar is obferv'd to make no Extraction, then pour off the Vinegar, and there will remain at the Bottom of your Vial a Crimfon colour'd Powder, fweeten this well with warm Water. This is the Tincture for the *Ruby* or *Hyacinth*

Then take black Flints, calcine them well, as has been already directed, in order to bring them to a good white Powder, and fift this thro' a Cambrick, take thereof, and of *Venice Borax*, of each one Ounce; of the forefaid Tincture Powder eight or nine Grains, mix it well together in a Crucible, and give it for half an Hour a gentle Fire, then augment it by degrees, till you fee your mixture in the Crucible as clear as Cryftal, and of a Crimfon Colour, then pour it into a Mould of what Shape you would have it

---

* The fix'd Nitre is thus made: Take a Piece of green Oak, about two Fingers thick, lay it upon an Iron Plate, into the middle of the top of the Wood put a little heap of Saltpetre, light it, and repeat it fo often till it burns through the Wood, and the Saltpetre runs upon the Iron. It turns at firft blue but afterwards greenifh, you muft keep it warm and dry, to prevent it from melting. In this manner one may make as much as one pleafes

To make a Ruby Palais

TAKE prepar'd powder'd Flint 3 Ounces, fix'd Salt-petre one quarter of an Ounce; Borax 3 Grains, some of the above mentioned Tincture Powder, of Copper and Iron 54 Grains, of prepar'd Manganese five Grains, mix it all together, and put it in a new Crucible, give it at first a gentle Fire till it begins to melt, then give it a strong Fire for two Hours and let it cool of it self.

To harden Bohemian Diamonds.

TAKE black Lead two Ounces, Gold Talk two Ounces, powder it fine, and mix it well together, then take of this Mixture, put it into a new Crucible, about half full, and place the said Diamonds upon that Powder, so as not to touch one another, then put of the Powder as much upon them as will fill the Crucible, cover and lute it, and set it in a Coppel with Ashes, so as to have the Ashes a hands breadth about the Crucible, then give it a slow Fire, and augment the Heat by degrees, in order to preserve the stones from breaking, till the Pan or Coppel, which holds your Crucible, begins to be red hot, continue it thus for 48 Hours, then let it cool, and take the Stones out of the Crucible, and you will find them look black, polish them with Ashes of Tin, they will not only have contracted a tolerable Hardness, but have also a finer Lustre, much resembling natural Oriental Diamonds.

A plain Direction concerning the Polishing of these Counter-feits, and also of Natural Gems.

IT is to be observ'd, that all Glass or artificial Stones may be cut and polish'd after one Method, namely, by strowing fine powder'd Emery upon a Leaden Plate, with Water, and holding the Stone firm, grinding it in what Form or Shape one pleases

If you fling grounded Tripoli, mix'd with Water, upon a Pewter-Plate, and add a little Copper Ashes among it, it will have the same Effect.

Pulve-

Pulverized Antimony ſtrow'd upon a ſmooth Plate of Lead, with *Tripoli* and Vinegar, poliſhes not only *Glaſs, Cryſtal, Granats, Calcedons, Agates* and *Amethiſt,* but all other natural Stones, except the Diamond The Diamond is only cut with the Diamond Powder itſelf. Any ſuch Diamonds, which can be touched by Emery, Lead, Copper or other Metals, or be cut therewith, are falſe, and this is a good Trial to know a real Diamond

All other Precious and hard Stones can be grounded or cut with Metal and Emery, but the poliſhing is different

The *Saphir* is after the Diamond the hardeſt, it may be poliſh'd beſt with Antimony and Vinegar, on Lead, or with calcin'd Flint-Stone and Water, upon Copper.

The *Ruby* is poliſh'd like the Saphir.

The Emerald and Turquoiſe is poliſh'd with Potter's Clay and Water, on Pear Tree Wood, or with *Tripoli* upon Wood, or with Emery upon Pewter.

The *Beryl* is poliſh'd with calcined Mother of Pearl or Muſcles, upon a Board covered with white Leather.

A *Pallas* is poliſh'd with Antimony, upon Copper.

The *Cornelian, Onyx, Agate, Calcedon* and *Jaſpis* upon Tin, with *Tripoli* or calcin'd Flint upon Pear Tree Wood; or with Antimony upon Lead

The *Amethiſt, Topaz, Turquoiſe* and other ſoft Stones, are poliſh'd upon a Board of Lime Tree Wood, upon a Plate of Tin, and upon a Board with Leather Firſt you poliſh it top and bottom, upon the Wood, the ſmall Diamond Cuts are done upon the Plate of Tin, and receive the laſt poliſhing Stroke upon the Board that's cover'd with Leather, with the following Powder.

A Powder for poliſhing ſoft Stones

TAKE Iron Scales, mix them with Vinegar and Salt, and let it ſtand thus infuſed for three or four Days, the longer the better, then grind it very fine, dry it, and put it in an Earthen Pot well luted, give it a good Fire, and it will be fit for Uſe.

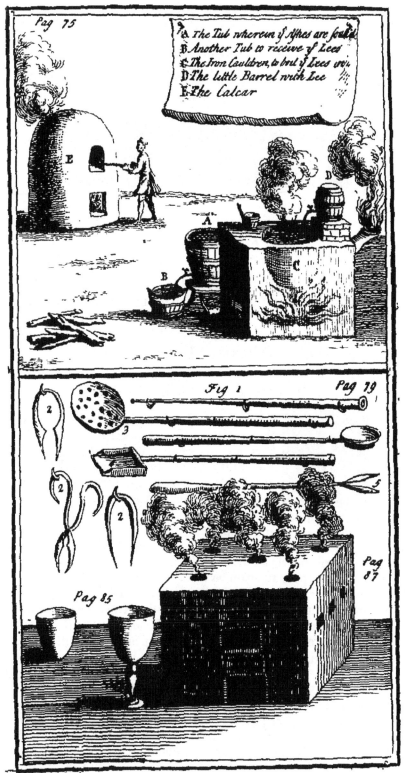

A. The Tub wherein ye Ashes are soaked
B. Another Tub to receive ye Lees
C. The Iron Cauldron, to boil ye Lees in
D. The little Barrel with Lee
E. The Calcar

Fig 1

Pag 79

Pag 87

Pag 85

Halett Sculp

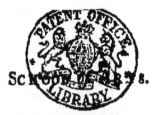
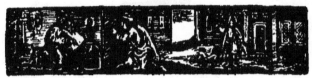

PART. III.

The Art of making GLASS Exhibiting withal the Art of Painting, and making Impreſſions upon GLASS, and of Laying thereon *Gold* or *Silver*, together with the Method of Preparing the Colours for POTTERS-WORK or DELFT WARE.

To prepare Aſhes for making of GLASS

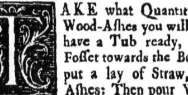

TAKE what Quantity, and what Sort of Wood-Aſhes you will, except thoſe of Oak, have a Tub ready, with a Spiggot and Foſſet towards the Bottom, and in this Tub put a lay of Straw, on which fling your Aſhes: Then pour Water upon them, and let the Aſhes ſoak thoroughly, till the Water ſtands above them Let it thus continue over Night; then draw out the Foſſet, and receive the Lee in another Tub, put under the Frſt for this Purpoſe. If the Lee looks heavy and troubled, pour it again on the Aſhes, and let it ſettle, till it runs clear, and is of an Amber Colour. This clarify'd Lee put by, and pour freſh Water on the Aſhes, let this alſo ſtand over Night; then draw it off, and you will have a weak Lee, which, inſtead of Water, pour upon freſh Aſhes. The remaining Aſhes are of great Uſe in Manuring of Land.

After you have made a ſufficient Quantity of Lees, pour them into an Iron Cauldron, brick'd up like a brewing or waſhing Copper, but let it not be fill'd above three Parts full On the Top of the Brick work put a little Barrel with Lee, towards the Bottom of which bore a Hole, and put a ſmall Foſſet in, to let the Lee run gently into the Kettle,

in a Stream about the Roundnefs of a Siaw But this
you muft manage according to the Quantity of the Lee,
for you ought to mind how much the Lee in the Kettle evaporates, and make the Lee in the little Barrel run proportionable, to fupply that Diminution. Care muft alfo be taken
that the Lee may not run over in the firft boiling, but if you
find it will not keep in the Kettle, then put fome cold Lee
to it, flacken the Fire, and let all the Lee boil gently to a
dry Salt. When this Salt is cold, break it out of the Kettle,
put it into the Calcar, and raife your Fire by Degrees, till
the Salt is red hot, yet fo as not to melt When you think it
calcar'd enough, take out a Piece, and let it cool, then
break it in two, and if it is thorough white, it is done enough,
but if there remains a blacknefs in the middle, it muft be put
in the Calcar again, till it comes out thoroughly white If
you will have it ftill finer, you muft diffolve it again,
filtrate it, boil it, calcine or calcar it as before The oftner
this is repeated, the more will the Salt be cleared from the
earthy Particles, and may be made as clear as Cryftal, and
as white as Snow, out of which may be made the fineft
Glafs you can wifh or defire

According to Mr *Merret's* Account, the beft Afhes
here in *England* are burnt from Thiftles and Hop-ftalks,
after the Hops are gather'd, and among Trees, the Mulberry is reckon'd to afford the beft Salt

The moft thorny and prickly Plants are obferv'd to yield
better and more Salt than others, alfo all Herbs that are
bitter, as Hops, Wormwood, &c Tobacco ftalks, when
burnt, produce likewife Plenty of Salt Notwithftanding
this, it is obferved that Fern-Afhes yield more Salt than any
other Afhes

Another Method to prepare Pott-Afhes for making of fine
Cryftal Glafs

TAKE Pot-Afhes, diffolve them in a clean earthen Veffel, in River- or Rain-Water. let them ftand over
Night, and fettle; The next Day pour off the clear Matter,
and filter the Settling through a Piece of Blanket, in order to
get a clear Lee: This boil in in Iron Kettle, till it becomes
a hard Mafs, then beat it in Pieces, and put it in a Calcar
to calcine. Diffolve it again in clear Water, filtrate and
boil it as before; and the oftner you repeat it, the clearer
and

and finer will be your Glass: But if it is for colour'd Glass once or twice doing it, will be sufficient.

To make the Glass Frit.

TAKE White-Silver Sand; wash it, and separate all the filthy Matter from it, and let it dry, or rather Calcar it. Of this take 60 pound, and of the prepar'd Ashes 30 pound; mix it well together Then set it in the melting Furnace; the longer it is melting, the clearer will be the Glass made thereof If it stands from Saturday Evening till Tuesday Morning, it will be fit to work with, or to tinge it with what Colour you please. Before you work it, add 40 pound of Lead and half a pound of Manganese to it.

Another Compound for fine Crystal.

TAKE Ashes, prepar'd as above, 60 pound; of prepar'd Silver Sand 160 pound, Crystalline Arsenick four pound, White Lead two pound, clear dry Saltpetre 10 pound, Borax two pound, mix all well together, and proceed as has been directed, and you will have a beautiful Crystal.

Another.

TAKE prepared Silver Sand 20 pound, clear and dry Saltpetre 30 pound, Borax six pound, Crystalline Arsenick eight pound, mix this well together, and put it in Fusion for four Days together, then add two pound of Manganese, and four pound of Borax.

Another.

TAKE prepared Silver Sand 38 pound, prepared Ashes 25 pound, Arsenick one pound, Saltpetre two pound, of Antimony and Borax four pound.

Another.

OF prepared Sand, take 40 pound, Saltpetre 13 pound and a half, Tartar six pound, Arsenick and Borax about one pound and a half.

Another.

PREPARED Silver Sand 10 pound, Afhes fix pound, Tartar three pound, Saltpetre four pound, Lime fix pound, Borax 12 ounces.

How to build a fmall Furnace, ufeful for Experiments in making of Glafs and to ferve on feveral other Occafions.

YOUR Furnace, muft be built according to the Situation, and Dimenfion of your Room, about a yard Square. At the Bottom you leave a hole, A, which is the Receiver of the Afhes, and alfo the drawer of the Wind to the Fire, which you may make as Fierce as you will, by expofing it either more or lefs to the open Air. B, is an Iron Grate, which is about a quarter and a half above the Hole A.

C, Are Holes over the Grate, wherein you put the Fewel; over the Grate is a brick'd Vault, wherein the Flames draw through the Hole D in the Upper Vault E.

F, Are two or more Holes, through which you put the Crucibles in, you may make one on each Side, and make Cakes of fuch Clay as the Glafs-makers ufe, to fet them before the Holes, and by this means mitigate the Flames, which fometimes may ftrike too fierce upon the upper Vault, and give them a little vent.

G, Is a Hole in the Upper Vault, which may be cover'd and uncover'd as far as you will, and thro' which the Flame may either go ftraight through the Funnel H, which at the top is provided with a Cover I, and which on fuch Occafion muft be taken off, or elfe in putting on the Cover I, you may convey a Reverberatory Fire through the Funnel K, into another little Reverberatory Furnace, which will be very ufeful for calcining and preparing feveral Matters, as may happen to be required

The Infide of this Furnace muft be lin'd fmooth, with fuch Potters Clay as the Glafs Makers ufe, two or three Inches thick. And having finifh'd it according to this Direction, you may place a good many Crucibles in at a Time, making the Holes through which you convey your larger Crucibles higher, fo that the Rim of the Crucible may come even with the Bottom of the Hole, and you may eafily convey a Ladle, Spattle, or any thing elfe through them. This

Fur-

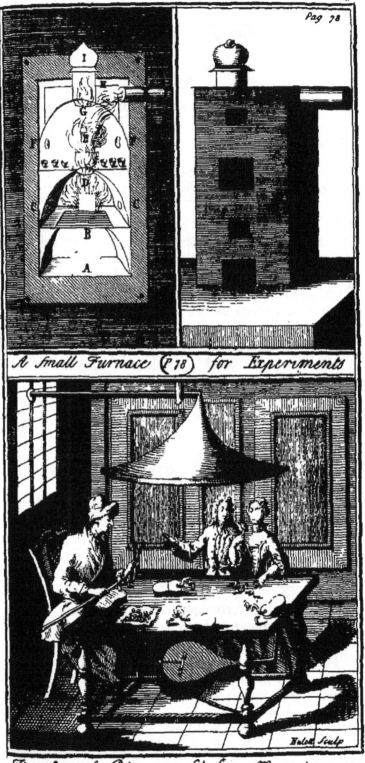

A Small Furnace (P 78) for Experiments

The Art of Blowing Glass in Miniature P 83

Furnace is the most compendious and useful, that can be contrived for a New Beginner in the Art of Glass.

The Principal Instruments that are used in making of Glass, are, 1 a hollow Pipe, for blowing the Glass, with a little Wooden Handle at Top, in order to manage it the better. Fig 1

2 The Scissars and Shears serve to cut and shape the Glass Fig 2

3 Iron Ladles, whose Handles at the end are covered over with Wood, these serve to take the Metal out of the large Melting Pot, and to put it into the little ones for the Workmen, for Scumming the Metal; to take off the *Alkalick* Salt; which swims on the Top, and for several other Uses Fig. 3.

4. Great and little Shovels or Peels, to take up Glass; to draw out the Ashes, &c. Fig. 4

5 Several Sizes of Forks, to carry the Glasses, when made, into the upper Oven to cool, for stirring the Matter; for conveying the Melting-Pots in the Furnace from one Place to another, and for other Purposes. Fig 5.

General Observations on the Art of Glass.

1. THE Principal Ingredients for making of Glass, are Stone and Salt.

2. The Stone is either *Tarso*, a Sort of Marble brought from *Tuscany*, and rekon'd by several Artists to be the best for making of Crystal Glass; or Black Flint Stones, which in every Respect are as good.   And where these are not to be had, clear Pebble or white Silver Sand, will, when rightly prepared, make also good Glass.

3. The next Ingredient is Salt, which, as has been said, is abstracted from Ashes, calcined and refined in the nicest and cleanest Manner possible

4. *Pulverine* or *Rochetta*, are Ashes made of certain Herbs, which grow in the *Levant*, and are amongst Artists allow'd to be the fittest to abstract the Salt for making of Glass; of the same kind is *Soda*, which comes from *Egypt* and *Spain* They prepare those Ashes thus. After the Herb has been dry'd in the Sun, it is burn'd on Iron Grates, the Ashes falling through it into a Pit underneath, made for that Purpose, where they grow into a hard Mass or Stone, and are laid up for use; but there is no occasion to fetch the

Ashes

Aſhes ſo far, when every Country produces ſufficient of its own Growth, Herbs, as well as Trees and Plants anſwer in every Reſpect the ſame purpoſe.

Pot-Aſhes and calcin'd Flint, Pebble, or Sand, will make good Glaſs Frit, after you have refin'd the Aſhes, by firſt diſſolving them in fair Water, and after they are ſettled, by boiling the clear Lees to a Salt, then nealing the Salt in a Furnace, diſſolving it again, and proceeding as at firſt, repeating it ſeveral Times, till it produces a Salt as white as Snow. Of this you may mix three parts to four of calcin'd Flint, or as you find it requiſite, in all which you will become more perfect by Practice than by Teaching.

5. Glaſs is alſo made of Lead, which firſt muſt be calcined; in doing this, you muſt obſerve that your Kiln be not too hot, but only ſo as to keep the Lead in Fuſion, or elſe it will not Calcine. When the Lead is melted, it yields at the Top a yellowiſh Matter, which take off with an Iron Ladle for that purpoſe. After the firſt Calcination you repeat it again, and give it a Reverberatory Fire, till it comes to a good yellow Powder, and is well calcined. Of the calcined Lead you take ſeven Pound, and of the prepar'd Aſhes ſix Pound. Care muſt be taken that no Settlement of Lead goes into the Crucible, but what is reduced to aſhes, elſe it will make its Way through it, bore or rent the Bottom thereof, and carry all the Metal along with it.

6. *Manganeſe,* when prepared as directed, is of great uſe to whiten your Glaſs, for without it, it will have a green Hue, but by mixing Manganeſe with the Frit, when melted, by little and little, and then quenching the Glaſs in a Pail of Cold Water, repeating this ſeveral Times, it will make it of a white and clear Colour.

To make Glaſs melt eaſy

PUT into the melting Pot a little of Arſenick that has been fix'd with Nitre, this will make the Glaſs mellow, and eaſy to fluviate.

To calcine Braſs, which in Glaſs makes a Sky or a Sea-green

BRASS, is Copper melted and mix'd with *Lapis Cala minaris,* which not only changes it into a Gold Colour, but increaſes it in Weight, which Augmentation gives a Sea
Green

Green or Sky Colour to Glaſs, when it is well calcined, to do this, obſerve the following Rules

Take Braſs Plate, cut in ſmall Slips, and put it into a Crucible, cover and lute it well, and give it a Reverberatory Fire in a Furnace, yet not a melting one, for if it melts, all your Labour will be loſt · let it ſtand in that Heat for four Days, by which Time it will be well calcin'd, then beit it to in impalpable Powder, and ſearce it, grind it fine on a Porphyre Stone, and you will have a black Powder, which ſpread on Tiles, and keep it on Burning Coals, or the round Hole in a Furnace, for four Days, clear it of the Aſhes that have fell upon it, pulverize and ſearce it, and keep it for Uſe. To try whether it is calcined enough, fling a little thereof into melted Glaſs, which if it ſwells, the Calcination is enough, but if not, then it is either not calcin'd enough, or elſe it is burn'd, and it will not colour the Glaſs near ſo well than when the Calcination is done to Perfection

To colour Braſs after another Manner, for a tranſparent Red Colour, or Yellow.

CUT your Braſs in ſmall Shreds, and lay it *ſtratum ſuper ſtratum* into a Crucible, with powdered Brimſtone; ſet it on a Charcoal Fire in a Furnace for 24 Hours, then powder and ſearce it. When this is done, put it covered into the Furnace Hole, for 10 Hours, to reverberate, and when cold, grind it again very fine, and keep it for Uſe

General Obſervations for all Colours

1 ALL the Melting Pots muſt be glaz'd with white Glaſs the inſide, elſe a new Earthen Pot that is unglaz'd will cauſe the Colours to look bad and foul, but the ſecond time of uſing theſe Pots they loſe their Foulneſs.

2 Obſerve that theſe Pots ſerve for one Colour only, and may not be uſed for another, for every Colour muſt have its own Pot, except they correſpond together.

3 Let the Powders be well calcined, neither too much, nor too little

4. Your Mixtures muſt be made in due Proportion, and the Furnace be heated with hard and dry Wood

5 You muſt uſe your Colours divided, ere part you muſt put in the Frit before it is melted, and the other after it is melted and become fine and clear.

G

To

To make Glaſs of Lead, which is the fitteſt to be tinctured with moſt Colours.

TAKE of calcin'd Lead 15 Pound, of *Rochetta* or pulveriſed Cryſtal Frit 12 Pound, mix it well and put it together into a melting Pot, then into a Furnace; and at the end of 10 Hours, caſt it into Water, clear the melting Pot of the Lead that may remain, and return the Metal into it, which after 10 hours Heat will be fit to work withal.

How to work the ſaid Glaſs.

BEFORE you take it upon the Iron, raiſe the Glaſs firſt in the Pot a little, then take it out to let it cool for a ſmall ſpace of Time, after which work it on a clean and ſmooth Iron Plate.

Blue Glaſs.

TAKE four ounces of calcined and pulveriſed Rock Cryſtal, two ounces of Saltpetre, one ounce of Borax, half a pound of Manganeſe, one pound of Indigo-Blue

A Chryſolite Glaſs.

TO one pound of Frit, take pulveriſed Verdegreaſe three ounces and a half, Red Lead one ounce

Saphir Green Glaſs

TO one pound of the above Compoſition or Cryſtal Frit take one ounce of good Zaffer, of curious fine Pin Duſt two pound

To make fine green Glaſs out of Tin.

TAKE the Filings or Shavings of Tin, nine parts, diſſolve it in Aqua Fortis, which is made of two parts of Vitriol, and three parts of Salt petre, ſweeten the Calx with clean Spring Water, then take 18 parts of nine times or more calcined Antimony its Calcination muſt be repeated 'till it has done evaporating Both theſe Calx melted together, makes a fine Chryſolyte or Emerald

This

This Glafs will melt upon Silver, like Enamel, and may be ufed on feveral Occafions, for Embellifhing fuch Things, as are proper for Ornuments

To make a Ruby Colour'd Glafs.

TAKE well fettled Aqua Fortis, made' with *Sal Armoniac* into *Aqua Regis,* four Ounces, fling into it by little and little thin Bits or Filings of Tin, one Ounce, and let it diffolve. Then take the fineft Gold, as much as you will, and diffolve it alfo in that *Aqua Regis*. Take a clean Glafs with clear Spring Water, and pour off the Solution of the Gold as much as you pleafe in it, the fame quantity put alfo to it of the Solution of the Tin, and the Water will turn in a moment to a fine Rofe Colour, with this Water moiften feveral Times your Glafs Frit, and let it dry, then proceed as you do with other Glafs in Fire, at firft it will come out White, but turn to a fine Ruby

The Art of Blowing GLASS in MINIATURE.

This Art is perform'd by the Flame of the Lamp in the following Manner

FIRST, provide your felf from the Glafs Houfes with feveral Pipes of Glafs, that are hollow the infide, of feveral Colours, and different Sizes, then you muft have a Table, as you fee reprefented in the Plate annexed. A is the Lamp, which is furnifh'd with Rape or other Oil, and a large Wick of twifted Cotton, below the Table is a Bellows, B When the Artift treads the Treadle faften'd to the Bellows, the Wind will be convey'd through the Pipes under the Table to the fmall pointed opening by C, directly againft which is plac'd the lighted Wick of the Lamp, D. The Smoak which iffues forth from the Lamp, is convey'd through a broad Funnel made of Tin or Wood E

The Wind which ftrikes in a fharp Point againft the Flame, occafions fuch a violent Heat that it will diffolve the moft ftubborn Glafs, and you may, after you have foften'd the End of your Pipe in the Flame, blow through the hollow thereof,

and

and form with small Plyers and other useful Tools whatever
you please. small twisted Noofes of Wire are very convenient
to hold your Work in, in order to shape and join different
Colours to one Piece   The whole Art depends chiefly upon
Practice

The Usefulness of such a Table answers several other
Purposes, as, for trying of Metal-Oar , in this Cafe put
some of it on a hollow'd Charcoal, &c and by directing the
Wind through the Lamp upon the Oar, the Heat will melt it
immediately, and shew what it contains   In Soldering it is
also very convenient , not to mention the Conveniency which
such a Table affords to Practitioners in Chymiftry.

How to lay Silver on Glass Utenfils, as Plates, Diffhes,
Salts, Drinking Cups, &c.

TAKE Silver, what Quantity you pleafe, and beat it very
thin, or corn it , then put it into a Matrafs, and pour
twice the Weight thereof of Spirit of Nitre upon it, and you
will prefently perceive the Silver to diffolve   When you
obferve its ceafing to work, put your Matrafs on warm Sand
or Afhes, and it will begin to work afrefh , let it thus
ftand fo long, till all your Silver is refolv'd   After this
pour the Solution out of that Matrafs into another, that
has a Head to it, with this draw off half the Spirit of Nitre
from the Solution of Silver, and let the Matrafs remain on the
Sand, till it is cool , then take it off, and let it ftand ftill for
four and twenty Hours, and the Silver will fhoot into white
Cryftals, from thefe pour off the Solution which remains,
and abftract from that again the half of the Spirit , then
put it up as before, to cryftallize, and this repeat, till near
all the Silver is turn'd into Cryftals , which take out of the
Glafs, lay it upon whited brown Paper to dry, and preferve
it for Ufe   The reft of the Silver that fhould remain in
the *Aqua-Fortis,* may be drawn out as has been directed
before

Of this Cryftal take as much as you will, and put it
into a Retort, pour upon it twice or three times as much in
Weight of the ftrongeft *Spiritus Salis Armoniari,* lute it
well, and put it in a gentle Warmth 8 or 14 Days to digeft,
and it will contract a blue Colour, pour it off, filter and
abftract in *Balneo Mariæ* almoft all the Spirits from it,
and there remains a grafs green Liquid, with this, draw
over your Glafs, and put it in a Glafs Furnace, or in any
gentle

gentle Heat, your Glaſs will look as though it were Silver Plate.

But in Caſe there ſhould be an Overſight, and the Spirit of *Sal Armoniac* be too much drawn off, and the Silver turn'd to a green Salt, then pour as much of that Spirit upon the Silver again to bring it into a green Liquid

A Curious Drinking Glaſs

TAKE two ſmooth Drinking Glaſſes, fitted cloſe into one another, ſo that the Brims of both may be even, then paint on the inſide of the larger Glaſs, with Oil Colours, what you will, either in imitation of Moſaick, or any other Invention, and when dry, you may with the Point of a Needle open fine Veins or other Embelliſhments, &c Then oil it all over with old Linſeed Oil, and before it is quite dry, and clammy, lay Leaf Gold upon it, preſs it cloſe down to the Glaſs with Cotton, and let it dry thoroughly The mean while take the other leſſer Glaſs, and lay a thin clear Varniſh on the Outſide thereof, and when moſt dry, lay on Leaf Gold, and the inſide of the Glaſs will look all over gilded. When this is dry, put it into the larger Glaſs, and make a Paſte of Chalk and Lack Varniſh, with this lute the Rims of the two Glaſſes, ſo that it may not be perceived, but look as if it were made out of one piece, let it thoroughly dry, and give it another lay of Lack Varniſh with a fine Pencil, and let it dry, then ſmooth it with Pumice Stone, and lay on a thin Varniſh, and when that is moſt dry, gild it with Leaf Gold, and give it two or three Lays of Lake Varniſh, and the Gold will remain ſecure

When inſtead of Painting with Oil Colours you only anoint the inſide of the Glaſs with old Linſeed Oil, and then ſtrew it over with *Spangles*, and put the inſide Glaſs gilded to join, it will have a ſingular Beauty This Leſſon will animate the Ingenious to try further Experiments of this amuſing kind

How to Quickſilver the Inſide of Glaſs Globes, ſo as to make them like Looking Glaſs

TAKE two Ounces of Quickſilver, one Ounce of Biſmuth, of Lead and Tin half an Ounce of each

Firſt put the Lead and Tin in Fuſion, then put in the Biſmuth, and when you perceive that in Fuſion too, then

let

let it ftand till it is almoft cold, and pour the Quick filver into it

After this, take the Glafs Globe, which muft be very clean, and the Infide free from Duft, make a Paper Funnel, which put in the Hole of the Globe, as near to the Glafs as you can, fo that the Amalgama, when you pour it in, may not fplatter and caufe the Glafs to be full of Spots, but pour it in gently, and move it about, fo that the Amalgama may touch every where. If you find the Amalgama begin to be curdly, and to be fix'd, then hold it over a gentle Heat, and it will flow eafy again. And if you find the Amalgama too thin, add a little more Lead, Tin and Bifmuth to it. The finer and clearer your Globe is, the better will be the Looking Glafs.

The Art of PAINTING upon GLASS.

THIS noble Art being the Admiration of all who have any tolerable Tafte of Defigning or Painting, it will not be improper to give the ingenious Enquirer after this Myftery fome few Leffons, in order, not only to fatisfy his Curiofity with the Nature thereof but alfo, if he is inclin'd, to lead him into the Practice thereof, which we fhall do in the plaineft and fhorteft manner poffible.

First then, Chufe fuch Panes of Glafs as are clear, even and fmooth.

2. Strike one Side thereof, with a clean fpunge or a foft hair Pencil, dipt in Gum Water, all over.

3. When it is dry, lay the clean fide of the Glafs on the Print or Defign you intend to copy, and with a fmall pointed Pencil (furnifh'd with a black Colour, and prepar'd for that purpofe, as fhall be directed) deliniate the Outlines or Capital Strokes, and where the Shades appear foft, work them by dotting and eafy Strokes one into another.

4. After you have finifh'd your Out-lines and Shades in the beft Manner you are able, take a larger Pencil, and lay on your Colours in their refpective Places, as a Carnation in the Face, Hands, &c. Green, Blue, Red, or any other Colour on the Drapery, and fo forth.

5. When you have done this, heighten the Lights of
your

your Work carefully with an unsplit stiff Pen, with which you take off the Colour by way of hetching, in such Places where the Light is to fall the strongest, and is also of particular Use to give the Beard or Hair a graceful turn.

6 You may lay all Sorts of Colours on the same Side of the Glass you draw your Design upon, except the yellow, which you lay on the other Side, in order to prevent its flowing and mixing with other Colours, and spoil your Work

Necessary Observations in the Baking of Glass after it is Painted

FIRST, your Furnace for baking Painted Glass must be, and is commonly built four Square, with three Divisions, as you see in the Print annex'd   The lower Division A, is for receiving the Ashes, and for a Draught for the Fire

2. The Middle Division is for the Fire, which has an Iron Grate below, and three Iron Bars cross the Top, to set the Earthen Pan upon, which contains the Painted Glass

The Third Division has the afore mentioned Bars at the Bottom, and a Lid at Top, in which are five Holes for the Exhalation of the Smoak and Flame

3   The Earthen Pan is made of good Potters Clay, according to the Shape and Dimension of the Furnace, about 5 or 6 Inches high, with a flat Bottom It must be Fire proof, and not larger than to have at least Two Inches Space all round, free from the Sides of the Furnace

The Figure here annex'd will better explain the Description

4. When you are going to bake your Glass, take Quick-Lime, which before-hand has been well neal'd or made red hot in a fierce Coal Fire   When cold, sift it through a small Sieve, as even as you can, all over the Bottom of the Pan, about half an Inch thick, then with a smooth Feather wipe it even and level, when this is done, lay as many of your painted Glasses as the Room will allow This continue, till the Pan is full, sifting upon every Lay of Glass a Lay of the mix'd Powder, very even, about the thickness of a Crown Piece   Upon the uppermost Lay of the painted Glass, let the Lay of Powder be as thick as at the Bottom The Pan thus fill'd to the Brim, put upon the Iron Bars in the middle of the Furnace, and cover the Furnace with a Cover made of Potters Earth, lute it very close all round, to prevent all Exhalation but what comes through the Holes

of

of the Cover-Lid. After you have order'd the Furnace in this Manner, and the Luting is dry, make a flow Charcoal or dry Wood Fire at the Entrance of the Furnace, increase it by Degrees, least by a too quick Fire the Glass should be subject to crack, continue thus to augment your Fewel, till the Furnace is full of Charcoal, and the Flame conveys itself through every Hole of the Cover, keep thus a very violent Fire for three or four Hours, and then you may draw out your Essays, which are Pieces of Glass on which you painted some yellow Colour, and place them against the Pin, and when you see the Glass bended, the Colour melted, and of a qualified yellow, you may conclude that your Work is near done, you may also perceive by the Increase of the Sparklings of the Iron Bars, or the light Streaks on the Pin, how your Work goes on. When you see your Colours almost done, improve the Fire with some dry Wood, and put it to that the Flame reverberates all round the Pin, then leave the Fire and let it go out, and the Work cool of itself. Take it out, and with a Brush clear your Glass from the Powder that may lay upon it, and your Work is done.

The Colours in use for Painting upon Glass, are next to be treated upon, and are as follow.

For a Carnation Colour

TAKE Meaning one Ounce, Red Enamel two Ounces, grind it fine and clean with good Brandy, upon a hard Stone. This, if you bake it sparingly, will produce a good Carnation.

A Black Colour.

TAKE Scales of Iron from the Anvil Block 14 Ounces and a half, mix with it two Ounces of White Glass, one Ounce of Antimony, Manganese half an Ounce, grind it with good Vinegar to an impalpable Powder.

2 Take Scales of Iron one Part, and *Recaille* one Part, grind it together very fine upon an Iron Plate, for one or two Days, when it begins to be tough, and looks yellowish, and cleaves to the Muller, it is a Sign that it is fine enough.

3 Take one Pound of Enamel, three quarters of a Pound of Copper Flakes, and two Ounces of Antimony, grind it as before directed, Or,

4 Take

4. Take Glass of Lead three Parts, Copper Flakes two Parts, and one Part of Antimony, proceed therewith as before

A Brown Colour

TAKE one ounce of white Glass or Enamel, half an ounce of good Manganese, grind it first with Vinegar very fine, and then with Brandy,

A Red Colour

ONE ounce of red Chalk, ground and mix'd with two ounces of grounded white Enamel and some Copper Flakes, will make a good Red, you may try with a little, whether it will stand the Fire, if not, add some more Copper Flakes to it

Another Red Colour.

TAKE red Chalk, that is hard and unfit to write withal, one part, of white Enamel one part, and one fourth part of Orpiment, grind it well together with Vinegar, and when you use it, avoid the Smoak, which is poisonous

Another

CROCUS Martis, or the Rust of Iron, Glass of Antimony, and yellow Lead-Glass, such as the Potters use, of each an equal Quantity, a small matter of Silver, calcined with Sulphur, grind it together very fine, and it will be fit to paint withal, and produce a good Red

Another

TAKE one half of Iron Flakes, one half of Copper Ashes, one half of Bismuth, a little Silver Filings, 3 or 4 Beads of Red Coral, 6 Parts of red Frit from a Glass House, one half of Litharge, one half of Gum, and 13 parts of red Chalk.

A Blue Colour for Glass Paint.

TAKE Burgundy Blue or blue Verditer, and Lead-Glass, an even Quantity, grind it with Water to a very fine Powder, and when you use it, lay the Flowers that are to be of a blue Colour, all over therewith, then raise the yellow

Parts

Parts open with a Pen, and cover them with a yellow Glaſs-Colour; obſerve, that blue upon yellow, and yellow upon blue, always makes a Green.

Another *Blue Glaſs Colour*

BLUE Verditer or Smalt, mix'd with Enamel, will make a good blue Paint

A Green *Glaſs-Colour*

GREEN Rocaille, or ſmall Beads of the ſame Colour, two Parts, Braſs File Duſt, ore Part, Menning two Parts, grind it together clear and fine, and you will have a good Green when it comes out of the Pan.

Another *Green.*

ÆS Uſtum 2 ounces, Menning 2 ounces, fine white Sand 8 ounces. Grind it to a very fine Powder, and put it into a Crucible, then lute the Covering and give it for one Hour a good briſk Fire in a Wind Furnace. After this, draw it off to cool; when cold, pound it in a Braſs Mortar, adding the fourth Part in Weight to the Powder, grind and mix it well together, and put it in a Crucible, then cover and lute it well, and give it a good Heat for two Hours in a Furnace.

A fine *Glaſs for a Yellow Paint*

IT has been found by Experience, that the beſt Yellow for Painting upon Glaſs is prepared out of Silver, wherefore if you will have a fine and good Yellow, take fine Silver, beat it into thin Plates, and diſſolve and precipitate it in Aquafortis, as has been directed, when it has ſettled, pour off the Aqua fortis, and grind the Silver with three times the Quantity of well burn'd Clay out of an Oven, very fine, and with a ſoft Hair Pencil lay it on the ſmooth Side of the Glaſs, and you will have a fine Yellow.

Another

MELT as much Silver as you pleaſe in a Crucible, and when in Fuſion, fling by little and little ſo much Sulphur upon, till it is calcined, Then grind it very fine on a

Stone

Stone, mix it with as much Antimony as the Weight in Silver, and when these are well ground together, then take yellow Oaker, neal it well, and it will turn to a Brown red, which quench in Urin, and take thereof double the quantity above specified, mix it all together, and after you have grounded it very fine, lay it on the smooth Side of the Glass.

Another Method

NEAL some thin Plates of Silver, then cut them into small Bits, put them with Sulphur and Antimony into a Crucible; when it is dissolv'd, pour it into clear Water, and thus mix't together, grind it very fine

A Pale Yellow.

STRATIFY thin Plates of Brass in an earthen Pipkin with powdered Sulphur and Antimony, and burn it so long till it yields no more Flame, then pour it red hot into cold Water; take it out and grind it fine   Of this Powder one part, of yellow Oaker, after it is neal'd and quench'd in Vinegar, five or six parts, let it dry; then grind it on a Stone, and it will be fit for Use.

How to deaden the Glass, and fit it for to paint upon

TAKE two parts of Iron Flakes, one part of Copper Flakes; three Parts of white Enamel, grind it all together with clear Water on a Marmor Stone, or upon a brass or Iron Plate for two or three Days, as fine as possible, with this rub your Glass well over, especially that Side you draw your Design upon, and you will finish your Work much neater

Some general Observations in the Management of Painting and Baking of Glass

FIRST when you lay your Glass into the Pan, let the painted Side be undermost upon the Lime, and the Yellow uppermost

2. Dilute all your Colours with Gum-Water.

3 Grind the Black and Red upon a Copper Plate, other Colours you may grind on a Piece of Glass, or a Stone

4. Glass-Colours ready prepared, are Glass Enamel, that's brought from *Venice* in Cakes, of most Sorts, also the small Glass Beads, that are brought over from *Germany*, especially

cially from *Franckfurt* on the *Main*. Old broken pieces of
painted Glafs are good for that purpofe, fo is the Green Glafs
of Potters, and the Glafs Drops that run from the Ware in the
Furnace

5 The Colours which are ufed by Potters, for painting on
earthen Ware, may alfo be ufed in painting upon Glafs

A particular *Way to paint upon a Drinking Glafs*

TAKE a fmall quantity of Linfeed, bruife it and put it
for four or five Days in a little Canvafs Bag, in Rain-
Water, and change the Water every Day, then prefs out the
Moifture, and you will have a clammy Subftance, like Glue,
with this grind your Colours as ufual, then paint or mark with
a Pencil what you pleafe upon the Glafs, and give it by degrees a thorough Heat, with the fame Glue you may alfo gild
upon the Glafs, before you put it to the Fire

A *fine Gilding upon Glafs*

TAKE Gum-Armoniac, diffolve it over Night in good
White-Wine Vinegar, and it will be as white as Flower,
pour off the Vinegar into another Veffel, and grind the Gum-
Armoniack and a little Gum-Arabick well together with clear
Water, when they are well incorporated and fine, then write
or draw upon your Glafs what you pleafe, and when almoft dry,
fo that it is but a little clammy, then lay on your Gold,
prefs it down with fome Cotton, and let it ftand over Night
rub the loofe Gold afterwards with a little Cotton gently off
the Glafs, and you will fee the Ornaments, Figures or Writing
in that Perfection as you defign'd them, then dry it flowly over
a gentle Heat, increafing it by degrees fo as to make it Red
Hot, let it cool of itfelf, and the Gold will look fine, and
ftand either Wine or Water

To Write or *Draw upon Glafs*

TAKE two parts of Lead, one part of Emery, and a
little Quantity of white Lead, grind it very fine with
clear Water, then temper it with Gum-Water, and with a foft
Hair Pencil lay it all over the outfide of your Glafs, and when
dry, you may with a Pen draw or write upon it what you pleafe,
then increafe the Fire from a gentle warmth to make the Glafs
red hot, let it cool, and you will fee your Drawing or Writing
fair upon the Glafs, which will not be defac'd either by cold or
hot Water.   The

✿✿✿✿✿✿✿✿✿✿✿✿✿✿✿✿✿✿✿✿✿✿✿✿

The Art of Glazing and Painting on fine Earthen, commonly call'd DELFT WARE.

POTTERS who paint with Colours on Earthen Ware, may be rang'd in the fame Clafs with Painters upon Glafs, fince they ufe almoft the fame Materials, and in many Refpeçts, the fame Method

What has already been faid under the foregoing Head, is fufficient, and may ferve Praçtitioners in Defigning and Painting as an Inftruction to paint Flowers, Landfkips, Figures or whatever elfe, upon Earthen Ware We fhall however here fet down fome Receipts that chiefly relate to the Glazing of Earthen Ware, but firft fhew,

How to prepare the Clay for fine Delft Ware

TAKE one part of Calcin'd Flint, one part of Chalk, and one part of Capital or the Cream of Clay, mix and Work it well to a proper Subftance

To prepare a White Glazing.

TAKE of Lead two pound, Tin one pound, calcine it to Afhes, as has been directed before Of this take two parts, calcined Flint or Pebble, one part, Salt one part, mix it well together and melt it into a Cake.

The Rotterdam fine fhining White

TAKE of clean Tin Afhes two pound, Lead Afhes ten pound, fine Venice Glafs two pound, Tartar half a pound, and melt it to a Cake

Or,

LEAD Afhes eight pound, Tin Afhes three pound, fine clear calcined Flint or Pebble fix pound, Salt four pound, melt it into a Cake.

Another

Another.

CALCINE eight pound of Lead and four pound of Tin into Ashes, of their take one Quart, Salt and Pebble of each one pound, and melt it into a Cake.

Another fine White for Earthen Ware.

CALCINE six pound of Lead, and three pound of Tin to Ashes, whereof take two parts, Salt three parts, Pebble or Flint three parts, and melt it into a Cake

Another White.

TAKE eight pound of Lead and four pound of Tin Ashes, among which mix six pound of Venice-Glass, and a handful of Rock-Salt, melt it into a Cake

Saltzburg White

TAKE three parts of Lead, six parts of Tin, or six parts Lead and three parts Tin, Salt three parts, Tartar one part, and Pebble five parts, &

Or,

TAKE five pound of Lead, one pound of Tin, three pound of Flint, three pound of Salt, &c

Another White

TAKE six pound of Lead, one pound of Tin, melt and burn it to Ashes, whereof take 12 Spoonfuls, 12 spoonfuls of Flint, and 12 of fine Wood Ashes

To lay a Ground upon Earthen Ware, on which the white Glass will better spread

TAKE calcin'd Tartar one pint, Flint and Salt of each one pint, mix it together, and use it for a Lay or Ground over your Earthen Ware, before you glaze it

The right Dutch Maſtırat for White Porcelain.

TAKE calcin'd Pebble, Flint or Sand, 100 pound, Soda 40 pound, Wood Aſhes 30 pound   This Mixture is by the *Dutch* call'd *Maſtırat*; of this take 100 pound, Tin and Lead Aſhes together 80 pound, common Salt 10 pound, and melt it three Times into a Cake

The Tin and Lead Aſhes are made out of 100 pound of Lead and 33 pound of Tin

The Common Ware is thus Glazed.

TAKE 40 pound of clear Sand, 75 pound of Litharge or Lead-Aſhes, 25 pound of Pot-Aſhes, and ten pound of Salt, melt it three Times into a Cake, quenching it each time in clear cold Water

Or,

TAKE clean Sand 50 pound, Lead Aſhes 70 pound, Wood-Aſhes 30 pound, Salt 12 pound, melt it to a Cake

With this Mixture they glaze fine and coarſe Ware, and ſet it in an Earthen glazing Pan, which is round, the Ware is let in them upon three corner'd Bars, that go through the like holes in the Pan, and the Ware is kept aſunder from touching one another.

The opening before, is only left in the Figure to ſee how the Ware ſtands, otherwiſe the Pan muſt be entirely clos'd up

Of Several Colours for POTTERS GLAZE WORK.

A Fine Yellow

TAKE Red Lead three pints, Antimony and Tin, of each two pound, melt it into a Cake, grind it fine, and melt it again   This repeat ſeveral Times, and you will have a good yellow.

Another.

Another.

TAKE 15 parts of Lead Oar, three parts of Litharge of Silver, and 15 parts of fine Sand

Another.

TAKE eight parts Litharge, nine parts of calcin'd Flint, one part Antimony, and a little Iron Filings, calcine and melt it into a Cake.

Fine Citron Yellow.

TAKE fix parts of Red Lead, seven parts of fine Red Brick-duft, two parts of Antimony, melt it into a Cake

A Green Colour

TAKE eight parts of Litharge, eight parts of Venice Glafs, four parts of Brafs Duft, melt it for ufe

Another

TAKE 10 parts of Litharge, 12 parts of Flint or Pebble, one part of *Æs uftum* or Copper Afhes,

Blue Colour

TAKE Lead Afhes one pound, clear Sand, or Pebble two pound, Salt two pound, white calcin'd Tartar, one pound, Venice or other Glafs 16 pound, Zaffer half a pound, mix it well together and melt it, quench it in Water, and melt it again, this repeat feveral times But if you will have it fine and good, it will be proper to put the mixture in a Glafs Furnace for one or two Days.

Another

TAKE Litharge four pound, clear Sand two pound, Zaffer one pound, calcin'd and melted together

Another.

TAKE 12 pound of Lead, one pound of Tin, and one pound of Zaffer, five pound of Sand, and three pound

of

of Salt, Tartar and Glafs one Pound, calcine and melt it
in a Cake.

Or,

TAKE two pound of Litharge, a quarter of a pound of
Sand, one pound of Zaffera, and one pound of Salt;
melt this as directed.

Or,

ONE part of Tartar, one part of Lead Afhes, one part
of Zaffera, one part of Sand, and two parts of Salt,
melt it as before

A Brown Colour.

TAKE of common Glafs, and Manganefe or Brown-
Stone, of each one part, Lead Glafs 12 parts.

A Flefh Colour.

TAKE 12 parts of Lead-Afhes, and one of white
Glafs

Purple Brown.

TAKE Lead-Afhes, 15 parts, clear Sand 18 parts, Manganefe one Part, white Glafs 15 Meafures, and one
Meafure of Zaffera

Iron Gray

TAKE 15 parts of Lead-Afhes, 14 parts of white Sand,
five parts of Copper Afhes, one of Manganefe, one of
Zaffera, and one of Iron Filings.

A Black.

TAKE Lead-Afhes 18 Meafures, Iron Filings three,
Copper Afhes three, Zaffera two Meafures, this, when
melted, will make a brown-black but, if you will have it
blacker, put fome more Zaffera to it

Brown on White.

MANGANESE two parts, Red Lead and white Glafs one part, melt it well together.

A fine Red

TAKE Antimony two pound, Litharge three pound, Ruft of Iron calcined one pound, grind it to a fine Powder.

To glaze with Venice Glafs.

WHEN your Ware is well dry'd, and ready to bake, ftrike it all over with White-Wine Lees, then lay on the Venice Glafs (ground fine and mixt with *Sal Tartar* and Litharge) and bake it as directed

A Green.

TAKE Copper Duft two parts, yellow Glafs two parts; melt it twice.

Or,

TWO parts of Copper Filings, one of Lead Afhes, and one of white Glafs; melt it to a Cake.

Yellow

MENNING three parts, Brick-duft two parts, Lead-Afhes two parts, Antimony two parts, Sand one part, of the above white Glafs one part, well calcin'd and melted

Or,

RED Lead four ounces, Antimony two ounces, melt it to a Cake

Gold Yellow,

TAKE of Antimony, Red Lead and Sand, an equal Quantity, and melt it to a Cake,

A fine

A fine Blue Glass to paint with.

TAKE Lead-Ashes one pound, clear Sand two pound, Salt two pound, white calcin'd Tartar one pound, Flint Glass half a pound, Zaffer half a pound, melt it together and quench it in Water, then melt it again, and repeat this several times

Zaffera finely ground by itself, makes good blue, to paint upon white-glaz'd Earthen Ware

A Brown.

ONE part of Manganese, one of Lead, and one of white Glass.

A Liver Colour

TAKE 12 parts of Litharge, eight of Salt, six of Pebble or Flint, and one of Manganese.

A Sea-Green.

TAKE five pound of Lead-Ashes, one pound of Tin-Ashes, three pound of Flint, three quarters of a pound of Salt, half a pound of Tartar, and half a pound of Copper dust

To lay Gold, Silver, or Copper on Earthen Ware, so as to resemble either of these Metals

MAKE an Utensil of fine Potters Earth, form and shape it thin, neat, and Silver Fashion, then bake it, and when bak'd, glaze it . but before you bake it again, if you will silver, gild or copper it, take a Regulus of Antimony, melt your Metal with it, and beat it to a Powder, grind it with Water very fine, and glaze it therewith. Then bake it, and when done, the whole Utensil will look like Silver; for when it comes in the Fire, the Antimony evaporates and leaves the Silver, &c. behind. But if you will silver or gild it only for Ornament sake, and keep it from any Wet coming to it, then you may lay on the Gold or Silver Leaves with Brandy, and afterwards polish and finish it in the best Manner, after the common Method.

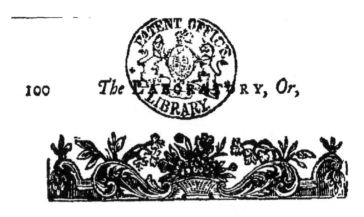
PART IV.

Several uncommon Experiments for *Casting* in
SILVER, COPPER, BRASS, TIN, STEEL, and other
Metals; likewise in WAX, PLAISTER of PARIS,
WOOD, HORN, *&c* With the Management of
the respective Moulds.

*To prepare Clay in such a Manner as to be fit to make all
manner of Moulds to cast Gold, Silver and other Metals
in them*

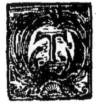AKE Clay, as much as you will, put it into
an Earthen Pot that's glaz'd, and cover and
lute it very close, then put it into a Potters
Furnace, and let it stand as long as other
Earthen Ware   After it is burn'd and
cold, grind the Clay upon a Colour Stone
very fine, sift it through a fine hair Sieve
into clear Water, and after it is settled, pour off the Water,
and grind the Clay once more upon the Stone, as fine as possible, then wash it again in fair Water as before, and set it
in the Sun or in a warm Place to dry

After this burn'd and wash'd Clay is thorough dry, take
thereof three pound, *Sal-Armoniac* two pound, Tartar two
pound, Vitriol one pound, mix this together, and put it in one
or two Pots, pour upon it about seven quarts of clean Water,
and boil this Composition for some time; then take this Water,
whilst it is warm, and mix your burn'd Clay therewith to
such a Substance that you may roll it into Balls; these lay
in a warm Place to dry, and when dry, put them into an
Earthen Pot as before, and give them another baking among
the Earthen Ware, and when cold, grind them fine, and that
Powder will be fit for Use

The

The Clay being thus prepared, take *Sal-Armoniac*, put it into a Glaſs with Water that holds about two Quarts, put ſo much of the *Sal-Armoniac* to the Water as it will diſſolve over a gentle Warmth, and let it ſtand one or two Hours cloſed up; then take your Powder of Clay, temper it with this Water to ſuch a Subſtance as to roll it into Balls, and make what Moulds you pleaſe thereof When you caſt your Metal, you muſt make your Mould red hot; and be alſo very nimble in the pouring out your melted Metal

To make Moulds of Clay to caſt Braſs or other Metals therein

TAKE good clear Clay, ſuch as the Pewterers uſe; take alſo Cloth Shavings or fine ſhort pluck'd Cotton, and fine clear Sand, and if the Sand is not fine enough, grind it on a Colour Stone, mix this with the Clay to ſuch a Subſtance as is fit to make or form your Moulds thereof Your Clay muſt not be made ſoft with Water, but with ſtrong Beer, and when you caſt, let your Mould be red hot

If you will have a fine and ſharp Caſt, ſift over your Clay ſome fine waſh'd Aſhes, before you make the Impreſſion.

To prepare Moulds, which need not be heated for caſting Metal in them

TAKE fine Sand, ſuch as the Goldſmiths uſe, mix it with Lampblack as much as you think proper, then temper it with Rape or Linſeed Oil, fit to make your Moulds thereof, whatever you caſt in them, comes not only out neat and ſharp, but you have no occaſion to heat your Mould, as is required in others This you muſt obſerve, that your Sand muſt be very dry before you temper it with the Oil

The Preparation of Mantua-Earth, for Moulds.

TAKE Mantua-Earth one part, and one part of Charcoal Duſt, burnt of Birch, and one part of Salt, then mix with it an equal Quantity of Tartar, boil it up together in a Copper Pan, and let it ſeeth or ebulate three times with this Water, which keeps always good, moiſten and temper your Earth, ſo as to form it into Balls between your Hands,

and

and when you will make your Mould, roll your Earth with a
Roller, till it is smooth and pliable, then you may form it
into what Fashion you please. In this Mould you may cast
before it is dry, and when you have cast, take off the Earth
which is dry'd through the Heat of the Metal, grind the
same again, and temper it as you did at first to use it again.

A Particular Sort of Mould, in which one may cast exceeding fine

TAKE Horse Mussels, or for want of them, Oyster-Shells,
let them be calcin'd in a Potters Furnace, then pulverize and temper them with Urine; of this make your
Moulds, and you will cast very fine and sharp

To Impress Bass Relievo or Medals, in Imitation of Ivory

TAKE of prepared Clay one pound, fine Plaister of
Paris eight ounces, white Starch eight ounces, mix
these together, and beat it up with the White of six or eight
Eggs, put to it three ounces of clear Gum Arabick, stir it
well together to a Paste, and put so much of the dry Mixture to it till you can knead it like Dough, then press it
into a Mould with the Palm of your Hand, and let it dry
in the Sun, observing thereby to lay the Paste side on a smooth
Board, and it will be clear and hard, like Ivory You may
impress all manner of Medals and Curiosities, and make
them of what Colour you please.

To cast Vegetables in Moulds, peculiarly prepar'd for Silver.

TAKE fine and clear Clay or Spalter, that s dry, and pound
it fine in a Mortar; then take a Copper or Iron Pan,
put in your Clay, and give it a brisk Fire, and after you have
heated it thoroughly, take it off and let it cool; then take
one part of this Clay, one part *Alumen Plumosum,* grind it
together, and cast it in little Tents, which put into a Fire
to neal, beat it very fine, and when you will form
your Plant, take one part of this Powder, and one part of
Alumen Plumosum, grind it together, and add as much of the
Clay Powder as the mix'd Matter doth contain, and mix
and grind it all together Then take some Potters Clay,
to make a Coffin round your Plant, spread it in what
manner you think proper, and after the Coffin is dry, anoint

the inside thereof, as also the Plant with good Brandy; dust the before prepared Clay and the Plant gently through a fine Cambrick, and when you have cover'd it all over as thick as it will bear, strike the rais'd Coffin a little with your Hand or Hammer, and the dust will settle closer to the Plant and make the Silver, cast in, come out the sharper.

After the Powder is well settled, and your Coffin closed, cover it first with dead Charcoal, and then lay some live ones over them; let the Fire gradually descend to the Coffin, and heat it by degrees to a strong Glue, then let it cool of itself with the Fire, take afterwards fine Clay, fine Sand and some Wool Shearings; mix this together, beat and knead it well in one another; then temper it with Glue, and fill your Coffin with it all over the Plant, leaving an opening at the Stalk for the Inlet, then put it again into the Fire and make it red hot, and with a pair of Bellows, first closed, draw out the Ashes from the Inlet, and it will be ready for Casting.

Then take Oil of Tartar, which is made of pounded Salt of Tartar, and scrape a little *Sal Armoniac* into it, to give it the Substance of a thin Paste, which is a good Flux for Silver; fling some of this upon your Silver when in Fusion, and it will cast fine and sharp.

After it is cast, anoint the Silver Plant with Oil of Tartar, lay it on live Coals, neal it, and then boil it in Tartar, to which you add a little Salt, and this will give it a fine bright Pearl Colour.

A curious Method to cast all sorts of Things in Gold, Silver, or other Metals.

FIRST pound Plaister of Paris, or Alablaster, to a fine Powder, sift it through a Cambrick, or very fine Hair Sieve, and put it into an Iron Pan, over a clear Coal Fire; stir it about till it begins to boil, and bubbles up like Water, keep it stirring; recruit your Fire, and continue this so long till you find it so thick as not to be able to draw it along with your Stick; then pour it into a Bowl and let it cool

Take also Brick-dust finely powder'd and sifted.

The Miners find sometimes a Matter in the Iron Mines, which they call Liver Oar, take this and wash it from the coarser Sand, and when dry, put it in an earthen Pot, cover it, set it to neal thoroughly, and when cold, pound and sift it. When it is right burnt, it will be of a Copper Colour, put all

the

thele different Powders in feveral Boxes, and preferve them from Duft and Soil, for proper ufe.

To caſt Vegetables and Inſects

FOUR parts of the above Plaifter of Paris, two parts Brick-Duft, and two parts Liver Oar, mix this well together, and fift it through a fine Hair Sieve, and when you are ready to form your Mould, pour clean Water to it, ftir it well together to the Thicknefs of a thin Pafte, but you muft be pretty nimble with this Work, elfe it will harden under your Hands, and be of no Ufe

The Mould you prepare thus .

TAKE the Plant you defign to caſt, and fpread the Leaves and Stalks not to touch one another, then make a Coffin either of Lead or Clay, put your Plant in it, fo as not to touch the Coffin, at the bottom you may lay a Piece of Paper, to keep the Stuff from fticking to the Board, but let your Stuff be neither too thick nor too thin, for if it is of a right Subftance it will force itfelf clofe to the Plants, and come out fharp, let the Stalks be carefully kept up for the Inlet, and when you pour this Stuff upon your Plants, do it gently, and part thofe Leaves which might clofe to one another, with a Needle, pouring all the while, to make the Mould the ftronger After it is harden'd, put it in a dry Place, and keep it till you have fome more ready to caft, but you muft fecure it from Froft.

If you will caft Infects, or any fmall Animal or Reptile, put them in what Pofition you will upon a little Board, brown Paper, or Pafte-Board, which firft muft be anointed with Oil, in order to make the Plaifter Stuff come off the eafier, about your Infect make a little Coffin, and if you can rife the Infect fo as to be free from the Board or Paper, it will be the better, which you may do by tying it with two or three hairs, faftening them at the Top of the Coffin, and by this means will hang in the middle thereof, when this is ready, pour, as before directed, your Plaifter gently upon it, and after the Mould is a little dry, put it alfo by for ufe

If you lay your Infect or other Creature on the Paper, and you muft make a Wall about and caft your Plaifter upon it, let it ftand a little, and when dry, take off your Wall, and cut the Plaifter round about the Infect, and taking the

Mould off the Paper, there will be an opening at the Bottom of the Mould where the Infect laid, turn this Mould and anoint it about the Opening and the Part of the Infect with Oil, then cafting fome frefh Plaifter upon that Place, your Mould will take afunder, and be very convenient to draw out the Afhes of the Infect, after it has been burn'd as is here directed.

Put your Mould upon fome warm Wood-Afhes, then cover it with Smallcoal, over the Smallcoal lay Charcoal, and then fling fome lighted Smallcoal over them to kindle the others, fo that the Heat may be convey'd to the Mould by flow degrees, and after it has glow'd fome time, and you think the Infect or Plant is confum'd to Afhes, let it cool of it felf with the Fire about it, to hinder the Air coming to it When your Mould is cold, open the Hole for the Inlet, and either with your breath, or with a little hand Spout that is moift, draw out the Afhes, and your Mould is ready

You may alfo burn thofe Moulds in a Muffle, if you clofe the Muffle to prevent the Air coming in, and lay the Coals on, and glow it as has been directed After you have taken out the Mould, put the fame in warm Sand, and having your Silver or other Metal ready melted, pour it in quick, but if you caft Silver, fling in the Flux a little *Sal Armoniac* and Borax, mix'd together After it is caft, let the Mould cool a little, then quench it in Water, and the Plaifter will fall off of it felf, brufh the Silver clean, and neal and boil it as has been already directed

To caft Vegetables or Infects in another Manner.

TIE your Plant, Sprig or Infect with a fine Thread to a little Stick, dip either of them into Brandy, and let it dry a little, temper your Plaifter of Paris, prepared as heretofore directed, with Water of *Sal Armoniac*, pretty thin, and dip your Plant or Infect in it all over, then put the little Stick in a Hole againft a Wall or any thing elfe, let it hang free, and in the drying you may difplay the Leaves of the Plant or the Legs of the Infect as you would have them, and when you have done this hang it in the Coffin; the little Stick may reft on each end of the Coffin, then pouring your Plaifter over, you will have an exact Mould, proceed then as directed before.

If

If you will have a small Insect to stand upon a Leaf, then dip the ends of its Legs in Turpentine, and put it on the Plant before you dip it. If it is a Spider or Graishopper, or any other Insect which you think will be too strong for the Turpentine, kill them first in Wine and Vinegar, and after this put their Legs in the Turpentine, and fix it to the Leaf of the Plant.

To cast Figures or Medals in Brimstone

MELT (in a glaz'd Pipkin) half a pound of Brimstone over a gentle Fire; with this mix half a pound of fine Vermillion, and when you have clear'd the Top, take it off the Fire, stir it well together, and it will dissolve like Oil, then cast it into the Mould, which you first anointed with Oil, let it cool, and take it out; but in case your Figure should change to a yellowish Colour, you only wipe it over with Aqua Fortis, and it will look like the finest Coral

How to form and cast all Manner of small Birds, Animals, Frogs, Fish, &c

TAKE an Earthen, Iron or Tin Ring, which is high and wide enough to hold the Animal you design to Cast, and set the Ring upon a clean Board or Paste-Board, then lay the Animal upon it, and cast the fine Mixture of Plaister pretty thick over it, the rest of the Vacancy you may fill up with a coarser Plaister, even to the Brim when this is done and pretty well dried, turn your Ring, and putting a little short Stick close to the Body of the Animal, cast a Crust on that Side, to cover that Part which lays close to the Board, and when dry, burn it, and go about the Casting as directed After you have burn'd or glow'd it thoroughly, you must draw the Ashes out of the Hole which is made by the little Stick, and this you may use for your Inlet.

❀❀❀❀❀❀❀❀❀❀❀❀❀ ❀ ❀❀❀❀❀❀❀❀

How to Caſt Images of *Plaiſter of Paris* , likewiſe
how to Caſt *Wax*, either ſolid or hollow, alſo how
to form Images in *Wax*, and caſt them afterwards
in any Metal, either ſolid or hollow

HOW to prepare the Mixture or the Moulds, has
been ſhewn before, for which Reaſon it is needleſs to
repeat it here again

If you will make a Mould to caſt an Image or Animal
in it, take clean Potters Clay, make thereof a Coffin
round about the Image, which you lay long ways on a Board,
and anoint over with Oil , then take your fine Plaiſter of Paris,
mix it with Water, and pour it all over the Image, ſo that it
may cover it every where; then give it a ſtronger Coat with a
Coarſer Sort, and when the Plaiſter is dry, take off the Coffin,
and cut that Side which is Caſt ſomething flat, making ſome
Notches or marks upon it , then turn it, and make a Coffin about it again, and Caſt that Side of the Image, after you
have anointed it with ſome Oil all over, ſo that the whole
may be intirely incloſ'd.

After the Plaiſter has been a Day or two upon the Image,
it will be quite dry; then with a Wooden Mallet beat
cautiouſly againſt the Plaiſter, till a piece thereof looſens,
which being taken off the reſt will come off eaſier; and after
you have diſmantled the whole, anoint the inſide thereof with
Linſeed Oil, with a fine Hair Bruſh Pencil, and let it dry in;
this do twice , and after they have lain two or three Days,
cut in an Inlet, where you think moſt convenient, and when
you will caſt with Plaiſter of Paris, before you do it,
anoint the inſide of the Mould, and after you have put all
the Pieces in their proper Places and tied them together, caſt
your Plaiſter, and let it ſtand half a Day; take the Pieces one
after another carefully off, in order to keep the Image intire,
but if you will caſt Wax in that Mould, put only the
Moulds for half an Hour before in Water, and the Wax will
not ſtick to it If you will have the Image hollow, then
mind that the Wax be not too hot, pour it into the Mould,
and you will eaſily ſee how thick it ſticks to it. When you think

it is thick enough, then turn your Mould about, and pour out the Wax that's remaining, and after you have for a little while laid it in Water, take off the Pieces of Moulding, and you will have the Image done to Perfection. You must observe, that before you break the Mould from the Image on which you form'd it, you must mark it all over with Crosses, Circles or Strokes, by which you may afterwards fix them right and exactly together to cast in again. If you will have the Wax Figures solid, then let the Mould with the Images lay for half an Hour or more to cool in fair Water.

To prepare the Wax.

TAKE one pound of white Rosin, that's not greasy, two pound of Wax, melt the Wax, in a Pan, strain it through a Cloath into a glaz'd Pan, and stir it about till it is cool.

To cast Medals and other Things in Bass Relievo.

LAY your Medal on a clean Piece of Paper or a clean Board, inclose it with a Wall of Clay or Wax, then pour the Plaister of Paris half an Inch thick upon it, when it is dry, take off the Medal, and anoint the Mould with clear Sallet Oil, both within and without, two or three times. If you will cast Plaister of Paris, lay the Mould first for a quarter of an Hour in clear Water, then cast your Plaister as thick as you please.

N. B. If you will polish some parts in the Plaister of Paris you have cast, you must do it with Soap Lees, and a Dog's Tooth, or some other smooth Tooth.

You must observe, that whenever you make a Mould of Plaister, let it be for Bass Relievo or Figures, you must always anoint it with Oil, two or three times, which will not only preserve them from the Damage they otherwise would sustain from the Water, but make the cast Pieces come out clear.

Medals and Figures in Bass relievo, how to cast them like Jaspis.

TO do this, you must have a Hand Spout, or a Glyster-Pipe, at the end whereof fix a Tin or Iron Blade, full of round Holes, some larger than others. In this Spout put a Paste, made of fine Chalk, of several Colours,

then

then forcing them out in small Shreds of mix'd Colours in one Piece, cut them with a fine edg'd Knife in thin round Slices, and put one into your Mould, pressing it down gently, then pour the Plaister of Paris upon it, and when dry, lay it first over with Fish-Glue, and after that varnish it, and it will be of singular Beauty

The Colours you may first dilute with Gum-Water, before you mix the Chalk with them

Another Method.

TAKE the above mention'd Chalk-Paste, and after you have mix'd it with a Variety of Colours, as Smalt, White Lead, Vermillion, Red Lead, Masticot, Verdegrease, Brown Red, &c. each Colour made separate into little Cakes, then (with a Rolling Pin) spread it thin like Pye-Crust, and when you have as many Colours together as you think proper, lay one Leaf upon another, and roll them together from one end to the other, and with a Knife cut thin Wafer-like Pieces, take these and cover your Mould with, press it close down with your Thumb, and pour your Plaister of Paris over it, after it is dry, do it over with Fish Glue, and then varnish or polish it with a Dog's Tooth

To Cast Animals, Fish, Reptiles, Fruit, or any kind of Thing, in a Pewter Plate or Dish.

TAKE a Pewter Dish that's finish'd, garnish the same with either Fish, Animals, Reptiles, Fruit, Plants, &c. dispose them in proper Order, as your Fancy directs you. Small Animals or Leaves of Plants fasten to the Dish with a little Turpentine, and when every Thing is in Order, wall it round, pour your Plaister of Paris over it, and strike upon the Table the Dish stands on, in order to make the Casting fix the closer about the Things, and after your Mould is dry, make the Mould for the back Part of the Dish, glow it, then fix these Moulds together for Casting, and having tied them round with Wires, and made them red hot, cast your Pewter, and in order not to make the Dish too heavy, convey some little Openings from the back part of the Mould to the Body or Hollow of the Animal, stopping the outside close up again, till your Cast is over, and as soon as you think the Pewter sufficiently struck or fix'd, then open
these

these Conveyances and pour out the Pewter which may remain in the Ingot melted

If you will cast it in Silver, then model your Leaves and Animals, Creatures, &c each separate and hollow, that they may be soldered on afterwards.

To cast Figures in Imitation of Ivory.

TAKE Izing-Glass and strong Brandy, and make it into a Paste, then take very fine grounded Egg-shells, and mix it together to a Mass You may give it what Colour you please, but cast it warm into your Mould, after you have oil'd it all over, leave the Figure in the Mould till it is cold, then set it in the Air to dry, and you will have fine Figures, like Ivory.

Another Mixture to cast Figures, in Bass relievo.

TAKE Flower of Chalk, that has been finely grounded, mix it with clear Glue well together, pour it into your Mould, press it with the Palm of your Hand, and it will come out very fine. You may do this in what Colour you please.

To cast with marbled Colours in Plaister

TAKE several Colours, as Vermillion, Dutch Pink, Yellow Oaker, Smalt, &c temper them with Water, and mix every one apart with Plaister Then take what Colours you please, and first sprinkle your Mould, which is best of Brimstone, with one or more of them, with a little Pencil or Feather, then pour a Colour different, from what you sprinkled, into the Mould, and after it is harden'd, give it a Gloss with Wax or Varnish, as pleases you best.

A Sand in which one may cast Things to the greatest nicety, whether flat, or in Bass Relievo

TAKE Fuller's Earth, put it into a Reverberatory Furnace, so long till it is red hot; then take *Sal Armoniac* about one pound, dissolve it in two Quarts of Water, with this Water moisten the burnt Earth, and when cool, put it into the Furnace into a red hot Dish; after it has glown there, take it out again, and after the Heat is a little over, sprinkle it with the Water again, till it is quench'd, then give it
ano

another Fire, and repeat this five or six times, the more, the better it will receive the Metal · then bring it to a very fine Powder, by grinding it; put it into the Frame, which may be either of Brass, Iron or Wood, but before moisten it a little with the fore-mentioned Water; then make your Impression near the Ingot, and after you have dried it before the Fire, while it is hot, cast your Metal, the Impression will be better the second Time than at first using it, but every time you use it, make it first red hot.

To make Horn soft.

TAKE one pound of Wood-Ashes, two pound of Quick-Lime, one Quart of Water, let it boil together to one Third, then dip a Feather in it, and if in drawing it out the *Plume* comes off, it is boil'd enough, if not, let it boil longer, when it is settled, filter it through a Cloath, then put in Shavings or Filings of Horn, let them soak therein three Days, and anointing your Hands first with Oil, work the Horn Shavings into a Mass, and print, mould, or form it in what Shape you please.

To cast Horn into Moulds.

TAKE Horn Shavings as much as you will, and lay 'em in a new Earthen Pot; take two parts of Wood Ashes, and the third part of Lime, pour clear Lee upon it, so as to cover it all over, boil it well, stir it with an Iron Ladle, till it has the Consistence of a Paste : if you will have it of a Red Colour, then take Red Lead, or Vermillion, as much as you think proper, temper it together; then cast it into a Mould, and let it dry, you may smooth it with a Knife, and it will be of one solid Piece, you may dry it thus of what Colour you will have it.

To cast Wood in Moulds, as fine as Ivory, of a fragrant smell and in several Colours.

TAKE fine Saw-Dust of Lime-Tree-Wood, put it into a clean Pan, tie it close up with Paper, and let it dry by a gentle Heat; then beat it in a Stone Mortar to a fine Flower, sift it through a Cambrick, and lay it, if you don't use it presently, in a dry Place, to keep it from Dust.

Then

Then take one pound of fine Parchment Glue, the fineſt Dragant and Gum-Arabick, of each four ounces, let it boil in clear Pump Water, and filter it through a clean Rag, then put into it of the ſaid Flower of Wood, ſtir it till it becomes of the Subſtance of a thick Paſte, and ſet it in a glaz'd Pan in a hot Sand, ſtir it well together and let the reſt of the Moiſture evaporate till it be fit for Caſting   Then pour or mix your Colours with the Paſte, and put in Oil of Cloves, of Roſes, or the like, to give it a Scent, you may mix it, if you will, with a little beaten Amber: For a Red Colour, uſe Braſil Ink, and for other Colours, ſuch as will be directed under the Article for Book-Binders   Your Mould will be better of Pewter or Braſs, than of Plaiſter of Paris; anoint it over with Oil of Almonds, and put your Paſte into it, let it ſtand three or four Days to dry and harden, then take off your Mould, and it will be as hard as Ivory, you may cut, turn, carve and plain it like other Wood, and be of a ſweet Scent, you may alſo, if your Mould will allow it, uſe ſeveral Colours in one Piece, leaving only in ſome Part the natural Colour of the Wood, in order to convince the Beholder what it is.   It is a fine and curious Experiment

Of the Mixture for Caſting MIRROURS, and other Things for OPTICKS.

WE find the Method for preparing theſe Mixtures preſcrib'd by ſeveral Authors, but after different Ways, wherefore I ſhall let down only a few which for the Generality are beſt approv'd of. And Firſt,

TAKE three Pound of the beſt refin'd Pewter, and one Pound of refin'd Copper. Firſt melt the Copper, and then add the Pewter to it, when both are in Fuſion, pour it out, and when cold, beat it to Powder. Then ſtrew upon it 12 Ounces of red Tartar, a little calcin'd Tartar, three Ounces of Salt petre, one Ounce and an half of Alum, and four Ounces of Arſenick. Mix and ſtir this together, and after it has done evaporating, pour out the Metal into

your

your Mould, let it cool, and when polish'd, you will have a fine Mirror.

This is the Composition which is commonly call'd the *Steel Mixture*

Some Artists will have the Arsenick omitted, it being of the Nature to turn the Mirror into a deadish blue Colour, and requires new polishing every Time one wants to use it, and think that Copper and Pewter are sufficient to answer that Purpose.

Another Method.

TAKE an Earthen Pan, that is not glaz'd, and has stood the Fire, put into it two Pound of Tartar, also the same Weight of Crystalline Arsenick, and melt it on a Coal Fire. When this Mixture begins to smoak, put to it 50 Pound of old Copper, and let it be in Fusion six or seven Hours, so that it may be well cleansed Then add to it 50 pound of Pewter, and let it melt together, after this take up some of the Mixture with an Iron, to see whether it is too hard and brittle, if so, then add a little more Tin, and when you have the right Temper, fling four Ounces of Borax over it, and let it stand in the Furnace till it is dissolv'd; then pour it into your Mould and let it cool, when it is cold, rub it first with Brimstone, and then with Emery, and after the Surface is made smooth and even, polish it with *Tripoli* or Tin Ashes, and give it the finishing Stroke with Lampblack.

Another.

TAKE Copper one part, Pewter three parts, and a very little Arsenick or Tartar These put together in Fusion, and let them incorporate

Some take of the Copper three parts, of Pewter one part, and a little Silver, Antimony, and white Flint.

Others do it with one part of Lead, and two parts of Silver

After the Metal is form'd and cast, it is requisite to have it smooth and well polish'd: The first is done with Emery, then with Powder of Brimstone or Tin Ashes, or else with *Tripoli*. The Polishing is done with pulverised Chimney Soot (of Wood Fires) and the Ashes of Willow or Cedar,

I   which

which will give it a fine Luftre. The Emery is ground to a fine Duft, and moiften'd with Water.

Another.

STEEL Mirrors are alfo made out of one pound of Pewter, and one third of Copper. When thefe are melted, put into it two Ounces of Tartar, and one Ounce of Orpiment, and when it is evaporated, pour it out into the Mould. The Cafting of a flat Mirror or Looking Glafs is done upon a flat Board, which muft be made dry and warm, and cover'd with Rofin or Pitch, by this means the Mirror is fix'd to the Board: When cold, rub it off with Sand and Water, then with Emery or Flower of Brimftone, and at laft polifh it with Tin-Afhes

Another Sort of a Steel Mixture.

TAKE good New Copper, of that Sort which is ufed for Copper Wire, eight parts, fine *Englifh* Pewter, one part; Bifmuth five Parts; put it together in a Crucible and melt it   Then greafe your Mould all over with Tallow, in order to caft your Metal in it, when it is in Fufion, dip a hot Iron into it, what fticks to it, let cool   If the Colour is inclining to white, it is right; but if to red, you muft add fome more Pewter, till it has its right Colour. Obferve, that whatever you put to the melted Metal, muft firft be made hot.   After this Manner you may form and caft whatever you pleafe

Another

MELT one pound of Copper, fling into it eight Ounces of *Spalter,* and ftir it, when the *Spalter* is in Flame with a Stick or Iron well together,   Then add five or fix Ounces of fine Pewter to it, pour it into your Moulds fmooth, and polifh it as you have been directed before, and you will have a fine and bright Mirror.

Peter Shot's *Metallic Mixture for Mirrors*

TAKE ten parts of Copper, melt it, and add fou parts of fine Pewter, ftrew upon it a fmall Quantity

c

of pulverifed Antimony and Sal Armoniac; ftir it well together, till the ftinking Smoak is evaporated · Then pour it out in the Moulds, and firft fmooth it with Sand and Water, and then proceed as has been directed

Thefe Mixtures for Mirrors are made different Ways, the Copper is the chief Ingredient, which muft be tempered with a whitifh Metal, in order to bring the Objects that are feen therein, to their natural Colour, and this is done by Pewter and Arfenick.

To caft a flat Looking Glafs, it will be beft to have two flat polifh'd Stones for a Mould, between thefe two Stones put on each End an Iron Wire, as thick as you would caft your Mirror, then tie or fcrew them clofe, and fill the Openings round about with Putty, leaving only an Opening to pour the Metal in. When that is dry and made thorough warm, pour the Metal in; and when 'tis cold, fmooth and polifh it as directed before. You may faften the one Side to a flat Stone with Plafter of Paris, and polifh the other with a fmooth Stone, and laft of all, give it the finifhing Stroke with a Piece of old Hat, and fine Tin Afhes.

If you will cafte a Concave Mirror, or Burning Glafs, have your Mould turn'd to Perfection, but if you cannot get it conveniently done, you may take a round Ball or Bowl, and proceed thus

Make a Cruft of Wax, roll it with a Roller to what Thicknefs you would have your Metal caft, and to make it of an Equality, you may fix a couple of Rules on each Side for your Roller to play upon. Then cut this Cruft of Wax into a round Circle, and form it clofe to your Bowl, and fet it in a cool Place to harden. In the mean Time prepare a fine Clay, by wafhing and pouring it out of one Pan into another, take the fineft of the Settling, and get it burnt in a Potter's Furnace to a reddifh Colour. When this is done, grind it with Sal Armoniac Sublimate and Rain Water, upon a Marmor Stone, very fine, and to fuch a Confiftence, that it may be laid on with a Pencil like Painter's Colour: With this paint the one Side of the Wax Mould over, and let it dry in a Shadow, when dry, lay on a ftrong Coat of hair'd Clay, of about two Finger's thick, and let this alfo dry in the Shadow. Then lay the Concave Side uppermoft, and do as before. Firft, with a foft hair'd Pencil paint the prepared

I 2 and

and burnt Clay all over, and when dry, lay it over with hair'd Clay, so as to cover the whole Mould of Wax; the Place where you design to cast your Metal, you may open after it is dry. Then fix the Mould, with the Hole downwards, upon a couple of Iron Bars, or a couple of Bricks, making a Charcoal Fire underneath and round the Sides of it, that the Wax may melt and run out at the Hole · you may catch some of the Wax, and set it by for another Use When thus the Mould is clear'd of the Wax, and is still hot, turn it up and put warm Sand round about it to the Top, to keep it firm, then put an Earthen-Ware Funnel into the Hole, and pour in the Metal, as soon as you begin to pour, fling into the Metal a little Rag dipp'd in Wax, and whilst it is in Flame, pour it out into your Mould: After the Metal in the Mould is cold, polish it carefully, so as to take no more off in one Place than in another, which, if you do, will prove a Detriment to the Mirror

The Polishing is best done after the Brasiers Manner, *viz.* with a Wheel, to which is fix'd a rough Sand Stone, to take off the coarse Crust, then, with a fine Stone and Water, bring it smooth, and with a wooden Wheel, cover'd with Leather, and laid on with Emery, polish it from all the Streaks or Spots, giving it a finishing Stroke with fine Tin-Ashes and Blood Stone, which you lay on to your Wheel, that is covered with Leather. continue this so long till it has a perfect Gloss. Keep it in as dry a Place as possible, to prevent its tarnishing, but if it should tarnish, you must polish it again with a Piece of Buck-Skin, dipp'd in fine wash'd Tin Ashes. After this same Manner you may also polish the Concave Side of the Mirror.

An uncommon Art of preparing a Mirror Mixture on Brass.

TAKE strong still'd white Wine Vinegar, one pound, fine Sal Armoniac, four Ounces, Quickfilver, four Ounces: Let this boil upon a hot Sand, till the third part of the Vinegar is boil'd away; this Liquid is the principal Ingredient for the Work· Then take a Brass Plate, polish it very bright with some Coal Dust, lay it into an Iron Pan on a gentle Coal Fire, and when it is pretty hot, dip a Rag into this Liquor, and rub your Plate with it for an Hour together, this lays the Foundation for what follows

Make

Make a Paste with one part of Quickfilver, and two parts of Soap-Tin, in this dip your Rag, and rub it into the Plate of Brafs, fo long till you have a Looking Glafs Colour.

These Plates, thus prepared, lay fo long in the Iron Pan upon a Coal Fire, till you fee they begin to turn to a reddifh Colour, which it will do in about a Minutes Time, with this Colour the Mercury flies away, and the Tin Colour remains on the Plate, then let it cool, and take a little prepared Emery upon a piece of Leather, and rub the Plate over with even Strokes, but not too long, for fear of rubbing with the Emery the Tin from the Brafs. You may inftead of Emery polifh it alfo with *Tripoli*.

N. B. If the Tin fhould make the Plate too white, you may ufe Lead inftead thereof, making a Pafte with that and Mercury, and proceed as above

By this Means you may make what Figures you pleafe, and cut them in what Shape you will; you may alfo ufe it for many other curious Experiments

To Caft *Iron*.

TAKE clean Filings of Iron, wafh them in Lee, and then in Water, mix them with as much Powder of Sulpher, put it into a Crucible, and give it a ftrong Fire, till it is in Fufion If you manage it right, it will caft clean and fmooth.

To Caft *Steel*

TAKE of the beft and fineft Steel, about one Pound, break it in Bits, put it in a good ftrong Crucible, and neal it to a bright red Colour. Then add 16 or 24 Ounces of good common Steel, and neal it thoroughly Add then 8 or 10 Ounces of * *Arfenic Glafs*, give it a violent Fire, and it will melt and fluviate, with which you may caft what you pleafe.

To

---

* *To Prepare the Arfenick* Take one Pound of white Arfenick, two Pound of good and clear Salt petre; put it in a new Pot, that is not glaz d, with a Cover that has a little round Hole in the middle, lute it well all round, then let it dry, and when dry, put the Pot in a Reverberatory Fire for three Hours, and there evaporates out of the Hole of the Cover a red

vene-

To Caſt Iron as white as Silver.

TAKE Tartar, Salt-petre, Arſenick, and clear Steel Filings, of each an equal Quantity; put it together into a Crucible, on a Charcoal Fire, when in Fuſion, pour it out into an Ingot, and you will have out of one Pound of Steel Filings about two or three Ounces of a white bright Maſs; clear the Top of the Droſs, and preſerve the Maſs for Uſe.

Another Method.

TAKE Tartar, Oil, and a little fix'd Salt-petre, and mix this into a Paſte; then put Iron or Steel Filings into a Crucible, ſet it in a Charcoal Fire, fling the Mixture upon it, and it will diſſolve and come out like Silver, but it is brittle, and apt to break

Another.

TAKE calcin'd Tartar, and mix it with Oil, of this take two Ounces, Steel-filings ſix Ounces, put it together into a luted Crucible, and ſet it in a Wind Furnace, ſo long, till you think it is melted. Then open the Crucible, and make a fierce Fire, till you ſee it riſe · Take it then off the Fire, clear it from the Droſs, and caſt it into an Ingot of what Shape you pleaſe, and it will be of a white Colour

---

venemous Fume, which you muſt take Care of, and keep at ſome Diſtance from it   The ſecond Hour, move the Fire nearer the Pot, and when the Fumes ceaſe, cloſe the Hole with ſome Clay At the third Hour put the Coals cloſe to the Pot, and give it a thorough Heat, then let it cool of itſelf, and at the opening of the Pot you will find a white, ſometimes a greeniſh white Stone, which put up in a dry warm Place, free from the Air, to prevent its melting Of this you take five Ounces, and of Borax three Ounces, grind it well together, and let it melt in a large Crucible till it is like Water, pour this in a refining Cup, and you will have a fine tranſparent Matter What is not uſed, you may preſerve from the Air, to keep it from diſſolving into Water.

How to Caſt Pictures with Iſing-glaſs, on Copper-Plates.

TAKE fine white Iſinglaſs, as much as you pleaſe, cut it fine, and put it into a Glaſs or Cup, pour on it ſo much Brandy as will juſt cover the Iſinglaſs, cloſe it well, and let it ſoak all Night; then pour ſome clear Water to it, and boil it on a gentle Coal Fire, ſo long, till when you put a Drop of it on a Knife, it is like a clear cryſtalline Jelly, ſtrain it then through a Cloth, and put it into a cool Place, where it will turn to a Jelly and be ready for Uſe

When you are about caſting a Picture, cut ſo much of the Jelly as you think you have Occaſion to cover the Copper Plate; diſſolve it in a clean Pipkin, or ſuch like Utenſil, over a ſlow coal Fire, and mix any of the hereafter mentioned Colours among it· Mean while your Copper Plate muſt be clean, to rub the Muſhel Gold or Silver into the Graving with a Hair Pencil, then wipe the Plate carefully with clean Hands, as the Plate Printers do, and when this is done, pour your diſſolved Iſinglaſs over it, but not too hot, ſpreading it with a fine Pencil very even every where, till your Copper Plate is covered: Set it then in a moderate warm Place to dry, and when you perceive it thorough dry, then, with the Help of a thin Blade of a Knife, you may lift it up from the Plate: If you find the Matter too thin, add more Iſinglaſs to it; but if too thick, add a little more Water

Of the Colours fit to be mix'd with the Iſinglaſs, for Caſting of Pictures

1. FOR red, mix with it ſome of the Liquid in which you have boil'd Scarlet Rags
2 For Blue, take Litmus diſſolv'd in fair Water.
3 For Green, take diſtill'd Verdegreaſe, grind it as fine as poſſible, and mix it with the above Matter
4. For Yellow, ſteep Saffron in fair Water.
5 A Gold Colour is made with the above Red and Saffron Yellow
6 Gold, Silver, or Copper, well ground, as is uſed for Painting, mix'd with the Matter, and pour'd quickly over the Plate If you firſt rub Printers Black in the Graving, the Gold and Silver will look the better

To Caft Plaifter of Paris on Copper-Plates.

FIRST rub the Colour, either Red, Brown or Black, into the Graving, and wipe the Plate clean, then mix as much Plaifter as you think you fhall have Occafion for, with frefh Water, to the Subftance of a thin Pafte, and having put a Border round the Plate of four fquare pieces of Reglets, pour the Plaifter upon, and move it fo as to flow even all over the Plate Let it ftand for an Hour, or longer, according to the Dimenfion of the Plate, and when you find it dry, and turn'd hard, take off the Riglets, and then the Plafter, and you will have a fine Impreffion of the Copper Graving You muft obferve, not to mix more at a time than you have Occafion for, for elfe it will grow hard before you can ufe it.

A Mixture which may be ufed for to make Impreffions of any Kind, and which will grow as hard as Stone.

TAKE clear and fine fifted Afhes, and fine Plaifter of Paris, of one as much as the other, and temper it with Gum-Water, or with Size of Parchment, knead it well together, and prefs it down into your Mould, but do not prepare more than what you ufe prefently, elfe it will harden under your Hands. You may give it what Colour you pleafe; in mixing it for Black, take Lamp Black; for Red, Vermillion; for White, Flake-White, for Green, Verdegreafe; for Yellow, Dutch-Pinck, &c

You may inftead of Gum or Size, ufe the White of Eggs, which is more binding

To Imprefs Figures in Imitation of Porcelain.

CALCINED and fine pulveriz'd Egg-Shells, work'd with Gum Arabick and the White of Eggs into a Dough, then prefs'd into a Mould, and dry'd in the Sun, will come out fharp, and look fine.

PART

PART V.

A Collection of very valuable Secrets, for the Use of Sᴍɪᴛʜs, Cᴜᴛʟᴇʀs, Pᴇᴡᴛᴇʀᴇʀs, Bʀᴀsɪᴇʀs, Bᴏᴏᴋ-Bɪɴᴅᴇʀs, Jᴏɪɴᴇʀs, Tᴜʀɴᴇʀs, Jᴀᴘᴀɴɴᴇʀs, &c.

I.

Choice Experiments in Iʀᴏɴ and Sᴛᴇᴇʟ.

To make Steel out of Iron.

TAKE fmall Iron Bars of the fineft Sort, powdered Willows or Beech-Coals, the Shavings of Horn, and Soot out of a Baker's Chimney; ftratify this in an earthen Pan, made for that Purpofe, with a Cover to it First make a Lay of the Mixture, about an Inch thick; then a Lay of Iron Bars, then again the Mixture, and fo proceed, till the Pan is full, the Top muft be of the Mixture then put the Cover upon it, lute it, and put it in a Wind-Furnace for 24 Hours, and give it a reverberatory Fire

To harden Sword Blades

SWORD Blades are to be tough, fo as not to fnap or break in pufhing againft any Thing refiftable, they muft alfo be of a keen Edge, wherefore they muft along the Middle be hardened with Oil and Butter, to make them tough, and the Edges with fuch Things as fhall be prefcrib'd hereafter, for hardening edged Inftruments This Work requires not a little Care in the Practife thereof

How

How to imitate the Damascan Blades.

THIS may be done to such a Perfection as not to distinguish them from the real Damascan Blades   First polish your Blade in the best Manner, and finish the same by rubbing it with Flower of Chalk, then take Chalk mixt with Water, and rub it with your Fingers well together in your Hand, with this touch the polish'd Plate, and make such Spots upon as please your self, and set it to dry before the Sun, or a Fire, then take Water in which Tartar has been dissolv'd, and wipe your Blade all over therewith, and those Places that are left clear from Chalk, will change to a black Colour, a little while after wash all off with clear Water, and the Places where the Chalk has been, will be bright, your Watering will be the more perfect, as you imitate it in laying on your Chalk.

How the Damascan Blades are hardened.

THE *Turks* take fresh Goat's Blood, and after they have made their Blades red hot, they quench them therein, this they repeat nine times running, which makes their Blades so hard as to cut Iron.

To perfume a Sword Blade, so as to retain always an odoriferous Scent.

TAKE eight Grains of Ambergrease, six Grains of the best Bisem, four Grains of right Cibeth, grind this together with a little Sugar-Candy, in a Glass or Agat Mortar, after this add to it four Scruples of the best Benjamin Oil, and mix it well together; then hold the Sword Blade over a gentle, clear Coal Fire, and when the Blade is well heated, dip a little Spunge in the forementioned Mixture, and wipe your Blade all over; this you do only once, and the odoriferous Scent will remain, although the Blade was to be polish'd again

A Steel and Iron Hardening, which will withstand and cut common Iron.

TAKE Shoe-Leather, and burn it to Powder, the older the Leather is, the better it is for Use, Salt, which is dissolv'd, and Glass-Gall powder'd, of one as much as the other

Then

Then take what you will harden, and wet it with, or lay it in Urin, and taking it out, ftrew it over with this Powder, or elfe ftratify it therewith in an earthen Pan, give it for five Hours a flow Fire to cement, and make it afterwards red Hot for an Hour together.

Several other Temperaments for Steel and Iron.

I.

IRON quench'd in diftill'd Vinegar, or in diftill'd Urin, makes a good Hardening

2

Vinegar in which Sal-armoniac has been diffolv'd, gives a good Hardening.

3.

So doth the Water in which Urin, Salt, and Saltpetre has been diffolv'd

4

Caput Mortis of Aqua Fortis, boil'd for an Hour in Water, and filter'd through a clean Cloath, makes a tough Hardnefs.

5.

Saltpetre and Sal-armoniac, of one as much as the other; mix it together, and put it into a Viol with a long Neck, then fet it in a damp Place, or Horfe-Dung, where it will turn to an oily Water, this Liquid will make Iron Work of an incomparable Temper and Hardnefs, if quench'd therein, when it is red hot.

6

A Lee made of Quick-Lime and Salt of Soda, or of Pot-Afhes (filtered through a Linnen Cloath) gives a very good Hardnefs to Iron, if quenched therein.

7. Dung

7

Dung of a Creature which eats nothing but Grass, tempered with Water and calcined Soap, and mix'd to a thin Paste, gives a good hardening to Iron, so that it will cut the same Metal that's not harden'd.

8.

Or, take Spanish Reddishes, grate them on a Gridiron, and press the Juice out of it, which gives a good Hardening when Iron or Steel is quench'd therein.

9

Take the Juice of Nettles, fresh Urin of a Boy, Ox Gall, Salt, and strong Vinegar, of one as much as the other, it gives an incomparable Hardening.

10

Red hot Iron or Steel, wip'd over with Goose-grease, and then quench'd in sour Beer, takes likewise a good Hardness.

A particular Secret to harden Arms.

MAKE a Mixture of the following Things, of each an equal Quantity. Take common Salt, Orpiment, burn'd Goats Horn, and Sal Armoniack, powder it, and mix it together, then anoint the Arms with black Soap all over, strew this Powder upon it, and wind a wet Rag about it, lay it in a fierce Charcoal Fire, and let it be thorough red hot, then quench it in Urin. If you repeat it, it will be the better.

To Temper Steel or Iron, so as to make excellent Knives thereof

TAKE clean Steel, quench it in five or six times still'd Rain or Worm-Water, and the Juice of Spanish Reddishes; the Knives made of such Steel will cut Iron

Take black or Spanish Reddishes, grate them on a Gridiron, Put Salt and Oil upon them, and let them stand two Days Then press the liquor out, and quench the Steel or Iron several times, and it will be very hard

To bring Gravers and other Tools to their proper hardness.

TAKE a little Fire Pan with live Coals, and put a couple of old Files, or any other small Bars of Iron over them, then lay your Gravers upon them over a gentle clear Charcoal Fire, and when you see them change to a yellowish Colour, it is a Sign that they are softer, after this Colour they change to a reddish, which shews them still softer, and if you let them turn to a blue, then they are quite soft and unfit for Use. After this Manner you may soften any Steel that's too hard.

General Rules to be observed in Tempering of Iron or Steel.

WE know by Experience, that the hardening of Iron is perform'd and executed several Ways, for every Operation requires a particular Method of hardening. The Tools that are used for Wood, require a different Temper or Hardness from those used in cutting of Stones or Iron, and therefore are prepared in the several Methods treated of before. An Artist ought therefore to acquaint himself by Practice of the Nature and Quality of the different Ingredients and Liquids that are here prescrib'd, and improve upon such as seem most agreeable: He is to observe the Degrees of Heat, which he is to give, and the length of Time he is to keep the Metal in the Liquid for quenching, for in Case the Iron is made so excessive hot, that it is not capable of receiving any more Heat, it cannot well be quenched, and will all be canker'd; but if it appears of a Saffron or reddish Colour, it is call'd Gold, and is fit to be quench'd for Hardening However, in this as well as most other Things, Practice is the best Teacher.

A Curiosity to hammer Iron without Fire, and make it red hot

TAKE a round Iron, about an Inch thick; at one End thereof fix a round Iron Nob, then begin gently to hammer it under the Nob, turning it quickly round, and by following your Strokes harder and harder, the Iron will heat of itself, and begin to be red hot, the Reason is, because the Nob remains untouch'd, and the heat on each of the Motions cannot dissipate

To

To soften Iron or Steel that's brittle.

1

ANOINT it with Tallow all over, neal it in a gentle Charcoal Fire, and let it cool of itself.

2

To neal it thus with human Excrement, softens it; but you must keep it in the Fire for two Hours.

3.

Or, take a little Clay, Lime, and Cows Dung, cover your Iron therewith, and neal it in a Charcoal Fire Then let it cool of itself

4.

Or, make Iron or Steel red hot, and strew upon it good Hellebore, and it will become so soft that you may bend it which way you please. This is very useful for those who cut in Iron or Steel

5.

Take Lead, put it into a Crucible, or Iron Ladle, and melt and pour it into Oil, this repeat seven times running. If you afterwards quench Iron or Steel in this Oil, it will be very soft, and after you have shap'd or work'd it in what you design'd it, you may harden it again by quenching it in the Juice of Onions

6.

Take Lime, Brick-Dust, and Venice Soap; with this anoint your Steel and neal it; then let it cool of itself.

7.

Take the Root of blue Lillies, cut it fine, infuse it in Wine, and quench the Steel in it,

8. Wind

8

Wind about the Steel some thin Slices of Bacon, and over that put Clay, let it neal for an Hour, and the Steel will be very soft

9

Take Quick-Lime and pulverized Soap, of one as much as the other, mix it together, and temper it with Ox's Blood; with this anoint the Steel, then lay a covering of Clay over it, and let it neal and cool of it self

10.

Take the Juice or Water of common Beans, quench your Iron or Steel in it, and it will be as soft as Lead

A particular Powder and Oil, to take off the Rust and Spots of Iron, and to preserve it from Rust for a long Time, very useful in Armories.

TAKE 32 Ounces Crucible Powder, of such as is commonly used for refining of Silver, and sift it through a fine Hair Sieve. Then take 64 Ounces of Emory, and one pound of Silver Oar, pound it all very fine, and sift it, put at last fine beaten Scales of Iron to it, and the Powder is ready.

To prepare the Oil for it.

TAKE three pound of *Lucca* Oil, and put it into a Copper Bason or Pot, then take three pound of Lead, melted, and pour it into the Oil, take it out, and melt it again, and repeat melting and pouring several times, the more, the better the Oil will be. After you have done this, and the Heat of the Lead has extracted both the Greasiness and Salt of the Oil, take the Lead out, and put the Oil into a Glass, fling three pound of Filings of Lead into it, shake it well together, pour it afterwards on a Colour Stone, grind it together as Painters do their Colours, put it again into the Glass, to preserve it for Use. The Lead will sink to the Bottom, and the Oil swim a top, which you may use in the following Manner

Take

Take some of it in a bit of Cloath, on which there is some of the before mentioned Powder, and rub the Moles or Spots upon Armour or any other Iron Work therewith, and it will take them clean off; and if afterwards you anoint the Arms or Iron Work with the clear Oil, it will keep it from Rust for a long Time

N. B The Emory which is used among the other Ingredients of the Powder, must be first calcined, which you do thus. Lay it on a Coal Fire, and when you see it of a red Colour, take it out and beat it in a Mortar, and it is fit to be mixt in the Rust-Powder.

Another Method.

FRY a middling Eel in an Iron Pan, and when brown and thoroughly fry'd, press the Oil thereof out, and put it into a Phial, to settle and become clear, in the Sun Iron Work, anointed with this Oil, will never rust, although it lay in a damp Place

To etch upon IRON-BLADES, either in ARMORY, or SWORD and KNIFE-BLADES.

To prepare the Etch Water

TAKE Mercury and Aqua-Fortis, put it together into a Glass, till the Mercury is devoured, and it is fit for Use.

To make the Ground

TAKE three Ounces Red Lead, one Ounce White Lead, half an Ounce of Chalk, all finely pounded, grind this together with Varnish, and anoint your Iron therewith, let it dry in the Sun, or before a slow Fire, and with a pointed Steel or Needle draw or write in it what you please, and then etch it with the above prepared Water.

Another

Another Water to etch with

TAKE two ounces of Verdegreafe, one ounce of burn'd Alum, and one ounce of Salt, which is diffolv'd, boil this in one Quart of Vinegar, till it is half boil'd away, and when you are ready to etch, warm it, and pour it with a Spoon or Glafs Cup over your Work, hold it over the Fire to keep it warm, and repeat this till you find it etch'd deep enough

To etch 100 *or more Knife Blades at once.*

GRIND Red Lead with Linfeed Oil or Varnifh, with this wipe your Blades all over, and let it well dry and harden, then write or draw with a pointed Bodkin whatever you will, then put them at fome Diftance from each other, into a Glafs or well glaz'd Pot or Pan, diffolve fome Vitriol in hot Water, pour it over the Blades, and lute the Glafs or Pot, fet it over a gentle Coal Fire, let it boil for fome time, and then cool, then take your Blades out, fcrape the Red Lead off, and you will find the Etching to your Satisfaction

To make blue Letters on Scimeters or Sword-Blades.

TAKE the Blade, hold it over a Charcoal Fire till it is blue, then, with Oil Colours write what Letters you will upon the Blade, and let it dry, when dry, take good ftrong Vinegar, make it warm, and pour it all over the Blade, which will take off the blue Colour, then wet your Oil Colour with frefh Water, and it will come off eafily, and the Letters drawn therewith, remain blue.

To harden Fifhing Hooks

AFTER you have (out of good Wire) made your fmall fifhing Hooks, you muft not put them into the Fire to harden, but lay them upon a red hot Iron Plate, and when they are turn'd red, fling them into Water, take them out again, and when dry, put them again on the hot Iron Plate, and when they appear of an Afh-Colour, fling them again in cold Water, this will make them tough, otherwife they will be brittle

K

To gild upon Iron or Steel.

TAKE common Salt, Saltpetre and Alum, of one as
much as the other, diffolve it in as little a Quantity of
warm Water as poffible, then filter it through a whited brown
Paper, put Leaf Gold, or rather thin beaten Gold to it, and
fet it in hot Sand, to make it almoft boiling hot, keep it in
that heat for 24 Hours, and if the Water evaporates, you may
fupply it with more, but at laft let it all evaporate, and it
will turn to a yellow Salt, this pulverize, put it into a Glafs,
and cover it with ftrong Brandy, or Spirit of Wine, two
Inches high above the Powder: Then ftop your Glafs clofe,
put it into a gentle Warmth, and the Brandy or Spirit will
extract all the Gold, and be of a beautiful Colour. With
this Water you may, with a new Pen or Pencil, write or draw
what you pleafe, upon a Sword-Blade, Knife, or any other
Thing made of Iron or Steel, and it will be gilded to a high
Colour.

A Ground for Gilding Steel or Iron.

TAKE five Ounces of Vitriol, two Ounces of Galiz-Stone,
two Ounces of Sal Armoniac, one Ounce of Feather
White, and a Handful of common Salt; beat all this together
till it is fine, and mix it well, put it into a glaz'd Pipkin, add to
it a Quart of Water, and give it a quick boiling; then take a
Knife, or any other Iron that is clean, and ftir it about, if it
is of a Copper Colour, it is right, but if of a Red Colour, it
is better.

If you have a Mind to gild with this Ground, put your
Steel on a flow Fire, and make it fo hot that you can't bear
it on your Hand, then take your Ground, and dipping fome
Cotton into it, wipe the Steel with it; take afterwards Quick
filver, and wipe your Ground over, then take the prepared
Gold, and lay it on fuch Places as you would have gilded,
After you have done this, lay it on a Charcoal Fire, till it turn
yellow, then wipe it over with Tallow, and take Cotton to wipe
your Blade, holding it all the while over the Fire, till it
inclines to a black, rub it with a woolen Cloath, till that
Colour vanifhes, and rub it again with Chalk, till you
bring it to a fine Glofs. If you will have the Ground
brown

brown or blue, hold it over the Fire, till it turns either to the one or the other Colour, then wipe it over with Wax, and polish it with Chalk

※ ※ ※ ※ ※ ※ ※ ※ ※ ※ ※ ※ ※ ※ ※ ※ ※ ※ ※ ※

II.
Of LEAD and PEWTER.

To make Pewter hard.

TAKE one Pound, or what Quantity you please, of Pewter, and let it melt in an Iron Pan, add to it some Salet Oil, let it well evaporate, and stir it continually, keeping the Flame from it; put to this some fine Wheat Flower, and stir it well about, then take all the burn'd Matter off the Top, and to each Pound of Tin add three or four Ounces of Plate Brass, cut in small Pieces, mix'd with Oil, and a few Ounces of pulveriz'd Bismouth, or Regul of Antimony; stir it all the while, and when all is melted and incorporated, you will not only have a Pewter that's harder and whiter, but also different in its Sound from common Pewter.

Another Method.

MELT Tin in an Iron Pan, strew Colophorni or Rosin, with fine Wheat Flower mix'd together, into it, and stir it gently about This takes off the Blackness, and makes it of a fine white Colour

If you will have it hard, add to each Pound of Tin one or two Ounces of pulveriz'd Regulus of Antimony and Veneris, this makes it white, hard, and of a clear Sound

Another Method to make Pewter as white as Silver.

TAKE clean Copper one Pound, and let it fluviate; add to it of the best English Pewter one Pound, and continue the Flux, to this add two Pound of Regulus Antimony and Martis, and let it still fluviate for Half an Hour, then cast it into an Ingot. Beat this in a Mortar to a fine Powder, and fling

thereof

thereof as much into the melted Tin as you think requisite
You will find (after you cast it) of a fine Silver Colour, it will
be hard, and give a fine Sound To make it fluviate the better,
you may add a little Bismuth.

Another Method.

MELT one Pound of Copper, add to it one Pound of
Tin, half a Pound of Zink, one Pound of *Reg.*
Antim and *Martis*, let it fluviate Half an Hour, and cast it
into an Ingot

N B. The *German* Author says, there are many more
Secrets relating to whitening and hardening of Pewter, but
thinks it not proper to divulge them, and adds, that he has
found by Experience, that the *Reg Antim.* and *Veneris* is
better for that Use, than the *Reg Antim* and *Martis*; because
the last will turn the Pewter in time to a dirty Blue, whereas
the former will make it continue white, hard, and of a good
Sound

To make Tin or Lead Ashes.

TAKE which Sort of these Metals you will, let it melt,
and fling well dry'd and beaten Salt into it, stir it well
together with an Iron Ladle or Spatula, till it separates, and
forms itself into a Powder.

Or,

AFTER the Tin or Lead is melted, pour it into fine dry
Salt, stir it together till it is fit for sifting Then put
this Powder into a Pan of clean Water, and stir it, pour off
the first Water, and put fresh to it, repeat this so often till the
Water comes off clear, and without the Taste of any Salt The
remaining Powder put into a melting Pot, set it in a rever
beratory Furnace, stir it well together, and you will have
fine white Tin-Ashes.

A Water to Tin all Sorts of Metals, but especially Iron

TAKE one Ounce of fine pounded Sal Armoniac, and put
it into very sour Vinegar, and when you will tin Iron,
wash it first with this Vinegar, and strew beaten Rosin over
it,

it; dip it into the melted Tin, and it will come out with a fine and bright Luftre

A Gold Colour upon Lead or Tin.

TAKE Saffron, as much as you will, and put it into ftrong Gum-Water, add to it a third Part of Vinegar, and let it foak over Night, then mix it with a little cla-ified Honey, ftir it well together, and let it boil till it comes to the Subftance of Honey, ftrain it afterwards through a Cloath, and it is ready for Ufe

Another

TAKE Linfeed Oil, which is fkimm'd over the Fire, and put Amber and Aloepatica in, of one as much as the other, fet it over a Fire, and ftir it till it is thick, then cover it all over with Earth for three Days If you anoint your Tin or Pewter therewith, it will have a fine Gold Colour

To make Tin which has the Weight, Hardnefs, Sound, and Colour of Silver

TAKE fine long Cryftal Antimony, beat it fine, and wafh it in Water till it becomes fleek, and let it dry again. Then take well dry'd Salt-petre and Tartar, of each an equal Quantity, beat it fine, and put it together into an earthen Pan, on which lay fome live Charcoal, and the Salt-petre and Tartar will foon begin to fulminate Then cover the Pan with a Lid, let the Matter burn out and cool, and you will find a yellow Salt. This Salt beat to Powder before it is quite cold, and put thereof into a Crucible one Pound, and of the wafh'd Antimony two Pound Mix it well together, and let it fluviate in a Wind Furnace for three quarters of an Hour. Then fling a few lighted Smalcoals in it, let them confume, and ftir it with a Stick well together Prefently after take the Crucible out of the Fire, beat it a little down to the Bottom, and let it cool of itfelf; then break the Crucible, and you will find a Silver colour'd Regulus, of three quarters of a Pound Weight

Take then two Pound of old Copper, cut it fine, neal it, and quench it, ten times running, in very ftrong Lee, made of the above Tartar and Rain Water. Take

it,

it, while wet, and put it into a Crucible, with one Pound of fine beaten Arſenick, *ſtratum ſuper ſtratum* When all is in the Crucible, pour as much Lindſeed Oil on it as will cover the Matter, then cover and lute your Crucible, put it into a new Pan, fill it all round with Sand, and ſet it three Hours in a Circle Fire. After it is cold, open it, and you will find the Copper to be ſpungy and of ſeveral Colours Of this take two Pound, and Plate Braſs two Pound, melt theſe together, add by degrees the Copper, and give it a quick Fuſion in a Wind Furnace. Then add two Pound of *Engliſh* Pewter, half a Pound of Biſmuth, and two Pound of the above Regulus, let it well fluviate, then pour it out, and you will have a fine Silver Mixture. This beat into a fine Powder, mix it with Lindſeed Oil to a Paſte, and with a Spatula add it to the melted Pewter Stir it well together, and you will have a fine Tin, which will reſemble the Silver in every Thing, except the Teſt.

To make Tin flow eaſy

TAKE Roſin and Salt-petre, of each an equal Quantity, beat it to Powder, and ſtrew it upon the Tin when it is in Fuſion.

A particular Method to make Tin reſemble Silver

MELT four ounces of fine Plate Braſs, add to it four ounces of fine clean Tin, and when it is in Fuſion, add four ounces of Biſmouth, and four ounces *Reg Antim* let this fluxuate together, and pour it out to an Ingot, then beat it to Powder, grind it with Roſin and a little Sal Armoniac, and with Turpentine form it into Balls; let them dry in the Air, and when you will uſe them, beat them fine, ſtrew the Powder thereof upon the melted Tin, ſtir it well together, and continue putting the powder d Balls upon the Tin, till you perceive it white and hard enough. Of this Tin you may draw Wire for Hilts of Swords, or make Buttons, it will always keep its Silver Colour

A Solder to Solder Tin with.

TAKE Tin and Lead, of each one Ounce, Biſmouth two Ounces, this melt, and pour it over a Plate to caſt it thin With this you may ſolder over a Candle or a ſmall Charcoal Fire.

Another

Another Solder for Pewter.

TAKE Rosin and Oil, let it melt in a Spoon, and fling into it a little Devil's Dung, then pour it out, and having new fil'd the two broken Pieces, anoint them with the Rosin, dust some fine fil'd Tin over it, and hold it over a Coal Fire, and when it flows, take it off and let it cool.

To make Tin Coat-Buttons, in Imitation of Work'd Buttons of Gold and Silk.

TAKE Lampblack, grind it with Oil of Spike, and mark the ground Work with a Pencil, when dry, draw it all over with the Varnish before describ'd The best Way to imitate worked Buttons is, to do them in a fine Mould, either stamp'd or cast, the Ground being first fill'd up with Black, Blue, Red or any other Colour, then the raised part wip'd very clean, and when dry, drawn over with the Varnish, which will make it look much finer than what can be done upon a plain Button

For a Brown Colour, take *Umber.*

For Green, take still'd Verdigrease, mix'd with other Colours, to make it deeper or lighter

For Gray, take white Lead and Lampblack

All your Colours must be ground with Oil of Spike

In this manner you may embellish some Pewter with a Coat of Arms, a Cypher, or Ornaments, I mean such Pewter Things that are not scour'd.

To gild upon Tin, Pewter, or Lead.

TAKE Varnish of Linseed Oil, Red Lead, White Lead, and Turpentine, put it together in a clean Pipkin, and let it boil, then grind it upon a Stone, and when you will gild Pewter, take a Pencil, draw the Liquid thin upon what you will gild, and lay your Leaf Gold upon it, or instead of that, Augsburg Metal, and press it with Cotton, to lie close.

Another Method to gild Pewter or Lead.

TAKE the White of an Egg, and beat it clear, with this wipe your Tin or Pewter, which must be first warm'd before a gentle

Fire

Fire, in such Places as you design to gild, lay on your Leaf Gold quick, and press it down with Cotton

The Juice of Nettles is also fit for that Use, and rather better than the Egg clear

Another Method to gild Pewter

TAKE Leaves of Staniol, and grind them with common Gold Size, with this wipe your Pewter or Lead over, lay on your Leaf Gold, and press it with Cotton: It is a fine Gilding, and has a beautiful Lustre.

A Method to gild with Pewter, or Lead Leaves.

THIS may be done several ways, but the best is, to take White Lead, ground with Nut-Oil, with this lay your Ground on what you design to gild, let it be Wood or any Thing else, then lay on your gilded Tin Leaves, press them down with Cotton, or a fine Rag, and let it dry, when dry, polish it with a Horse's Tooth or Polisher, and it will look as if it had been gilded in Fire

To gild Lead

TAKE two Pound of Yellow Oaker, half a Pound of Red Lead, and one Ounce of Varnish, with which grind your Oaker, but the Red Lead grind with Oil, and temper them both together, lay your Ground with this upon the Lead, and when it is almost dry, lay on your Gold, let it be thorough dry, then polish it.

III.

Some Experiments relating to COPPER and BRASS.

To melt Copper and Brass, and give it a quick Fusion

TAKE Saltpetre, Tartar, and Salt, beat it together very fine, when you see that your Metal begins to tink with the Heat, fling a little of this Powder into it, and when melted, fling again a little into it, and

after

after you fee it in Fufion, like Water, fling a little again, the third time To 25 pound of Metal fling about a Walnut full of Powder, and your Copper or Brafs will caft eafy, and be of a malleable Temper.

To make Brafs malleable that's Brittle, and apt to rent in the working of it

TAKE Tartar, Saltpetre, and Sulphur, pulverife it together, and after you have made your Brafs red hot, ftrew it all over it, and let it cool of it felf

A Solder for Brafs.

TAKE one Grain and a quarter of Silver, three Ounces of Brafs, one Ounce of Zink, and melt it together, when melted, fling a good quantity of *Venice* Borax upon it.

To make Copper as white as Silver

PUT your Copper in a ftrong melting Pot, in the midft of a Quantity of Glafs, and fet it in a Glafs Furnace to melt, let the Copper be all over cover'd with Glafs, and the Glafs will contract the Greennefs of the Copper, and make it look white. If you repeat this feveral times, your Copper will be the whiter.

Another Way

TAKE old Copper, that has been much ufed, or been long in the open Air and Weather, melt it in a ftrong Crucible before a Smith's Forge, or in a Wind Furnace, but take Care of the Smoak, let it melt a Quarter of an Hour, or longer, and clear it from the Scales that fwim a-top Then pour it through a Wifk or Birtch Broom into a fharp Lee, made either of Quick-Lime and Wine-Branch-Afhes, or of Salt of Tartar, or *Caput Mortis* of diftill'd Spirit of *Nitre*, or fuch like, and the Copper will corn fine and nice. Then take it out of the Lee, and let it melt again as before · Repeat this four Times running, in order to purify the Copper, and when the Copper is well purified, melt it over again; when it is in Fufion, fling two Ounces of Cryftalline Arfenick in, by little and little, but take Care of the Smoak, and

tie

tie a Handkerchief, moiſtened with Milk, about your Mouth and Noſe: After it has evaporated, or rather before it i quite done, fling into it two Ounces of Silver, and when that is melted, granulate it again through a Wiſk, and mel it again for Uſe. It will be fit to make any Thing in Imita tion of Silver.

Another.

TAKE white Arſenick half a Pound, Salt peter eight Ounces, Tartar eight Ounces, Borax four Ounces Glaſs-Gall four Ounces, pulverize each very fine, then mix and put them together in a Crucible, and let it fluviate i a Wind-Furnace for an Hour or more, then pour it out, and you will have a whitiſh yellow Subſtance

Then take one Part of old Copper, and one Part of old hammer'd Braſs, both cut in ſmall Pieces, neal theſe well and quench them in a Lee made of a Quart of Urine, an Handful of Salt, four Ounces of white powder'd Tartar, and two Ounces of Alum · Boil it up together, and repeat it 10 or 12 Times.

When thus you have cleanſed the Copper and Braſs, put it together in a Crucible, and give it a ſtrong Fire in a Wind Furnace, or before a Smith's Forge, let it well flu viate, and then fling of the above Compoſition (which muſt be pulveriſed) one Spatulo full after another into the Cru cible, ſtirring it ſometimes about with a Stick, to one Ounce of Copper you take an Ounce and half of Powder When all is infuſed and incorporated, then fling a few Pieces of broken Crown Glaſs into it, and let it melt, then draw it out again with a Pair of Tongs, and fling *Sal Armoniack* into it, of the Bigneſs of a Walnut, and when it is in thorough Fuſion, pour it out into a Caſting Pot, and your Copper will be of a fine White.

If you take of this Copper 24 Ounces, and melt one Ounce of Silver among it, letting it well fluviate with Sal Armoniac, you will have a fine Maſs, which may be work'd what Shape, or into any Utenſil you pleaſe, and it will hardly be diſtinguiſh'd from real Silver Plate

When the Silverſmith works this Compoſition, he muſt obſerve always, when melting, to fling ſome *Sal Armo niack* into it, to make it malleable And in hammering he muſt often neal it, and let it cool of it ſelf ; then hammer it gently, till it is as thin as he would have it , for if it is beat quick in the Beginning, it will be apt to crack

The more this Metal is neal'd and gently hammer'd, the better it will be When the Work is done, neal it , then rubbing it with Charcoal, and boiling it afterward, three times in a ſtrong Lee of Tartar, your Work will be like Silver.

IV.

Choice Secrets for Bᴏᴏᴋ-ʙɪɴᴅᴇʀꜱ.

To prepare a Lack Varniſh for Book binders, for French Bindings

FIRST, when the Book is cover'd, either with Calf or Sheep Skin, or with Parchment, it is ſtruck over with a Varniſh, and ſpotted with ſuch Colours as are taught under the Article of imitating Tortoiſes on Ivory or Horn Some will ſpot the Leather before they lay on the Varniſh, and after they have ſprinkled their Colour (which they commonly make of Umber) they lay the Varniſh over, and poliſh it with a Steel Poliſher, after which they give it one Lay of Varniſh more, which is the finiſhing Stroke

French Leather for Binding of Books.

MAKE Choice of ſuch Leather that's wrought ſmooth and fine, and ſtrain it on a Frame , then having your Colours ready at Hand, take firſt of one Sort in a Pencil made of Hogs Briſtles, and with your Finger ſprinkle the Colour out thereof upon the Leather, and when you have done with one, you may take another Colour, and proceed with as many Colours as you think proper . If you will imitate a Tyger's Skin, you dot your Colours upon the Leather with a Stick that's rough at the End, or a Pencil, and after it is well dry'd, you lay it over with a *Spaniſh* Varniſh, which you make in the following Manner   Take

Take a Pint of high rectified Spirit of Wine, of clear Gum *Sandarac* four Ounces, clear Oil of Spike one Ounce pound the *Sandarac*, and put it in the Spirit of Wine, and then into the Oil of Spike, let it stand till it is diffolv'd and fettled

To prepare Parchment that refembles Jafpis or Marmor.

HAVE a Trough, made in the Nature as will be directed under the Article of making Marbled Paper let it be fill'd with warm Water of Gum Tragant, and having your Colours ready prepar'd (as will be directed) ftir the Gum Water with a Stick, and bring it to a quick circular Motion In the Interim dip your Pencil with Colour in the Center thereof, the Colour will difperfe and form it felf in Rounds, as it is carried by the Motion of the Water Then ftir it round in another Place, and with a different Colour proceed as you did with the firft, till your Trough is covered with Varieties of Colours When all is ready, and the Water fmooth and without Motion, then lay on your Parchment (which before has been laid between damp Paper or Cloaths) and proceed therewith as you do with the marbled Paper, hang it up to dry, then fmooth and glaze it, in the Manner you do colour'd Parchment

A Green tranfparent Parchment

WASH the Parchment in cold Lee, fo long till it comes clear from it, then fqueeze out the Wet as much as poffible, and if you will have it of a fine green Colour, take ftill'd Verdigreafe, ground with Vinegar, and add a little Sap Green to it, temper it neither too thick nor too thin, then foak your Parchment with this Colour thoroughly, a whole Night, rinfe it afterwards in Water, ftrain it immediately on a Frame, and fet it to dry, then take clear Varnifh, lay it on both Sides; fet it in the Sun to dry, after this cut the Parchment out of the Frame into Leaves, as large as you pleafe, and lay them in a Book under a Prefs, to keep it fine and ftreight The Virtue of this Parchment is, that it magnifies a fmall Letter, when put over it, as big again, and is a great Preferver of the Eyes, to thofe who read much by Candle Light.

The

The Varnish must be prepared of Linseed Oil, and boiled in Frankincense, *Mastick* and *Sandarac*.

If you will have the Parchment of a clear, transparent, and white Colour, you only wash, strain, and varnish it, as above

If you will colour it yellow, steep your Parchment, after it has been wash'd, in a yellow Liquid, made of Saffron; for which purpose tie Saffron in a thin Linnen Rag, hang it in a weak Lee, and let it warm over a slow Fire, and when you see the Lee tinctur'd yellow, it is fit for Use.

For *transparent Red,*

TAKE Brasil, as much as you will, put it in a hot Lee, which is clear, and not too strong, and it will tincture the Lee of a fine red, then pour in about half an Egg-shell full of clear Wine, draw the Parchment through the Colour, and when it is as deep as you would have it, strain it, as before.

For *a Blue,*

TAKE *Lombard* Indigo, grind it with Vinegar on a Stone, and mix *Sal Armoniac* among it, to the Quantity of a Pea, with this wet your Parchment, and proceed as has been directed for the Green

For *a Violet or Purple*

TEMPER two thirds of the above red, and one third of the blue, and use it as before directed.

For *a Black Colour.*

TAKE Roman Alum, beat it to Powder, and boil it in Rain-Water, till a fourth Part is boil'd away, then add Roman Vitriol or Atrament, with some Roman Gall, and boil it together, with this stain your Parchment twice or three times over, and when dry, lay the *Spanish* Varnish over it.

N B. With these transparent Parchments you may make curious Bindings, one Sort, used at *Rome,* is made thus. Lay the Board or Paste-board over with Leaf Gold, Leaf Silver, Stagniol, Metal Leaves, &c. Then binding the Parchment over it, it will give it an uncommon Lustre and Beauty.

To

To make red Brafil Ink.

YOU muſt firſt obſerve, that when you boil Brafil for Ink, you ought to do it when the Weather is fair, and the Sky without Clouds or Wind, or elſe your Ink will not be ſo good

Take Quick-Lime, pour Rain-Water on it, and let it ſtand over Night   In the Morning pour the clear from off the Top, through a Cloath, and to a Quart of this Water take one Pound of Brafil Shavings, let them boil half away, and put to it two Ounces of Cherry Gum, one Ounce of Gum Arabick, and one Ounce of beaten Alum, then take it, when all is diſſolv'd, from the Fire, pour it off the ſhavings, and put it up for uſe, you may alſo add to it a little clear Chalk

To prepare Brafil Ink without Fire.

TAKE a new glaz'd Pipkin, in which put two handfuls of Brafil Shavings ; pour half a Pint of Vinegar on it, and let it ſtand over Night, then put to it half an Eggſhell full of Alum, with a little Gum , take alſo Chalk, ſcrap'd fine, about an Eggſhell full, or more, put it gently by little and little into the Pipkin, and ſtir it well together with a Stick, and it will begin to boil, as if it was upon the Fire You muſt ſet your Pipkin in a clean Earthen Diſh, before you put your Chalk in, for as ſoon as the Chalk is in, it will boil over, and you cannot hinder it   when this Ebullition is over, then put it again into the Pipkin, let it ſtand a Day and a Night, and you will have a fine Brafil Ink.

To prepare Brafil Ink in Sticks.

TAKE Brafil Shavings, or Chips, put them in a Pan, and proceed in every reſpect as directed in the foregoing After the Brafil is thus made fit for Writing, pour it into Shells, and ſet it in the Sun, where no duſt can come to it, to ſtand a full Hour : Then take other Shells, pour the Top of the Brafil out of the firſt Shells into them, and fling the ſettling away, ſet theſe Shells alſo in the Sun, and after they have ſtood an Hour, proceed as before , this do ſo long till it is quite purified, then boil it as dry as Wax,

put

put it up into a Nut-fhell, or in a piece of Parchment, and you may dilute it with a little Wine or fair Water, in a little Cup, as much as you have occafion for, and write or paint therewith, it is a fine Colour, and very fit for Colouring Maps or Prints

By mixing the Brafil Ink with a little ground Indigo, you have a Crimfon or Purple, and if with a little white Lead, you will have a Rofe Colour.

To prepare or extract all manner of Lakes out of Flowers.

TAKE Flowers, of what Sort or what Colour you will; if they ftain white Paper, when rubb'd againft it, they are good With thefe Flowers fill a common, but large Head, upon a common cucurbit, that's fill'd with Aqua Vitæ ; put a receiver to it, and lute it well, then ftill it over a gentle Fire, and the fubtil parts of the Spirits will fly up into the Head, extract the Tincture out of the Flowers and Herbs, and fall into the Receiver. This colour'd Spirit, if diftill'd in another Still, will pafs without any Colour, and may be ufed again for the like Purpofes, but the Tincture or Colour will remain at the Bottom of the Still, which you take out and dry at a gentle warmth. In this Manner you may make the beft Lake fit for Painters ufe.

Directions for Extracting all Sorts of Colours out of Wood, Flowers and Herbs

WHEN Mariners are fent in fearch of Dyers Drugs, Wood, or Plants, they are advifed by the Merchants to try thefe Commodities by chewing them, and fee whether they colour the Spittle, which if they do, it is a Sign they are good, and fuch Tryals may alfo be made on white Paper or Linnen.

The Drugs or Plants that are known to be good for Extraction of Colours, are among many others thefe, *Lignum Nephriticum*, or *Fufticks*, is good for yellow and green Colour, *Compegiana* and *Sylveftre*, &c.

To gild Paper.

TAKE yellow Oker, grind it with Rain Water, and lay a Ground with it upon the Paper all over, when dry, then take the White of Eggs, beat it clear with White Sugar Candy, and strike it all over, then lay on the Leaf Gold, and when dry, polish it with a Tooth

Some take Saffron, boil it in Water, and dissolve a little Gum with it, then strike it over the Paper, lay on the Gold, and when dry polish it.

To prepare Blue Ink.

TAKE Elderberries, press the Juice thereof into a Glass and put powder'd Alum into it, add to it about the Quarter Part of it of Vinegar, and a little Urin, then dip a Rag into it, and try whether the Colour is to your liking, you may if it is too pale, add a little more of the Juice, and if too dark, of the Vinegar to it

To make good Writing Ink

IT must first be observed, that according to the Quantity of Ink you design to make, the Weight and Measure of the Ingredients must be either augmented or lessen'd Thus for Example If you would make 10 Quarts of Ink, you ought to take four Quarts of Water, six Quarts of White Wine Vinegar, three Quarts of White Wine, and proportion the rest by Weight accordingly

Good Ink for Paper.

TAKE one Pint of Water, one Pint and a half of Wine, one Pint and a half of White Wine Vinegar, and mix it all together, then take six Ounces of Gall powdered and sifted thro' a fine Hair Sieve, put it in a Pot or Bottle by itself, and pour on it one half of your mix'd Liquor, take also four Ounces of Vitriol powdered, put it into a Bottle by itself, and pour half the remaining Liquor upon it To the rest of the Liquor put four Ounces of Gum-Arabick, beaten fine, cover these three Pans, or Pots, or Bottles, let them stand three Days, and stir every one of 'em three or four times a Day, on the fifth Day put the Pan with the Galls upon the

Fire,

Fire, and when you see that it is most ready to boil, keep the Gall down, and whilst it is warm, pour it into another Vessel through a Cloath, don't squeeze or wring the Cloath, but let it go through of itself, then add the Liquor which is in the two other Vessels to it, stir it well together, let it stand three Days, stirring it every now and then, the fourth Day, after it is settled, pour it through a Cloath into a Jar or Bottle, and you will have good Writing Ink

Ink for Parchment,

IS prepared in the self same Manner as the foregoing Receipt directs, only to a Pint of Water, take half a Pint of Wine and half a Pint of Vinegar, which together will make one Quart of Ink.

Another.

TAKE three or four Ounces of powder'd Galls, and three or four Ounces of Gum Arabick, put it together in a Vessel with Rain Water, and when the Gum is dissolv'd, then strain it through a Cloath, and add to it near half an Ounce of powder'd Vitriol

Another

TAKE one Pint of Beer, put in it one Ounce of powder'd Gall, let it boil till you see it of a reddish Colour. Then add six Drams of green Vitriol powder'd to it, and let it boil again, when you take it off the Fire, add six Drams of Gum-Arabick, and of Alum the Bigness of a Pea, both powder'd; stir it till it is cold

Another Receipt for Writing Ink.

TAKE five Ounces of Gall, six Ounces of Vitriol, four Ounces of Gum, and a fresh Egg, a little Powder of Walnuts, two Gallons of Beer, and put it into an Earthen Pot; add a little *Sal Armoniac*, to keep it from moulding.

Another.

TAKE for one Quart of Ink, one Pint and half a Quartern of Water, half a Quartern of Wine, half a Quartern

L   of of good Vinegar, four Ounces of Vitriol, four Ounces of Gall, both powder'd by itself, then mix it together in a glaz'd Vessel, and pour the foresaid Matter upon it, stir it often, during six or more Days, and when settled, pour it into a Bottle, and you will have very good Ink.

To prepare Red Ink

TAKE two Ounces of fine Brasil Chips, the White of 12 Eggs, and the Quantity of a Hazel Nut of Alum, beat the White of the Eggs clear, put it all together in the Sun, or before the Fire, stir it sometimes about, strain it through a Cloath, and let the Juice dry well, then keep it from Dust, and when you will use it, only temper it with fair Water.

Or,

TAKE the best Fernambuck, put it into a Cup or Pot that's glaz'd, pour good Wine Vinegar over it, let it stand three or four Hours to soak, then take Beer that's clear and bright, mix it with clear Pump Water, about an Inch above the Chips, let it on a middling Fire, let it boil, and take Care it does not run over, after it has boiled some Time, add Alum, the Quantity of a Walnut, powder'd, to it, and as much Gum Arabick, let it again upon the Fire, and let it boil, after it has boil'd a little, take it off, and strain the Liquor from the Chips, put it into a Glass, close it up, and you will have a fine red Ink.

If instead of Alum you put a little Sal Armoniac to it, it will make the Ink look bright.

Yellow Ink

TAKE the Leaves of yellow Cowslip Flowers, that grow common in the Fields, squeeze out the Juice, and mix it with Allum.

Or,

MIX a little Alum to some Saffron and Water, which makes a very good yellow Ink.

To Write Letters or any Thing else either with Gold or Silver

TAKE Flint Glafs, or Cryftal, grind it to Powder, temper it with the White of an Egg, Write with it, and when it is dry, take a Gold Ring, or a Silver Thimble, or any Thing of either of thofe Metals, rub your Writing therewith gently over, and when you fee the Gold or Silver ftrong enough, glaze it over with a Tooth

To Write with Gold out of a Pen

TAKE 16 Leaves of the fineft Gold, put it upon a Colour-Stone, fprinkle a little Vinegar over it, and let it lay for a little while, then grind it with your Muller to a fine Powder, put this into a Mufcle Shell, with as much clear Water as will fill it, mix it together with your Finger, then let it fettle, and after that pour off the Water, and fupply it with clear Water again, ftir it well with your Finger, as before, this repeat fo long till you fee the Water comes off from the Gold as clear as when put on, after you have thus clear'd your Gold, temper as much as you have occafion for prefent ufe, with a little clear Gum Water, till you fee it will eafily flow from your Pen, after your Writing is dry, glaze it gently with a Tooth

Fine Red Ink, of Vermillion

TAKE Vermillion, grind it fine with clear Water, and put it up to keep it from Duft, when you ufe it, take as much as you think you fhall have occafion for, and dilute it with a little Gum Water.

Another.

TAKE half an Ounce of Vermillion, or prepared Zinnaber, put it into a Galley Pot, take a little powdered clear Gum Arabick, diffolve it in Water and temper therewith your Vermillion, you may add a little of the White of an Egg to it, which you beat up till all becomes a Scum, and when you let it ftand, the Settling will be like clear Water, which is fit for Ufe.

An

An Artificial Water for writing Letters of Secrecy.

TAKE Vitriol, finely powder'd, put a little thereof into
a new Ink Horn, pour clean Water on it, and after it
has stood a little, write therewith either on Vellum or Paper, and the Writing cannot be seen any other Way, than by
driving the Letter through a Water, which is thus prepar'd. Take a Pint of Water, put into it one Ounce of Powder'd Gall, temper it together, and strain it through a
Cloth, put the Water into a Dish that's wide enough, and
draw your Writing through it, and you will read it as plain
as you do other Writings, and to make the secret Contents
less liable to Suspicion, you may write on the contrary Side
of the Paper or Parchment with black Writing Ink, Matters
of less Consequence.

*Another Secret, to write a Letter white upon white,
which cannot be read but in fair Water.*

TAKE clean Alum, beat it to a fine Powder, mix it
with Water, but not too thin, then take a new Pen,
and with this Mixture write what you please upon Paper, and
let it dry. Then let him, who is to read it, lay the Letter into
a flat Bason or Dish, that's fill'd with clean Water, and in a
Quarter of an Hour the Letters will appear white upon
white, so that they may be plainly seen and read.

Another.

TAKE the Juice of Onions, write with it, he who would
read it, must hold it over the Fire, and the Writing will
turn of a reddish or brownish Colour.

The Manner of marbling Paper or Books.

TAKE clear white Gum Tragacanth, put it into an Earthen Pan, pour fresh Water to it, till it is two
Hands nigh o'er the Gum, cover it and let it soak
24 Hours, then stir it well together, add more Water to it,
keep it often stirring for a whole Day, and it will swell,
keep it standing several Days, according as you find your
Gum is fresh or stale, for the fresh will dissolve sooner than

that

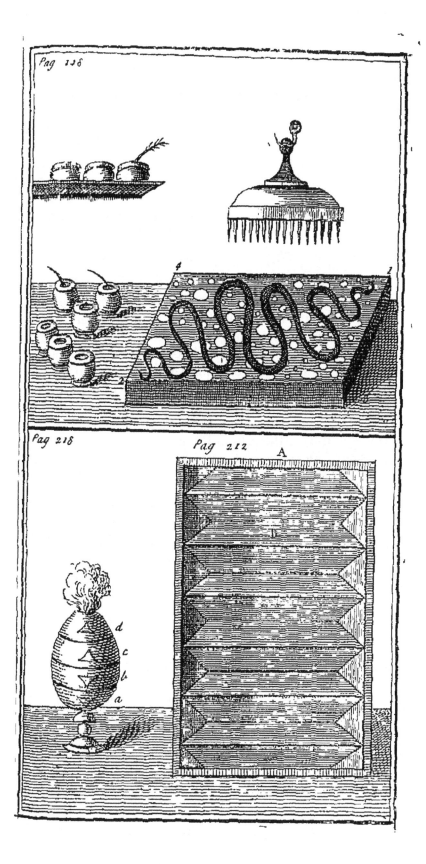

Pag. 116

Pag. 218   Pag. 212

that which has laid by a long time. Keep it low and then stirring, when you find it well diffolved, pour it through a Collender into another Pan, add to it more Water, and after it has flood a little, and been ftirr'd about, ftrain it through a clean Cloth into another clean Pan, keep it well covered, to hinder the Duft or any other thing from coming to it. This Water, when you go to make ufe of in Marbling your Paper or books, muft be neither too thick nor too thin; you may try it with your Comb, by drawing the fame from one end of the Trough to the other, if it fwells the Water before it, it is a Sign that it is too thick, and you muft add in Proportion a little more Water.

Your Trough muft be of the largenefs of your Paper, or rather fomething wider, and about four Inches deep.

After you have fil'd your Trough with the foremention'd Water, and fitted every thing for the Work, then (before you lay on your Colours) take a clean Sheet, and draw the Surface, which will be a thin fort of a Film, off on't, then have your three Colours, namely, Indigo mixt with White Lead, yellow Oaker, and Rofe Pink, ready prepared at Hand, and for each Colour have two Galley Pots, in order to temper them as you would have them in different Shades.

All your Colours muft be ground very fine with Brandy.

The blue is eafily made deeper or lighter, by adding more or lefs White Lead.

The Yellow ufed for that Purpofe, is either yellow Orpiment or *Dutch* Pink.

For Blue, grind Indigo, and White Lead, each by itfelf, in order to mix that Colour either lighter or darker.

For Green, take the forefaid Blue and White, add fome yellow to it, and temper it darker or lighter, as you would have it.

For Red, take either Lake, or Rofe Pink.

Every one of thefe Colours are, as we faid before, firft ground very fine with Brandy, and when you are ready to go to Work, add a little Ox or Fifh Gall to them, but this muft be done with difcretion, and you may try them by fprinkling a few drops upon your Gum Water, if you find the Colour fly and fpread too much about, it is a Sign of too much Gall, which to remedy, add more of the fame Colour which has none, but when you fee the Colour fpread and detract it felf again gently, it is right.

L 3   When

When thus you have your Colours and all Things in good order, then take a Pencil, or the end of a Feather, and sprinkle or put first your red Colour, then the Blue, Yellow, Green, &c begin your red from N° 1, and go along your Trough to N° 2, also the Blue from N° 3, all along to N° 4　The yellow and green you put here and there in the vacant Places, then with a Bodkin or a small Skewer, draw a Sort of a Serpent Figure through the Colours, beginning from N° 1, to N° 2. When this is done then take your Comb and draw the same strait along from N° 1, to N° 2. If you will have some Turnings or Snail Work on your Paper, then with a Bodkin give the Colours what Turns you please

Thus far you are ready in order to lay on your Paper, which must have been moisten'd the Day before, in the Nature as the Book Printers do their Paper for Printing, take a Sheet at a time, lay it gently upon your Colours in the Trough, press it slightly with your Finger down in such Places where you find the Paper lays hollow, this done, take hold at one end of the Paper, and draw it up at the other end of the Trough, hang it up to dry on a Cord, when dry, you glaze it, and it is done　You may if you will embellish your Paper with Streaks of Gold, by applying Muscle Gold or Silver tempered with Gum-Water, among the rest of the Colours.

To prepare Ink, so that what is wrote therewith cannot be read but in a dark Place

TAKE half a pint of Goat's Milk, a sweet Apple, pealed and cut, a handful of Touch Wood, which in the Night time appears to be lighted, put this and the Apple into a Mortar, beat them together, pouring now and then a little of the Goat's Milk to it, after it is well beaten, pour the rest of the Milk to it, stir it well together, then wring it through a Cloath, with this Liquor write what you please, and if you will read it, go into a dark Cellar or Chamber, and the Writing will appear of a fiery or Gold Colour.

To make fine red Paper

TAKE a Pin full of Water, put some Quick Lime into it, to make it into a Lee, and let it stand over Night,

Night, then put Brasil Chips into a clean Pot, about half full, fill it with the Lees, and boil it to half, and when it is just hot, add to it a little Alum. When you go to use it, mix it with a little Gum or Size, and then with a pretty large Pencil lay your Colour on the Paper with an even Hand.

To prepare Ink for drawing of Lines, which when writ upon, may be rubb'd out again

BURN Tartar to Ashes, or till it is calcined to a white Colour, take thereof the bigness of a Hazle Nut, and lay it into a Cup full of Water to dissolve, then filtrate it: To this Solution mix as much fine grounded Touch Stone as will colour it black enough to write with: With this Ink you rule the Lines to write upon, when you have done writing, you only rub it over with the Crumb of a stale Roul, or with Crumbs of Bread, the Lines will vanish and the Paper be as clean as it was before This may be made useful for Schools

To Write so that the Letters appear White, and the Ground of the Parchment Black.

TAKE clean Water, temper it with the White of Eggs so as to write therewith, with this write upon your Vellum or Parchment what you please, let it dry and draw it through Ink, so that it may take every where, or strike it over with a Pencil to make it of a good black, when it is thorough dry then scrape it gently off with a Knife, and draw it carefully through fair Water, let it dry, and your Writing will appear as white as the Parchment was, before you wrote upon it

To make Oil Paper

TAKE the Shreds of Parchment, boil them in clean Water, so long till the Water is clammy and like a strong Glue, pour it through a Cloth, and with a large Pencil strike it over the Paper, when dry, varnish it over with a Varnish of Turpentine, or the *Spanish* Varnish mentioned in the First Article under this Head

V Choice

V.

Choice Secrets for CABINET-MAKERS and TURNERS.

To prepare a black Colour for staining Wood

PUT two Ounces of Iron Filings into a new earthen Pan, add to it one Ounce of Sal-armoniac, diffolv'd in a Quart of Vinegar, and let it ftand 12 Days, the longer it ftands the better it will be, then take rafp'd Logwood, and three Ounces of Gallnuts, pounded fine, infufe this in a Quart of Lee made of Lime, let this alfo ftand the fame time as the above

When you have occafion to ufe it, warm both thofe Liquids over a flow Fire, and with the Lee firft ftrike the Wood over you defign to dye, and then with Vinegar, repeat this till you fee the Wood black enough to your likeing, after which, wax the Wood over with Bees-Wax, and rub it with a woolen Rag, and it will look bright and fine

To imitate Ebony Wood

TAKE clean and fmooth Box, boil it in Oil till it turns black, Or,

Take fmooth plain'd Pear-Tree Wood, ftrike it over with Aqua Fortis, and let it dry at a fhady Place, in the Air, then wipe it over with good black Writing Ink, let it alfo dry in the Shade, repeat and wipe the Ink over it, fo long till the Black is to your likeing Then polifh it with Wax, and a Cloath Rag

Another, but more coftly Method

DISSOLVE one Ounce of fine Silver to one Pound of Aqua Fortis, add a Quarter of a Pint of clear Water to it, with this ftrike your Wood over, repeat it fo long till you perceive it to be as black as Velvet, then polifh it with Wax

Another

Another Way to imitate Ebony

TAKE what Sort of Wood you will, as Box, Cedar, Mulberry, Pear-Tree, and the like, steep it for three Days in Allum Water, in a warm Place, or if in Summer, by the Sun; then boil it to Oil, in which mix some Vitriol and Sulpher; the longer you boil it, the blacker will be the Wood, however you must not let it boil too long, least it should be scorch'd.

Another.

STRIKE your Wood over with Spirit of Vitriol, hold it over a Coal Fire, and repeat this till it is black enough; then polish it

Another.

IRON Filings steept in Beer and Urin, makes a good black

Another

PUT one Pound of rasp'd Brasil in a clean Pan, boil it in three Pints of strong White-Wine Vinegar, till the half is boil'd away, then pour it clear off Take also one Pound of bruised Gallnuts, put them into another Pan with Water, and let them stand for eight Days in the Sun to soak, then put to it eight Ounces of Vitriol, stir it together, and let it stand for two or three Days, pour it off clear, and add to this Liquid the fourth Part of the prepared Brasil, and with this strike your Wood over 20 or 30 Times running, letting it every Time dry in the Shade.

Then take fine Silver, as much as you please, dissolve it in common Aqua Fortis, add to it twice the Quantity of Spring-Water, with this strike over the dy'd Wood once or twice, set it in the Air to dry, and it will be of a fine Coal Black, after which polish it as before directed

To dye Wood of a Red Colour.

TAKE one Handful of Quick-Lime, two Handfuls of Ashes, put it together into Rain Water, and let it soak

for

for half an Hour, till it is well settled, and you have a good Lee. Then take a new Pan, in which put one Pound of Fernambuck, pour on it the said Lee, and after it is soak'd for half an Hour, let it boil, and when it is cool, pour it off into another clean Pan, and fling one Ounce of Gum-Arabick into it, take another earthen Pan with Rain-Water, put into it two Ounces of Alum, boil your Wood in it, and after it is well soak'd, take it out, let it cool a little, warming the mean while the red Colour, and striking it over your Wood, repeat this till your Colour is deep enough to your likeing, then polish it with a Dog's Tooth.

Another Red, for Dying of Wood.

TAKE rasp'd Brasil, boil it till you see it of a fine red Colour, then strain it through a Linnen Cloath.

The Wood you design to dye, you colour first over with Saffron Yellow, and after it is dry, you strike it over with the red Colour, so long till it is deep enough, then polish it with a Tooth. If you put a little Allum to the Brasil-Colour, it will turn it to a Brownish Hue.

To marble upon Wood.

TAKE the Whites of Eggs, beat them up till you can write or draw therewith, then with a Pencil or Feather draw what Veins you please upon the Wood, after it has dry'd and harden'd for about two Hours, then take Quick-Lime, mix it well together with Wine, and with a Brush or Pencil paint the Wood all over, after it is thorough dry, you rub it with a scrubbing Brush clear off, so that both the Lime and the Whites of the Eggs may come off together, then you rub it with a Linnen Rag till it is smooth and fine, after which you may lay over a thin Varnish, and you will have a fine marbled Wood.

Another.

GRIND White Lead or Chalk together with Water upon a Marble very fine, then mix it up with the Whites of Eggs well beaten, wherewith you may paint or marble as you think proper, when dry, you strike it over with a Lee made of Lime and Urin, this will give the Wood a brown-red Colour,

Colour, upon this Colour you may, when dry, marble again with the Whites of Eggs, and again when dry, give it another Brush with the Lee, after you have with a scrubbing Brush rub'd off the Marbling Whites of Eggs, then you may strike it once more all over with the Lee, and your Work when dry and polish'd, will look very pleasant and of a fine Marbling

A Gold, Silver, or Copper Colour on Wood

TAKE Crystal, beat it in a Mortar to Powder, then grind it on a Marble with clean Water, and put it into a clean new Pot, warm it, and add to it a little Glue, with this strike or paint over your Wood When dry, take a Piece of Gold, Silver or Copper, and rubbing it over therewith, you will have the Colour of any one of those Metals upon the Wood, which you afterwards polish

To colour Wood of a Wallnut Tree Colour

TAKE the Bark of Wallnut Trees, or the Green Shells of Wallnuts, dry them in the Sun, mix, as much as you have occasion for, with Nut-Oil, boil it up, and rub the Wood over therewith

To stain Wood a fine Green

TAKE green Nut-Shells, put them into a Lee made of Roman Vitriol and Alum, in which let them boil an Hour or two To this Lee add some Verdegreafe, finely grounded with Vinegar, then take your Wood, after you have foak'd it for two Days in strong white Wine Vinegar, and boil it therein.

Another

TAKE the finest Verdegreafe, grind it with sharp Wine Vinegar, add to it a little Tartar, let it stand over Night, the Verdegreafe will settle, and you will have a fine Green ; with this strike over your Wood for several Times If you will have it Grass-Green, then put a little Sap-Green among it

A Red Colour for Wood

TAKE Quick-Lime, pour Rain Water upon it, let it stand over Night, and filter it through a Cloath, then add more Rain-

Rain-Water to it, and put clear and fresh Brasil-Chips in, together with the Wood you intend to dye, and boil it so long till the Colour is to your Mind. The Wood is first to be thoroughly soaked in Alum-Water

Another Method

POLISH your Wood-Work, after you have finish'd it with your Plain, and then lay on it Muscle-Gold or Silver, diluted with size or with the White of an Egg, marbling it in the Manner above directed in marbling of Wood, and when dry, you strike it over for several Times with the following Colour

Take fine rasp'd Brasil, pour on it, or infuse it in Oil of Tartar, and it will extract a fine red Colour This colour'd Oil you pour off, and put fresh to the Brasil, to extract more Colour These Extractions you let gently dry, then draw it off again with Spirit of Wine, and you will have a fine Red for your Use

A Violet Colour for Wood.

TAKE four Ounces of Brasil, and one Ounce of Indigo, infuse it together in a Quart of Water, and boil your Wood therein.

To adorn Wood with Ornaments of Silver or Tin

FIRST you carve or hollow your Ornaments out upon your Wood in the best Manner, so as to undermine the Edges on both Sides of your Strokes Then make an Amalgama of Tin, by dissolving it over a gentle Heat, and putting into it the same Quantity of Quicksilver, which, before you have heated, stir with a Stick well together, and pour it into a Pan of cold Water, when dry, you grind it upon a Marble with Water very fine, tempering it with clear Size, and fill up the carv'd Figures, smoothing it with your Hand, and when dry polish it To make it more of a Silver Colour, rub it over with an Amalgama of Silver and Quicksilver, and polish it with a Dog's Tooth

Instead of Tin, you may also use Bismuth grounded fine with Water

To Emboss or Trace all Manner of Ornaments on a gilded smooth Pannel, the Gold being laid over with Black or any other Colour

FIRST gild your Pannel or other Wood Work, as you are directed under the Article of Gilding, and when thorough dry, paint it all over smooth and even with Lampblack, ground with Linseed and Nut-Oil, add to it an equal Quantity of Umber, in order to dry it the better, after you have let it for two or three Days, or according to the Conveniency or the Time of the Year, to dry, then, before it is quite hard, draw or pounce what you design to emboss upon, and with a blunt pointed Bodkin, Horn, or Wood, you trace into the black Lay, down to the Gold, opening those Places, and making the Gold appear in the best Manner you can. In birds, Plants, Cattle, and such like, you must observe to take the Heightenings out clear, and leave the Shade, by Hatching into the Black, agreeable to your Design, the fine and soft Shades of the Hair, &c you may finish with a fine Pencil, with the black Colour, upon the Gold, and when you have done, let it thoroughly dry for three or four Days more, then lay over it a clear Varnish, which you may, after it is dry'd, repeat a second Time, and your Work will look beautiful.

To do this upon a blue Ground

AFTER you have gilded your Work, then take Alum which is not too coarse, mix it with Water on a Marble Stone, adding to it the White of an Egg, with this and a little Water mix your Smalt, and strike it fine and even over the Gilding. Then, when it is almost dry, sift through a fine Sieve some of the finest Smalt over it. You may, if you will, mix it with Spangles of several Colours, and when thorough dry, wipe off what sticks not to it, and proceed in tracing up your Figures you design for Gold. The fine falling Strokes upon the Gold because they cannot well be done with Smalt, you may use *Prussian* Blue or Indigo mixed with White Lead. You may, if you will, varnish it, but it will look better without.

Vari-

Varieties of GLUES and CEMENTS, for joining not only *Wood*, but alſo *Stone*, *Glaſs*, and even *Metals*.

An excellent Glue for Wood, Stone, Glaſs, and Metal.

TAKE good Glue four Ounces, ſoak it over Night in diſtill'd Vinegar, then boil it up with Vinegar, take a Clove of Garlick, beat or bray it in a Mortar, add to it one Ounce of Ox-Gall. This Juice wring through a Linnen Cloath into the warm Glue, then take Maſtic and Sarcocollæ, of each one Dram, Sandarac and Turpentine of each two Drams, grind the Sandarac and Maſtic fine, and put it together with the Sarcocollæ and Turpentine into a little Phial, pour one Ounce of the ſtrongeſt Brandy upon it, and let it ſtand three Hours in a moderate Heat, well ſtopp'd up, giving it now and then a Shake, put this alſo to the warm Glue, then ſtir or beat it together with a wooden Spatula, till ſome of the Moiſture is evaporated, and the Glue is grown cold. When you have occaſion to uſe it, then take as much or little as your Work requires, ſoak it in ſtrong Vinegar, till it is diſſolv'd. If you uſe this Glue for Stones, you mix it with Tripoli, or with ſome powdered Chalk, and if for Glaſs, you mix, beſides a little Tripoli, fine ground Venice Glaſs, and if you will uſe it for Metals, as Iron, Braſs, Copper, you put to it ſome of the fineſt Filings, you may alſo add a little Iſinglaſs. And if you will have this Glue hold out or ſtand the Water, you mix it up with a ſtrong Varniſh as much as preſent Occaſion requires.

A good Stone Glue or Cement for Grotto Work.

TAKE two Parts of white Roſin, melt it clear, add to it four Parts of Bees Wax, when it is melted together, add Stone-Flower of the Stone you deſign to cement, two or three Parts, or ſo much as will give the Cement the Colour of the Stone, to this add one Part of Flower of Sul-

phur,

pher firſt incorporate all together over a gentle Fire, and afterwards knead it with your Hands in warm Water With this you cement the Stones, after they are well dry'd and been warm'd before a Fire, in order for to receive the Cement the better.

A Wood Glue, which ſtands the Water

COMMON Glue mix'd up with Linſeed Oil or Varniſh, applied to the Places to be glued together, after they have been warm'd, when thorough dry, it will laſt and ſtand the Water

Another fine Glue.

TAKE Iſinglaſs and common Glue, ſoak it over Night in ſtrong Brandy, then diſſolve it over a Coal Fire, and mix with it a little fine powder'd Chalk, it will make a very ſtrong Glue

Another extraordinary Glue

TAKE Sal Armoniac, Sandarac and Gum Lacca, ſoak and diſſolve it in ſtrong Brandy, over a gentle Heat, put in it a little Turpentine, when all is diſſolv'd, then pour it over Iſinglaſs and common Glue, and in a cloſed up Veſſel, diſſolve it over a ſlow Fire, add to it a little Glaſs-Duſt, and when it is of a right Temperament, uſe it

A good Water Cement.

TAKE one Part Menin or Red Lead, and two Parts of Lime, mix it well together with the Whites of Eggs.

Stone Glue, wherewith you may glue either Stone or Glaſs.

TAKE white Flintſtone Powder, which is dry and finely ſearched, then take white Roſin, melt it in an Iron or earthen Panniken, ſtir the Powder in it, till it is like a thick Paſte, warm the Glaſs, or what you deſign to glew together, ſtrike it over, and after you have laid your Stone or Glaſs together, gild the Places or Joinings, and it
will

will add a great Beauty   This has been made ufe off in the
Embellifhment of Cabinets, and other Things

A Cement for broken Glaffes

BEAT the white of an Egg very clear, mix with it fine
powdered. Quick Lime, with this join your broken
Glaffes, China and earthen Ware,

Or,

TAKE old Varnifh, glue therewith your Pieces together, tie it clofe, and fet it to dry at the Sun, or a
warm Place, when dry, fcrape off the Varnifh that's prefs'd
out at the Sides, and it will hold very well

To join broken Amber

ANOINT the Pieces with Linfeed Oil, join and hold
them clofe together over the Fire

An excellent Glue or Cement to mix with Stone, Glafs, Marble, &c in order to make Utenfils, Images and other Things therewith

TAKE Fifh Glue well purified, four Ounces, Maftick two
Ounces, powdered Sealing Wax fix Ounces, fine ground
Brick duft one Ounce, put the Fifh Glue into a glaz'd Pipkin upon a flow Fire, and after you have mix'd your Ingredients, put it together into the Pipkin, boil it up, and what
hangs together ufe If you mix it up with fine powdered Glafs,
of any Colour, you may form it to what Shape you will,
and when cold and dry, it will be as hard as a Stone.

Another Cement which dries quickly.

TAKE Pitch, as much as you will, melt it, and mix it
with Brick Duft and Litharge, and to make it harder,
moiften the Brick-Duft firft with fharp Vinegar, and take a
larger Quantity of the Litharge, it will be as hard as
Stone.

Good

Good Glue Sticks, or Spittle Glue, fit for Book-binders

TAKE two Ounces of Isinglass, half an Ounce of Sugar-Candy, and half a Dram of Gum Dragant. Then take half an Ounce of flips or bits of white Parchment, pour on it a Pint of Water, and let it boil well, take that Water, strain it through a Cloath, and pour it over the two other Ingredients, mix'd with a little Rose Water, let it boil away above half, then take it off the Fire, and cast it into little flat Sticks, or in any Shape you please.

A Water Cement, which, the longer it is in Water, the harder it grows.

TAKE Mastick, Incense, Rosin, and fine cut Cotton, of each an equal Quantity, melt, and with some powder'd Quick Lime, mix it up into a Mass.

A Cement as hard as Iron.

MELT Pitch, then take ground Sand, which comes off the Smiths or other grind Stones, stir it well together, boil it up, and it is fit for Use.

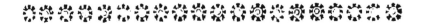

Several curious Secrets relating to IVORY, BONE, and HORN

To whiten Ivory that's turn'd to a reddish or yellow Colour.

PUT Alum into fair Water, so much as to colour it pretty white, then boil it up, in this put your Ivory for an Hour to soak, rub it with an Hair Cloath, and wipe it over with a clean Napkin or Linnen Rag, which is moistened before, in this let it lie, till it is dry of itself, else it would be apt to split.

Another

Another Method to whiten Green Ivory.

BOIL the Ivory in Water and Quick-Lime, fo long till you fee it has a good White

To marble upon Ivory.

MELT Bees-Wax and Tallow together, or elfe yellow and white Bees-Wax, and lay it over your Ivory; then with an Ivory Bodkin, you open the Strokes that are to imitate Marbling, pour the Solution of fome Metal or other on them, and let it ftand a little while, then pour it off, and when it is dry, cover thofe Strokes again with Wax, and open fome other Veins with your Bodkin for another metallick Solution, and this you repeat to the Number of Colours you defign to give it

The Solution of Gold gives it a Purple; of Copper, a Green, of Silver, a Lead Black, of Iron, a Yellow and Brown Colour Thefe Solutions well manag'd, and apply'd on Ivory, will intirely anfwer the Satisfaction of the Artift.

By this Method you may imitate Tortoife Shell, and feveral other Things on Ivory.

To ftain Ivory of a fine Green.

TAKE to two Parts of Verdegreafe one third of Sal Armoniac; grind it well together, pour ftrong white Wine Vinegar on it, and put your Ivory into it; let it lie covered, till the Colour is penetrated, and deep enough to your likeing If you will have it marbled or fpotted, fprinkle or marble it with Wax

And thus you may colour your Ivory with any other Colours, if you prepare them in the Manner directed, *viz.* With Sal Armoniac and Vinegar.

To dye Ivory or Bone of a fine Coral Red

MAKE a Lee of Wood-Afhes, of which take two Quarts, pour it upon one Pound of Brafil, in a Pan, to this add one Pound of Alum, two Pound of Copper Filings, and boil it for half an Hour; then take it off, and let

it

it stand In this put the Ivory or Bone, the longer it continues in this Liquor, the redder it will be.

To stain Ivory or Bone of a Black Colour.

TAKE Litharge and Quick-Lime, of one as much as the
other, warm it in Rain-Water, till it begins to boil. In
this put the Bones or Ivory, stirring them well about with a
Stick; and afterwards when you see the Bones colour, take
the Pan from the Fire, stirring all the while the Bones, till
the Liquor is cold.

To make Horn soft.

TAKE Man's Urin, which has been put by and cover'd for
a Month, in this boil one Pound of Weed-Ashes, or
the Ashes of Wine-Stalks, two Pound of Quick-Lime, eight
Ounces of Tartar, and eight Ounces of Salt, after it is
boil'd, pour it through a Cloath, and filter it thus three times
running Keep this Lee covered, and soak the Horn therein
for eight Days, and it will be soft.

Another

TAKE Weed-Ashes and Quick-Lime; of this make a
strong Lee, filter it clear, and boil the Shavings or Chips
of Horn therein, and they will be like a Paste You may
colour it of what Colour you please, and cast or form it in
any Thing you intend

To prepare Horn Leaves in Imitation of Tortoise-Shell.

TAKE Quick-Lime one Pound, and Litharge of Silver
eight Ounces, mix it with some Urin into a Paste, and
make Spots with it, in what Form or Shape you please, on
both Sides of the Horn, when dry, rub off the Powder,
and repeat this as many times you will Then take Vermillion,
hich is prepared with Size, lay it all over the Horn, as also
on the Wood, to which you design to fasten it
For Raised Work, you form the Horn in a Mould of what
Shape soever; put it by to dry, and with the aforesaid Paste
and the Vermillion give it the Colour, then lay on a clear
Glue (neither too thick, nor too thin) upon both the Horn

M 2

and

and the Wood on which it is to be fixed, and clofe it toge
ther, do this Work in a warm Place, and let it ſtand over
Night, then cut or file off the Shag, or what is ſuperfluous
about, rub it over with a Coal, and poliſh it with Tripoli
and Linſeed Oil

The Work made in this Manner looks very beautiful and
natural, and may be uſed by Cabinet Makers for Pillars,
Pilaſters, Pannels, or any other Embelliſhment in Cabinet
Work.

Another Method to Counterfeit Tortoiſe-Shell on Horn

TAKE good Aqua-Fortis two Ounces, fine Silver one
Dram, let the Silver diſſolve, and after you have
ſpotted or marbled your Horn with Wax, ſtrike the Solu
tion over it, let it dry of itſelf, and the Horn will be in
thoſe Places, which are free from Wax, of a brown and
black Colour. *Or,*

Lay the Wax all over the Horn, then with a pointed
Skewer or Iron draw what you will, laying the Figure you
draw open on the Horn; then pouring on the above
Solution, let it ſtand a little, and after you have pour'd it
off, either ſcrape or melt the Wax, wipe it with a clean
Rag, and poliſh it

Inſtead of the Silver Solution, you may boil Litharge of
Silver in a ſtrong Lee made of Quick Lime, ſo long till it
turns res black Or, inſtead of Silver you may diſſolve
Lead in Aqua Fortis

To ſolder Horn together, after it has been lin'd with proper
Foyles or Colours

TAKE two Pieces of Horn, made on Purpoſe to correſ
pond together, either for Handles of Knives, Razors,
or any thing elſe, lay Foyles of what Colour you pleaſe on
the Inſide of one of the Horns, or inſtead of Foyles painted or
gilded Paper or Parchment, then fix the other Piece upon
it, lay a wet Linnen Fillet, twice doubled, over the ſide
Openings, and with a hot Iron rub it over, and it will
cloſe and join together as firm as if made out of one Piece

T

To dye Horn of a Green Colour

TAKE two Parts of Verdegreafe, one third Part of Sal Armoniac, grind it well together, pour on it strong white Wine Vinegar, and it will be tinctured of a pleasant Green, then put your Horn into it, let it lay therein till you fee it dy'd to what Height you wou would have it

Another Method

TAKE the Green Shells of Walnuts, put them into a ftrong Lee, with a little Vitriol and Alum, let it boil to two Hours, and lay the Horn for two Days in ftrong Vinegar, then put half an Ounce of Verdegreafe, ground with Vinegar, into the Lee, boil the Horn in it, and it will be of a fine Green

To die Horn of a Red Colour

TAKE Quick Lime, pour Rain Water upon it, and let it ftand, filter it through a Cloath, and put to it one Quart of clean Water, and two Ounces of ground Brafil, lay the Horn into it, then boil it, and you will have a fine Red, if before you have foak'd it for a While in Alum Water

To ftain Horn of a Brown Colour

TAKE Quick-Lime, flacken it with Urin, and ftrike it over the Horn, then take Red Curriers Water, wafh the Horn therein, and it will turn to a Green Colour, wipe it over again with the faid Lime, and when dry, wafh it with Lee, let it lay therein a whole Day, it will be of a fine Chefnut Colour

To dye Horn of a Blue Colour.

TAKE a Brafs Bowl, and when you have made it red hot, wipe it over with Sal Armoniac, then pour Lime Water upon it, ftir it together, and you will have a Blue Water, in which lay your Horn, the longer you let it lay, the deeper will be the Colour.

Of

VI.

Of VARNISHING or JAPANNING on WOOD, &c.

A white Varnish

TAKE ten Ounces of rectified Brandy, and fine pulve riled Gum Sandarac two Ounces, clear Venice Turpentine two Ounces, put it together into a Glafs, and cover it clofe with wax'd Paper and a Bladder, then take a Pot with Water, put it on a Coal Fire, and when it begins to be warm, put fome Hay on the Bottom of the Pot, on which fet your Glafs, then let it Boil for two or three Hours, and the Sandarac and Turpentine will diffolve, and unite with the Brandy Then pour your Varnifh boiling hot through a clean Hair Cloath, and put it up in a clean Phial for Ufe. This is an excellent Varnifh, fit to be ufed for Varnifhing light Colours, as White, Yellow, Green, Sky, Red, alfo fuch Things which are filver'd or gilded

Another Varnifh fit to mix with red or dark Colours, and to Japan the Work over therewith

TAKE rectified Brandy which will ftand Proof, that is, when pouring fome of it on Gun Powder, it will light it, or, when a Linnen Rag being dipt into it, and lighted, it will confume it, one Pound, of clean Gum Lacca a quarter of a Pound, grind it fine, and put it into a Phial then pour the Brandy over it, let it ftand for two Days (fwinging and fhaking it about once every Hour) the third Day hang it over a gentle Heat of Coals till it is well diffolv'd, then ftrain it through a Hair Bag and put it up for Ufe

Another Lac Varnifh.

TAKE of the beft and ftrongeft Brandy one Quart, calcined Tartar one Pound, let the Brandy ftand upon the
Tarta

Tartar, clofe covered, for one Day, in a gentle Warmth, then pour off the Brandy and filtrate it through a Paper, of this take one Pound, white Amber fix Ounces, Sandarac fix Ounces, Gum Lacca two Ounces (the Amber muft not be of the Drofs, or Powder, but pick'd out of clear Pieces) grind all fine together, put it into a Phial or Matrafs, then pour on it three Pound of the filtrated Brandy your Phial muft be but about half fill'd, then fwing and fhake it about for an Hour together, keep it in the Matrafs for two Days, giving it a Shake about once every Hour, when fettled, pour it through a Hair Cloath, and it is fit for Ufe

What Settling there remains in the Phial, may be ufed in making another fuch Quantity of Varnifh, adding to it but half the Quantity of frefh Ingredients.

Another Lac Varnifh

TAKE high rectified Brandy one Pint, Gum Lacca four Ounces, Sandarac two Ounces, white Amber one Ounce, white Frankincenfe one Ounce, Powder thefe in a Stone Mortar very fine, and put it together, with the Brandy, into a Phial or Matrafs, ftopping it very clofe, fet it in the Heat of the Sun, or in Winter Time in a warm Place, and after it has ftood three or four Days, fet it on Afhes over a Charcoal Fire, boil it foftly for two Hours, and when you fee the Brandy of a yellow-brownifh Colour, and of a thickifh Confiftence, pour it hot through a Hair Cloth, and preferve it in a clean Phial for ufe.

A White or clear Lac Varnifh.

TAKE Gum Elemi, Gum Animæ, white Frankincenfe, and white Amber, of each one Dram, grind it fine, put it into a Glafs, and boil it in diftill'd Vinegar, then pour off the Vinegar, and wafh the Settlement with clean warm Water, and it will be of a white Colour; dry it, and grind it fine again, add to it one Dram of Gum Dragant, two Drams of white Sugar-Candy, both finely grounded, put it by little and little into a Matrafs, wherein you have before hand put two Pound of high rectified Brandy, and after you have put all the Ingredients into it, fhake it about for an Hour together, then put it into a *Balneum Marie*,

M 4   and

ard when it begins to boil, keep it so for two Hours, then let it cool, and after you have let it stand for three Days, pour it off in o a clean Phial, stop it close, and save it for Use.

A other Method

TAKE the above specified Ingredients, boil them in Vinegar as directed, and after you have put to it the Gum Dragant and Sugar Candy, take of clear Oil of Spike or Turpentine one Pound, Cyprian Turpentine six Ounces, put it together into a strong Matrass, and set it, provided with a Leaden Ring, in a Balneum; when the Balneum begins to boil, and the Turpentine is dissolv'd and becomes pretty warm, then add the other fine grounded Ingredients to it, stir them with a Wooden Spatula well together, and let it stand in the boiling Balneum for three or four Hours, then take it out, and when cold, and has stood two or three Days, pour it into a clean Phial, and you will have a fine Varnish.

A fine Varnish for Blue and other Colours, which will make them bright like a Looking Glass

IF your Table is to be of a blue Colour, then paint it first over with Indigo and White, ground with Oil, and a little Turpentine, when dry, you may give it another Lay and heighten and deepening it to your liking and when this is thorough dry, then varnish it with the following Varnish.

Take clear Cyprian Turpentine half an Ounce, Sandarac one Ounce, Mastic two Ounces, grind the Sandarac and Mastic very fine, then take Oil of Spike two Ounces, Oil of Turpentine one Ounce, put it into a Glass, and dissolve it over a gentle Heat, add to it the pulverised Gum, set the Glass or Matrass in a Pan with Water, and let it boil over a slow Fire for an Hour, and all will be dissolv'd and united, then let it cool, preserve it in a Phial well clos'd up for Use.

When you use it, first wipe your painted Table, and clean it from all Dust, then take some fine and light Smalt in a Cup, or upon a Plate, according to what Quantity your Piece requires, temper it with the above Varnish, and with a large Hair brush. Pencil glaze it quick all over, let it dry in a clean Place that's free from Dust, which will be in about

about three Hours Time, then glaze it over again, the more you repeat it, the brighter will be your Table, and if you will have it of an exceeding fine Luftre, glaze it over 12 or 15 Times.

A Chinefe Varnifh for all Sorts of Colours

PUT into a Matrafs a Pint of Brandy, one Ounce of Gum Animæ, two Ounces of Maftic, two Ounces of Sandarac or Juniper Gum, powdered together fine in a Mortar, when you have put all together into the Matrafs, clofe it up, and hang it in hot Weather in the Sun for 24 Hours, or fo long over a Fire, till the Gum is diffol'd, and the Brandy is tinctur'd therewith, then filter it through a fine Cloath, and keep it in a Phial clos'd up, you may ufe it with what Colour you pleafe. For Red ufe Vermillion, for Black ufe Lampblack or Ivory Black, for Blue ufe Indigo and White, *Pruffian* Blue or Smalt and White Lead, &c.

How to Varnifh Chairs, Tables, and other Furniture, to imitate Tortoife-Shells fo as not to be defac'd by Oil or ftrong Water

FIRST lay your Work over with a Lac Varnifh, of which you have been inftructed before, then lay it over again with Red Lead and yellow Pink, well grounded and mix'd up with the faid Lac-Varnifh, you may do it twice or three times over, letting it be thorough dry every time before you do it. After which rub it with *Dutch* Rufhes, fuch as the Joiners and Cabinet Makers ufe.

Then take Dragons Blood, which is a red Gum, and may be had at the Druggifts, beat it very fine in a Mortar, and temper it with this Varnifh if you will be very nice, wring it through a fine Cloath, and put it up in a Phial for ufe, the longer it ftands the finer will be the Colour. With this you may Cloud your Table or other Work in the beft Manner you can. If you go over Clouding it again, you muft have a darker Shade, and to deeping your Clouds, you may add to your Varnifh a little Ivory Black, Umber, or Indigo, and work the Colours in one another, as your own Mind will beft direct. When you have done your Work, and it is thorough dry, then take fome Pumice Stone,

make

make it red hot, and beat it to a fine Powder, and with this and *Dutch* Rushes, soak'd in Water, rub it smooth and even, and then rub it with a clean woolen Rag, and holding it over a gentle Heat, give it five or six more Lays of Varnish, but be careful you heat it not too much, least it should blister, and spoil your Work, after it is thorough dry, then take Tin Ashes and sweet Oil, and with the rough Side of *Spanish* Leather, polish it, and give it the finishing Stroke with some Tin Ashes and the Palm of your Hand, wiping it so long till it has a fine Lustre.

From this Direction the Ingenious will make further Improvements.

A very fine Indian Varnish

TAKE four or five Quarts of good Brandy, distil and rectify it to the highest Degree, that when you light a Spoonful, it will consume itself in the Flames, and leave nothing behind. Having this ready, take Gum Lacca, beat it fine, and put it to the Spirit into a Phial or Matrass, let the Spirit be four Fingers high above the Gum, close the Glass, by tying a treble *Bladder* over it, then put it on a hot Sand, and let it stand till the Spirit and Gum is well united and boil'd, but be careful to see whether you perceive some blisters drive up to the top of the Glass, and as soon as you perceive them, take a Needle and prick the Bladder, in order to give it Vent, else your Glass will be in danger of bursting.

After which filtre it through whited brown Paper into another Glass, and keep it clos'd up for Use

If you will use this Varnish with Colours, let them be first grounded with the rectified Brandy, and then temper as much as you have occasion for present use, with the Varnish, and lay it on your Work, and when you think you have laid your Varnish thick enough, smooth it, when dry, with *Dutch* Rushes, then polish it with Tripoli and sweet Oil; give it one Lay or two of clear Varnish, and it will be fine.

To Japan with Gold, Glass, or any other Metal Spangles

FIRST lay on your Work with Lac Varnish, then grind Coln's Earth and Gumboge with the same,
this

this Varnish muſt be bright and clear· with that Colour lay your work alſo once or twice over, let it dry, and then do it over with Varnish only, and ſift the Gold Duſt, or what elſe you deſign to do it over with If your Work or Table is large, you lay the Varniſh on one Place after another, for the Varniſh would dry in one Place before you have done ſifting the other   And after you have ſifted your Work all over, and it is thorough dry, then give it 12 or 16 Lays more of clear Varniſh, after which ſmooth and poliſh it as directed.

A very fine Varnish for a Violin.

TO make this to Perfection, you muſt have three Glaſſes before you· In the firſt you put of the fineſt Gum Lacca eight Ounces, Sandarac three or four Ounces, both very finely pulveriz'd, upon this pour of the beſt rectified Spirit of Wine, ſo much till it ſtand four Inches above the Ingredients when diſſolv'd, ſtrain it through a Cloath, and put it cloſed up in a ſtill Place to ſettle, in a few Days the Top will be clear, which decant off into another Glaſs, and preſerve it from Duſt

In the ſecond Glaſs put of Dragon's-Blood five Ounces, and of Red Wood three Ounces, diſſolve and extract it with the ſame Spirit of Wine

In the third Glaſs diſſolve of *Colophoni* three Ounces, *Aloe Succotrine* two Ounces, *Orleni* 3 Ounces, and when altogether is extracted, then pour the Matters of the three Glaſſes into one, cloſe it up, and let it ſettle, then pour off what's clear at Top, and filter the reſt through a brown Paper If you find the Varniſh too thin, exhale it a little over a gentle Heat, and you will have a fine Red Varniſh, which will gild Pewter, and be of extraordinary Uſe for varniſhing of Violins, &c

A choice Varnish which cannot be hurt by Wet.

TAKE Gum Capall, as much as you pleaſe, beat it fine, put it into a Glaſs, and pour of high rectified Brandy four Inches high over it, then cloſe the Glaſs with a Bladder, ſet it for 24 Hours on a warm Oven for the Gum to diſſolve, after which put the Glaſs in *Baln Mar*. till the Spirit and the Gum is united.

A fine

A fine Marbling on Wood, or Japanning

TAKE of the best transparent yellow Amber what Quantity you please, beat it to a Powder, put it in a clean Crucible which is glaz'd within, let it melt over a gentle Charcoal Fire, and stir it well, to keep it from burning, then pour it upon a smooth, clean Marble Table, let it cool, and beat it again to Powder Take afterwards clear Turpentine, and in a Glass warm it in hot Sand, put in it the beaten Amber, let it boil and dissolve gently together, till it is of a Consistence fit to be used with a Pencil, strain it through a Cloath and you will have the finest Lac Varnish that can be had, and although it is of a brownish Colour, yet when laid on, it h is a fine clear Gloss

The Colours wherewith you marble, are the following, Lampblack, Brown red, Oker, Vermillion, these four are ground with Linseed Oil Venice White Lead is ground with Nut Oil

For a White, lay your first Ground with Linseed Oil, and if there are any Holes in the Wood, fill them up with Calk, tempered with Size For a black Ground lay it first with Lampblack and Size, when the Ground is dry, mix the Vermillion with the before describ'd Lac Varnish, and with a Brush Pencil lay it on with an even and quick Hand, repeat this three or four times, till it is bright and fine, and lay the Varnish by it self over it twice or thrice Then mix your other Colours with the Varnish in an Oister Shell, or in little Cups, and with them Marble upon what ground you have prepared, in Imitation of whatever you design.

A fine Gold Varnish, wherewith one may gild silver'd or tinn'd Things, with so much Lustre as if done with Gold

TAKE of the finest Gum Lacca in Grains eight Ounces, clear Gum Sandarac two Ounces, Dragon's Blood one Ounce and a half, Colophormium or black Rosin one Ounce and a half, beat all together into Powder, and put it into a Quart of high rectified Spirit of Wine, which is strong enough to light Gunpowder, put it in warm Sand over a Smallcoal Fire, let it boil for two Hours (if you can do it in a *Baln Mar* it is better) or so long till it is dissolv'd as much as possible, then let it cool, wring it through a Cloath into a Glass, so as to separate the Dross that might have been in the Ingredients, this you lay on over any Thing that has either been silver'd or tinn'd, three or four times, and it will resemble the brightest Gold. If you will have the gold Colour still higher, you only add about two Grains of Gurgummi, two Grains of the best Aloeparica, and one Grain of the finest Dragon's Blood, boiling it up, and straining it through a Cloath into another Glass.

When you use it, put the Glass into a Bason with Water over a gentle Charcoal Fire, in order to make the Varnish fluid, it is also requisite to warm the Work before you begin to varnish it.

Of CORAL WORK.

To make Red Coral Branches, for the Embellishment of Grotto's

TAKE clear Rosin, dissolve it in a Brass Pan, to one Ounce thereof add two Drams of the finest Vermillion, when you have stirr'd it well together, and you have chose your Twigs and Branches, peal'd and dry'd, take a Pencil and paint these Twigs all over, whilst the Composition is warm, and shape them in Imitation of natural Coral of a black Thorn, when done, hold it over a gentle Coal Fire, turn the Branch with your Hand about, and it will make it be all over smooth and even, as if polish'd.

In the same Manner you may with white Lead prepare white, and with Lampblack, black Coral.

A Gentleman may with very little expence build a Grotto of Glass Cinders, which may be easily hid Pebbles, or Pieces of large Flint, and embellish it with such counterfeit Coral, pieces of Looking Glass, Oster, Muscle and Snail-Snells, Moss, pieces of Chalk, Oar, &c. The Cement to bind and Cement them together, you have Direction now to prepare under the Article of Cements.

P A R T

PART VI.

The Art of Preparing Colours for PAINTER' LIMNERS, &c.

I Of BLUE-COLOURS

To make or prepare Ultramarine.

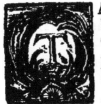 AKE of Lazur-Stone or *Lapus Lazuli* the blue Veins, calcine them in a Crucible on a Charcoal Fire, and quench them in Vinegar, this repeat twice, then grind them on a fine hard Stone to an impalpable Powder

When it is thus grounded, then take white Rosin, Pitch, new Wax, Mastick and Turpentine, of each six Ounces, Frankincense and Linseed Oil, of each two Ounces, let it altogether dissolve over a gentle Fire, stir it well with a wooden Spatula, in order to unite them together; then pour it into clean Water, continually stirring it, take it out, and preserve it from Dust for Use

When you go to prepare your Ultramarine, take to each Pound of the pulveriz'd Ultramarine 20 Ounces of the Mass. The Mass you dissolve before a gentle Warmth by Degrees, in a Pipkin, and fling the Powder in it by little and little, whilst it is dissolving, after your Powder is all in, and well incorporated with the Mass, then pour it into a Pan with cold Water, form it into little Tents or Drops, but to prevent its sticking to ones Fingers, you must anoint them with Linseed Oil, those Tents or Drops you lay again into fresh cold Water for 15 Days, shifting the Water every other Day.

Then

Then take and put them in a clean earthen well glaz'd Cup or Bason, and pour warm Water on them; when that cold, pour it off, and put fresh warm Water to it, this you repeat till the Tents or Drops begin to diffolve, which will then turn the Water into a blue Colour.

When the Water is of a fine blue Tincture, and cold, then pour that into another clean earthen Cup or Bason, and pour more warm Water upon the remaining Tents, when that allo is colour'd, pour it off, and fresh on, repeating this till the Water receives no more Tincture

Let the tinctur'd Waters stand for 24 Hours to settle, after which you will see a Greasiness on the Surface, which, with the Water together you pour off gently, and put fresh clean Water upon the Settling, stirring it well together, and pouring it through a fine Hair Sieve into a clean Bowl, the Sieve will attract some of the slimy or greasy Matter, that might remain in it, and after you have wash'd your Sieve, and repeated the next Settling, pouring it through with clear Water, three Times running, then let it settle, pour off the Water, and let it dry of itself. Thus you will have a fine Ultramarine.

To prepare a curious Blue Colour, little inferior to Ultramarine, out of Blue Smalt.

TO do this you grind your Smalt very fine, and proceed in every Respect as you have been taught before, in preparing of Ultramarine

To prepare a curious Blue Colour out of Silver

HAMMER Silver very thin, neal it thoroughly, and quicken or anoint it a little over with Quickfilver; then put of the sharpest distill'd Vinegar, in which you have dissolv'd some Sal Armoniac, into a Glass; hang the Silver Slips over it, so as not to touch the Vinegar, cover it very close, and put it into a warm Place, so that thereby the Fumes of the Vinegar may be raised a little, which extract out of the Silver a most beautiful Ultramarine, and hangs itself upon the Silver Slips, wipe them off into a Shell, and hang the Silver Slips over the Vinegar again, well closed; repeat this till all the Tincture is drawn out of the Silver.

Another

Another Method to extract a fine Blue out of Silver

TAKE of the finest Silver as much as you will, 7 or 8 Ounces, and dissolve it in a clear and strong Spirit of Nitre, then draw off Half of the Spirit of Nitre, and set the Glass in a damp and cool Place, and the Silver will over Night shoot in fine Cryftals, not unlike Saltpetre, then pour the Spirit of Nitre clear from it, put the Cryftals into Glass Plates, and let them ftand in a warm Place till they fall into Flower, then grind it with as much clear Sal Armoniac, which is fublim'd over common Kitchin-Salt, fet it together in the open Air, till you fee the Mafs turns of a blue or greenifh Hue, then put it together into a Cucurbit with a large Head to it, and fublime it, and the Sal Armoniac will carry the *Anima Lunæ* up along with it; after this grind the Silver that's left at the Bottom of the Matrafs with frefh Sal Armoniac, and fublime it as before, this repeat till all the Animus, or the fine blue Tincture is drawn out of the Silver. The Water you evaporate over a gentle Fire, and you will recover your Sal Armoniac again, the Tincture you dry and preferve. It is a fine and beautiful Colour, fit to be ufed for the moft curious Painting or Limning.

Another Method

TAKE of the fineft Silver as much as you will, beat it very thin, and with four Times as much Quickfilver make it into an Amalgama, wring it through a Leather, and drive all the Mercury afterwards from it, thus you will have a fine Silver Calx, which diffolve in clear Aqua Fortis, the Quantity whereof muft be as little as poffible, when it is diffolv'd, let the Water evaporate, and the Silver will remain at the Bottom like damp Afhes, pour over it fome Sal Armoniac mix'd with fharp white Wine Vinegar, let it fettle and clear; then pour off the Vinegar, and keep the Settling at the Bottom for a Month well clos'd up, to prevent the leaft Evaporation, and you will find a very curious blue Colour.

To prepare a Blue Colour out of Verdegreafe

TAKE Sal Armoniac and Verdegreafe, of each fix Ounces, mix it with Water of Tartar well together into

a Pafte

a Paste, put this into a Phial, and stop it close; let it stand for several Days, and you will have a fine blue Colour.

Another Method

TAKE Sal Armoniac one Part, Verdigreafe two parts, beat them both to a Powder, and mix it with a little white Lead , then incorporate it together with Oil of Tartar, put it into a Glafs and close it well , put it afterwards in a Loaf and bake it in a Baker's Oven; as soon as the Loaf is bak'd enough, your Colour will be ready

Another Method to prepare a fine blue Colour.

TAKE Quickfilver two Parts, Sulphur three Parts, Sal Armoniac four Parts, mix and beat it all well together, temper it with Water, put it into a well glaz'd Pipkin into a Furnace, over a Coal Fire, and when you fee a blue Smoak arife, take it off and let it cool, then break the Utenfil, and you will find a fine Sky Blue, not unlike *Ultramarine.*

To make Venice Sky Blue

TAKE Quick Lime one Pound, mix and work it with fharp White-Wine Vinegar into a Dough , let it stand for half an Hour, and when hard, pour more Vinegar to it, in order to make it foft, when done, add to it two Ounces of pulverifed fine Indigo, mix it first well together, set it into a Glafs Veffel for 20 Days under a warm Mift, after which time fee whether it is of a fine Colour ; if not, fet it again as long as before in the Mift, and it will then come to its Perfection.

II. Of feveral RED COLOURS.

To make fine Lake out of Cochineal

TAKE Cochineal eight Ounces, Alum one Pound, fine and clean Wool eight Pound, fine powdered Tartar half a Pound, Bran of Rye eight Handfuls , boil the Bran in about three Gallons of Water, more or lefs, it is no great Matter, put it over Night to settle, and pour it through a Flannel to have it clear and fine, then take a Copper Kettle, large enough to contain the Wool, pour half of the Bran Water and half clean Water to so much as you think sufficient to boil the Wool in it, let it boil, then add the above Tartar and Alum to it, and put in the Wool, let it also boil for two Hours, turning all one while the Wool up and down, in order to cleanse it thoroughly. after it has boil'd that Time, put the Wool into a Net, to drain out the Wet. Take then the other half of the Bran Water, and pour to it as much clean Water, and let it boil, after it is well boiled, put in Cochineal, which before must be ground very fine with four Ounces of white Tartar, you must stir it continually about, whilst it is boiling, to prevent its running over, then put in the Wool and let it boil for an Hour and a half, keeping it all the while turning about, after the Wool has attracted the Colour, put it again into a Net, let the Wet drop off, and you will have it of a Scarlet Colour.

This Colour may indeed be done in another Manner, and of a brighter Lustre, in a Pewter Kettle, with Tin and Aqua Fortis, but the above Method is sufficient for the purpose design'd, and may be made by Anybody, without the Implements which are requir'd to dye it the other Way.

To extract the Lake out of the Scarlet Wool.

TAKE clean Water about six or seven Gallons, dissolve therein as much Pot Ashes as will make it a good sharp Lee, filtrate it through a Felt or Flannel Bag to make it very clear, in this put the Wool, let it well boil in a Kettle, till it is white again, and the Lee has contracted all the Colour, then pour it again through a clean Felt or Bag and squeeze out the Wool, take then two Pound of Alum let it dissolve in Water and pour it in the colour'd Lee, stir it well together and it will curdle and turn to a thick Substance of a Pulp, pour it again into a clean Bag, and the Lake will remain in the Bag, but the Lee will run clear from it, and in case it should still an colour'd from it, you must let it boil with a little of the dissolv'd Alum, which will wholly curd it, and keep the Lake back.

When the Lake in this Manner is in the Bag, you pour clear Water over it, in order to clear it from the Alum or Salt that might still remain in it, and take a Plate of Plaister o

Put

Paris, or Chalk, pour the Lake through a Paper Cone that has a small opening at the Point, in little Drops or Tents upon it, and when dry, put them up for Use.

You must observe, that in Cafe the Liquid should fall short in boiling the Wool, you must recruit it, not with cold, but with warm Water

If you can get the Sharings of Scarlet Cloath, you will save your self much Trouble, by only boiling them in the Lee, and proceeding is has been directed

Another Method.

TAKE Lee of Ashes or Tartar, to this put a little diffolv'd Alum, and pour it in a wide Glafs Utenfil; then take Cochineal, put it into a clofe Linnen Bag, and swing it backwards and forwards in the Lee, till all the Colour is extracted, then take lukewarm Alum Water, pour as much into the Lee as will curdle it, pour the curdled Lee through a Flannel, fweeten it off with clear Water, then you dry the Colour on a Piece of Plaifter of Paris, as before directed.

To make fine Vermillion

TAKE two Parts of Quickfilver, and one third of Sulpher, put it into a Pipkin, and melt the Sulpher and the Quickfilver together, when it is cold, then grind it well upon a Stone, and put it into a Glafs, which beforehand has been laid over with a Coat of an Inch thick; then make a Coffin of Clay for the Glafs to ftand in, fet this on a Trivet, firft over a flow Fire, put a Cover of Tin, with a little Hole in the Middle upon the Glafs, and lute it all round, put an Iron Wire through the Hole, for to ftir it about, augment your Fire by Degrees, and watch your Glafs carefully, for you will fee feveral colour'd Smoaks proceed from the Matter in the Glafs, but keep on augmenting your Fire, till you fee the Smoak comes out of a red crimfon Colour, then it is enough, take off the Fire, let it cool, and you will have a fine Vermillion

Before you ufe it to paint or write therewith, take as much Vermillion as you will, and grind it well with good White-Wine on a Stone, and after that with the White of Eggs, add a fmall Matter of Aloepatica to it, make it up in little Cakes, and when dry, put them by for Ufe. When you ufe them, grind or dilute them with clear Pump-Water, and a little White of Eggs, and if it will not flow readily from the Pen, mix a little Myrrh among it.

How to purify Vermillion.

THE Vermillion being made of Mercury and Sulpher, the Impurities which it has contracted of thofe Minerals muft be fubftracted, and this is done in the following Manner

Grind the Pieces of Vermilion with Water upon a Stone, and put it on glaz'd Plates to dry, then pour Urin upon it, and mix it thoroughly with it, fo that it may fwim over it, let it thus ftand, and when the Vermillion is fettled, pour off that Urin, and put frefh upon it, let that ftand over Night, repeat this four or five Days fucceffively, till the Vermillion is well cleanfed; then pour the White of Eggs over it, mix it up therewith, and ftir it well together with a Spatula of Nut-Tree, let it ftand again, when fettled pour it off, and put frefh on, repeat this three or four Times, covering your Utenfil every Time clofe, to keep the Duft from falling into it, which elfe would take off the Beau'y of the Colour When you ufe this Vermillion, dilute it with Gum-Water.

Another Method

GRIND the Vermillion with the Urin of a Child, or Brandy, and fet it to dry in the Sun

If you will hive the Vermillion of a high Colour and free from its black Hue, then put into the Brandy or Urin a little Saffron, and grind your Vermillion with it

To make a fine Purple Colour

MELT one Pound of Tin, after which put two Ounces of Quickfilver to it, ftir it fo long together, till it is an Amalgama, then take Sulpher and Sal Armoniac, of each one Pound, grind it fine, and mix it up with the Amalgama, in a Stone Mortar, or wooden Bowl, put it into a Glafs, which is well coated with Clay, fet it firft over a

gentle

gentle Fire, and augment it by Degrees, so as to keep it in one Motion; stir the Matter with a Stick, and when you perceive it to be of a yellow Colour, take off the Fire, and let it cool, and you will have a fine Gold Colour, besides a beautiful Purple

III. Of all Sorts of COLOURS extracted from Flowers, &c

How to extract a Yellow, Blue, Violet, and other Colours

PREPARE a middling sharp Lee out of Lime, and Soda or Pot Ashes, in this boil the Flowers or Leaves of single Colours, over a slow Fire, so long till the Tincture of the Flower is quite extracted, which you may know when the Leaves turn pale, and the Lee is of a fine Colour. This Lee put afterwards in a glaz'd Pipkin or Pan, and boil it a little, putting in some Roach Alum; then pour the Lees off into a Pan with clean Water and you will see the Colour precipitate to the Bottom, let it well settle, then pour that Water off, and pour on fresh, this you repeat till the Tincture is entirely cleans'd from the Lee and Alum, and the freer it is thereof, the finer will be your Colour. The Settlement is a fine Lake, which you spread upon Linnen Cloaths, and lay them on clean Tiles in the Shadow to dry

You may dry your Colours upon a Plate of Plaister of Paris, or for Want of that on a Piece of Chalk, either of them will do better, and dry the Colours quicker than the Method teached before

To the Receipt for extracting the Tinctures out of Flowers, Leaves, Herbs, and Plants, by Distillation, which has been already inserted p 143 I only add, that it will be adviseable to preserve the first Droppings of the Extraction that fall into the Receiver, by themselves, they yielding the finest and most beautiful Colour. Care must be also taken, not to bruise the tender Leaves of the

Flowers

Flowers, elfe the coarfe Juice will diftill along with the Tincture, and make it of an unpleafant Hue. Such Leave that are firm and ftrong, require not that Care.

Mr Kunkel's *Method of extracting the Colours out of Flowers, &c*

I Take, fays he, high rectified Spirit of Wine, which is without any Phlegm, and pour it over a Herb or Flower wch I will, and if the Leaves of Plants are large and coarfe cu them fmall, but I leave the Leaves of Flowers whole, as foon as I perceive the Spirits tinctur'd, I pour it off and put on frefh, when that is tinctured, and I find both Colours of in I quality, I put them toge her, but if the differ, I put each feparate by itfelf, after which I diftil the Spirit of Wine from it, to a very little, fo that I may take it out of the Cucurbit, and then put it into a China Tea Saucer, a Glafs Cup, or a fmall Matrafs, and let it evaporate over a flow Fire till it comes to fome thicknefs, or, if you will, quite dry, but this muft be done very flowly, on Account of the Tendernefs of the Colour.

Some Flowers will change their Colours and produce quite different ones, and this the blue Flowers are moft fubject o, to prevent which, one muft be very flow and careful in diftilling them. I have never had fo much Trouble with any other colour'd Flowers as the Blue ones, and yet, I cannot boaft that I have obtain'd a blue Colour from Flowers to my Satisfaction. The whole Matter depends chiefly upon Care, Practice will be the beft Teacher.

By this Method one may prefently fee what Flowers or Plants are fit for Ufe, for by only infufing fome in a little Spirit of Wine, it will foon fhew what Colours they will produce.

IV. Of Green Colours

How to make good Verdegrease

TAKE sharp Vinegar, as much as you will, clean Copper Flakes, one Pound, three Quarters of a Pound, red Tartar eight Ounces, Sal Armoniac two Ounces, Leven twelve Ounces, but which is to be beaten to a fine Powder, and mix it all with the Vinegar well together, put it into a new well glaz'd Pan, cover it with a Lid, and lute it with Clay, then bury it for 14 or 20 Days in Horse Dung. Take it out again, pour off the Vinegar gently, and you will have good Verdegrease.

Another

TAKE a well glaz'd Pan or Pot, put into it good sharp Vinegar, then take of thin Copper Slips a pretty large Quantity, put them into a Crucible, and let the same into the Pan with Vinegar, so that the Vinegar may not touch the Copper, then lute the Cover well with Clay to keep out the Air; thus put the Pan into Horse Dung, or into a warm Place, for 25 Days, then take it out again, open it, and you will find the Verdegrease hanging to the Copper Slips, scrape the Verdigrease with a Knife off the said Slips, and let it fall into the Vinegar, after which, close up the Pan again as you did before, put it into the Dung or a warm Place, and thus repeat it till the Copper is all consum'd. The Verdigrease will settle at the Bottom of the Pan, which, after you have gently poured off the Vinegar from it, you may put up for Use.

Another easier Method to make Verdegrease.

TAKE a Copper Kettle or Bowl, put into it good sharp Vinegar, set it in the Heat of the Sun to dry, and you will have fine Verdegrease, after you have taken it out of the Kettle or Bowl, you may pour more Vinegar, and repeat it as often as you think proper.

T

To make a fine Verdegreafe for Dyers

FIRST take four Pound of Tartar, two pound of Salt, one pound of Copper-Afhes, one pound and a half of good Vinegar, then take a Crucible or an unglaz'd Pan, take an Handful of Tartar, and fling it into the Crucible, alfo one Handful of Salt, and a Handful of Copper Afhes, fling all in one after another, till the Crucible or Pan is full, then pour on the Vinegar, and ftir it well together, till the Ingredients are thorough wet, and are turned to a black Colour, cover the Pan, and lute it clofe with Clay, to prevent the Air coming to it, put it for a Fortnight or three Weeks in hot Horfe-Dung, and you will have good Verdegreafe. If you will have it dry, hang it up in a Bladder in the Air.

Another Method.

TAKE Vinegar in which has been fteep'd fome Copper, and one Pound of fearc'd Salt, mix the Salt with fo much Vinegar as to make it of a Subftance; then put it into a Copper Veffel, clofe it up, and put it in a damp Place, and after it has ftood fome Days, you will have a good Verdigreafe.

Another Method

TAKE an old Kittle or Copper, and fcour it clean with Sand, then take Vinegar and Honey, of each an equal Quantity, mix it together, and ftrike it all over the Infide of the Kittle, then take fearc'd Salt, and fprinkle it upon the Honey, fo as to ftick to it, have a Board, made with a good many Holes, and cover the Kittle therewith, then turn your Kittle with the Board upon hot Horfe Dung, cover it all over with the Dung, and let it ftand for eight Days together, and you will find a fine Verdegreafe.

A fine Verdegreafe for Limners.

TAKE Copper Slips or Filings, put them into a ftrong Copper-Box, with a Cover to it, pour fome Vinegar mix't up with a little Honey, into it; fet it in the Sun, or in a warm Place for fourteen Days, and the Vinegar will be

turn'd

turn'd Blue, which pour into a Glaſs, and cloſe it well up; then put more Vinegar and Honey upon the Copper-Filings, and proceed as before, till they don't tincture the Vinegar: What you have gather'd up in Glaſſes, put in the Sun or a warm Place, till it becomes of a proper Thickneſs, then grind it on a Stone, and temper it with a little Gum-Water: if you will have it of a Graſs-Green, mix it with a little Sap Green.

How to make Sap-Green

ABOUT a Fortnight or three Weeks before *Michael-mas* take as many Slows as you pleaſe, maſh them a little, and put them into a clean glaz'd Pan, ſprinkle them well over with powder'd Alum, and let them ſtand in a hot Place for 24 Hours, then pour upon them a clear Lee, put it upon a Fire, and give it a ſlow Boiling, ſo long till it has boil'd away a good Quantity, then take it off the Fire, let it cool, and pour it through a Cloath, what comes through it, put up in a Bladder, and hang it in the Air to dry, afterwards keep it always hanging in a dry Place, or in the Chimney-Corner, and when you have occaſion to uſe it, take as much as you want and dilute it with clear Water If it ſhould turn too much upon the Yellow, mix it with a little Indigo.

Another finer Sap Green

TAKE of blue Lilies that Part of the Leaf which is of a fine blue Colour, for the reſt is of no uſe, and ſtamp them well in a Stone-Mortar, then put upon them a Spoonful, or according to the Quantity of the Leaves, two or more Spoonfuls of Water, wherein before has been diſſolv'd a little Alum and Gum-Arabick, and work it well together in the Mortar, then ſtrain it through a Cloath, put it in Muſcle-Shells, and ſet them in the Sun to dry.

Another Method

AFTER you have proceeded as before, fling ſome powder'd Quick Lime over it, before you ſtrain it in a Cloath, and put it up in Muſcle-Shells

A.o ber

Another Method.

BEAT the blue Leaves of Lilies in a Stone Mortar, strain it through a fine Cloath into Muscle-Shells, and fling some powder'd Alum over it, to one more than another, in order to make the Colour of different Shades

To prepare a fine green Colour

TEMPER Indigo and yellow Orpiment with Gum Water, grind it fine, and mix with it a little of Ox o Fish Gall, and you will have a pleasant Green You may shade it with Indigo or Sap Green, and heighten it with *Dutch* Pink.

V. Of WHITE COLOURS.

To make fine White Lead

TAKE some cast Sheet-Lead, cut it into Plates of about two Inches wide, and six or eight Inches long, make thro' each of them a Hole, to draw a String through, then have an oaken Vessel, about two Foot high, into this put two Quarts of good Vinegar, and a Handful of Salt, hang your slitted Leads over the Vinegar in the Vessel, and cover it, set it over a gentle Coal Fire, so long till it is boiling hot, then take it off, and put it for ten Days in a warm Place, then take off the Cover, take out the Leads, which will be covered with a white Colour on both Sides, a Finger's thick, which you scrape off with a Knife, put it into a clean Bason, then hang the Leads again in the wooden Vessel, and proceed as before, scraping the Colour once every ten Days, grind the Colour in a Stone Mortar with clean Water to a Paste, and put it up in clean Pans to dry

Another

Another Method to make White Lead

TAKE long and flat Pieces of Lead, hang them in a glaz'd Pan, or rather in an earthen square Vessel, which is pitch'd the Inside, but before you hang the Lead in the Vessel, pour in it good Vinegar, heated, cover it close, lute it to keep out the Air, and put it in a warm Place for a Month or five Weeks, then take off the Cover, and scrape the White Lead which hangs about the Lead, this you repeat every Fortnight or three Weeks, and you will have good White Lead

To prepare another white Colour

TAKE Quick-Lime, mix with it calcined Egg Shells, grind these two Ingredients with Goat's-milk very fine, and it is fit to paint withal

A good white Colour

TAKE Crown Glass, and beat it to an impalpable Powder, take also fine pulveriz'd Sulpher, mix it together in a Pan with a Cover to it, lute it close, and put it upon a Charcoal Fire, so as to make the Pan red hot all over When it is thus heated, take off the Fire, and let it cool, then take off the Cover, grind the Matter upon a Stone with clear Water, and temper it with either Oil or Gum-Water: It will give a good white Colour

A fine white Colour, for Painting in Miniature

TAKE four Ounces of good Bismuth, and beat it fine; then dilute it in eight Ounces of the best clarified Aqua Fortis, pour the Dissolution into a Glass, and put a little Salt-Water into it, and the Bismuth will precipitate to the Bottom, in a Snow white Powder, pour off the Water, sweeten the Powder well with clean Water from the Sharpness of the Aqua Fortis, then dry it, and keep it carefully from Dust When you use it, dilute it with Gum-Water.

How to refine White Lead extraordinary fine

TAKE fine White Lead, grind it upon a Stone with white-Wine Vinegar, and it will turn black, then take an earthen Dish full of Water, wash your grounded White Lead well, and let it settle, then drain the Water gently from it, grind it once more upon a Stone with Vinegar, and wash it again, this repeat three or four Times, and you will have a curious fine White, that's fit for the nicest Work, both in Oil and Water Colours.

How to prepare the Egg Shells for White

SOAK the Egg-Shells three or four Days in good sharp Vinegar, then wash them in clear Water, dry them in the Heat of the Sun, beat them to a fine Powder, and grind them on a Stone.

IX. Of several BLACK COLOURS.

To burn Lampblack, in order to make it finer, and of a better Colour.

TAKE a Fire-Shovel, hold it so long in the Fire till it is red hot, then fling your Lamp-black upon it, and when it has done smoaking, it is enough

How to make a finer Lampblack than what is ordinarily sold in Colour or Chandler Shops

HAVE a Lamp with a large Wick of Cotton, stor'd plentifully with Oil, fix over the Lamp a Sort of Canopy, made of Tin or Iron, the Smoak which settles to it, sweep off with a Feather, and preserve it from Dust When you use it, temper it with Oil or Gum Water.

To make a Black of Trotter-Bones

TAKE as many Trotter-Bones as you pleafe, burn them in a clean Crucible, and quench them in damp Linnen Rags, grind them with fair Water, before you ufe Gum with it This Black is fit to be mix'd with Lake and Umber for Shades, in Carnation or Flefh Colour.

To make Ivory-Black.

TAKE the Shavings or Rafpings of Ivory, which you may eafily have at the Comb-Makers, mix them up with a little Linfeed Oil, put them into a Pan or Crucible, and lute it clofe, leaving only a little Hole in the Middle of the Cover, fet it in a Coal Fire, and let it ftand till you perceive no more Smoak, then take it off, and fet it in Sand, putting another Pan or Crucible that's entire, over it, when cold, you will have the fineft black Colour that can be prepared.

Another Method to burn Ivory either Black or White.

FILL a Crucible with the Waftes of Ivory, or Harts-Horn, lute it well, and put it in a Fire, and when the Phlegm, Spirit, Oil, and fluid Salts have left them, they will be of a very fine black Colour, but if you keep them longer in the Fire, they will turn as white as Snow.

A Cherry-Stone-Black

FILL a Crucible with Cherry-Stones, cover and lute it well, let them firft dry by Degrees, then burn them to a Coal, afterwards beat them to Powder, and moiften it with Gum Dragrant Water, form it into little Balls, and they are ready to be ufed when Occafion ferves, either for Oil or Water-Colours.

Several

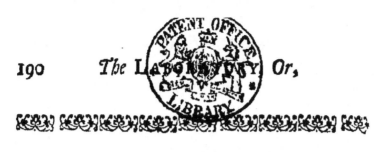

Several Methods of GILDING.

*A particular Way of Gilding, for such Painters or Gilders as are oblig'd to perform it in the open Air
where the Leaf Gold cannot be manag'd, on Account
of the Wind*

TAKE thin Pewter Leaves, strike them over with
Gold Ground, or Gold Size, and when you are
oblig'd to gild any Thing that's high, and you have
no shelter to keep off the Wind, you lay only the Size on
your Work something stronger, in order to make the Pewter gilded Leaves stick on the better

*How to gild upon Wood, Picture Frames, or any other
Sort of Work.*

THE Wood must be first well smooth'd, then twice or
thrice struck over with Size made out of the Shreds o
Glove Leather, and grounded nine or ten Times over with
Chalk, when it is dry, rub it well over with *Dutch*
Rushes, to make it even and smooth, then with a soft Hair
Pencil lay it over with Size Water, after which lay on the
Gold colour'd Ground, twice or three times, when it
is thorough dry, rub it over with a Linnen Rag, till it
looks polish'd, then have your Leaf Gold ready cut upon
Leather Cushion, and when (with a large Pencil, dipp'd in
the strongest Brandy you can get) you have gone over your
Work, be quick to lay on the Gold; when it is quite dry
polish it with a Tooth

How to prepare the Size for the Use just now mention'd

TAKE two Pound of Cuttings or Shreds of white Glove
Leather, let it soak for some time in fair Water, and
then boil it in a Pot with 10 Quarts of Water, let it boil to
two or three Quarts, then strain it through a Cloath into a
clean earthen Pan. You may try whether the Size is strong
enough

enough, by taking a little between your Fingers, to see whether it is of a gluish Substance, and whether it will stick.

To prepare the White Chalk.

WHEN you have made the Size, then take white Chalk, scrape it fine with a Knife, or grind it upon a Stone, and when you have diffolv'd your Size over a Fire, and it is made hot, put in so much Chalk, as will make it of the Substance of a thick Paste, keep it standing for a quarter of an Hour, and then stir it well about with a hard Brush Pencil, add to this White Colour some more Size, and after you have mix'd it well and brought it to a proper Temperature, lay it on your Wood which you design to gild, by daubing it all over with a broad Pencil; and when you have done, let it thoroughly dry, before you lay on another Ground. This you must repeat 10 or 12 Times

When you have done laying on your Gold Ground then with a soft broad hair Pencil, moisten'd with clear Water, go it all over, in order to smooth your Ground, and when dry, rub it over with *Dutch* Rushes, or a Piece of new Linnen, smooth and fine

How to Bronz or Metallize Images of Plaister of Paris.

TAKE Isinglass, steep it in very strong Brandy, put it well closed in the Warmth, and it will dissolve, add to it a little Saffron, and mix it up with Metal Powder in a Muscle or Oyster shell, this strike over your Image with a soft Hair Pencil, but before you do this, you must first strike it over with Size-Water, mix'd with a little Red Lead.

How to prepare the Northern Metal Powder of mix'd Colours, which gives a beautiful Lustre when strew'd upon Writings or Letters

TAKE the Filings of Copper, Brass, Iron, Steel, or any other Metal, serce it through a fine Sieve, and put it into a clean Bason or such like Utensil, wash it well with a clear and sharp Lee, and when you have pour'd that off, wash it with clean Water, so long till you have cleans'd it from all its Soil

After

After your Filings are thus cleans'd and dry, then take a smooth Plate, either of Iron or Copper, lay it upon live Coals, and put one Sort of the Filings upon the Plate, stirring it continually about with an Iron Spatula As soon as the Metal is touch'd with the Heat, it changes into varieties of Colours, and that which suffers the greatest Heat, will contract the darkest Colour, each Metal a different Sort

When you thus have done one Sort, proceed in the same Manner with another, by which means you will have varieties of Colours.

Then take a Platting-Mill, such as the Silver Wire Drawers use, or those who are employ'd in plating of Gold, Silver or Copper Plate, which must be fitted with a Sort of Funnel a-top, through which the Filings may be convey'd to the Platting Rolls, which ought to be very exact and parallel to each other, made of the finest Steel, and polish'd like a Looking Glass. When you are thus prepared, work it with Carefulness between the Rolls, and you will have a most beautiful Powder, which sparkles with all manner of Colours.

The Filings of Brass produce a bright Gold Colour , the Copper a fine red Fire Colour, Iron and Steel all manner of Shades of Blue, Pewter, Marcasit, and Bismuth, produce a white Colour.

To spot a White Horse with Cole black Spots.

TAKE Letharge three Ounces, Quicklime six Ounces, beat it fine and mix it together , put it into a Pan, and pour a sharp Lee over it, then boil it, and you will have a fat Substance swim a-top, with which anoint the Horse in such Places you design to have black, and it will turn to that Colour immediately

It has the same Effect in changing Hair that's red into a black Colour, with only this Difference, *viz* Take an equal Quantity of Lime and Letharge, and instead of boiling it with Lee, boil it only with fresh Water; what swims a top, is fit for Use, and will answer your Expectation; what Hairs you anoint with it in the Evening, will be black the next Morning.

How

How to dapple a Horse.

TAKE in the Spring the large Buds of young Oak-Trees, mix it among the Horse's Provender, and give it him three or four times to eat, and he will be appled, and continue so a whole Year, the Buds of young Elm Trees will have the same Effect

PART VII.

Of the Nature and Growth of SALTPETER.

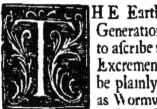THE Earth being naturally inclin'd for the Generation of Saltpeter, there is no Occasion to ascribe the Growth thereof to the Urin and Excrements of certain Animals; for this may be plainly seen in some particular Vegetables, as Wormwood, &c. which although it grows in such Places, where there has been none of such Excrement and Urin, when the Juice thereof is pressed out, will of itself shoot into Saltpeter, as is often experienced by Apothecaries and Chymists However, it must not be disown'd that the Urin and Excrements, particular that of Sheep, contributes not a little to the Growth thereof.

Saltpeter is of such an increasing Nature, that whatever Place is once impregnated therewith, its Ferments are multiplied to Admiration, and like unto a little Acid or Bitter, will diffuse its Qualities among a large Quantity. Whosoever considers this, will easily conjecture how to assist Nature in the Growth of Saltpeter Even ocular Demonstration will prove this, for if one only takes a Silver Calx that's taken out of Aqua Fortis, and puts it into a glaz'd Earthen Plate, and therein sweetens it

O   with

with clear Water, one will find that the Trifle of Spirit of Nitre which remain'd in the Calx, and is drawn from it by washing it in clear Water, impregnates the Earthen Plate fo, that although the moft remairs in the Water, yet it ferments in fuch a Manner, that in a little Time it grows all over and out of the Plate, and caufes the Glafing to fcale and fall off.

We know, that when Aqua Fortis is ftilled of common Salt, the Dreggs thereof will turn into good burning Saltpeter; and more, if for Example you diffolve common Salt in Aqua Fortis or Spirit of Nitre, warm, and let it afterwards to ftand in the cold, it will fhoot into Saltpeter. From which fundamental Experiments one might try a Fermentation, whereby Saltpeter might be in greater Quantity generated, as indeed fome, not without good Succefs, have made Attempts that Way, and that in different Methods. Some have affifted the Saltpetre Earth, after it has been boiled out, with trifling Means, that in a fhort Time the Earth has grown rich thereof again, which was, by mixing the Earth, when laid up again, with the Skimming of what was boiled out.

Others dig one or more large Pits in the Earth, and with the Earth flung up, wall it round, for to prevent the Floods of Rain running into it, for which Reafon they cover it alfo with a Roof, to keep it from Rain, but leave it open to receive the Sun Beams and the Air, without Interception. In fuch Holes they fling all their Sweepings, Afhes of which Lee has been made, as well as others that feem ufelefs, the Remains or Afhes of burnt Straw, Soot out of Chimnies, the Sweepings of Poultries, Pidgeon-Houfes, all Sorts of bitter and fharp Vegetables, as Wormwood, Wolfs-Milk, Nettles, Flee-Grafs, Sea Beans, the fallen Fruit in Autumn, or rotten Fruit, the Excrements of Men and Beafts, and any Dung, the Outcafts from Slaughter-Houfes, as Hair, Claws, Horns, the Paunch with Dung, Guts and Blood, all Manner of Urin, Suds that have been ufed in wafhing, and the like, till the Pit is full, there let it rot for fome Years, daily flinging upon it Urin, Brine of Herrings or Meat and fuch like, till it is rotten, then they ceafe from flinging any Moifture upon it, and let it lie dry, till they boil the Saltpeter out of it, then they fling the Remains again into the Pit, pouring upon it the Liquor that will not fhoot, and fo let it lie a confiderable Time before they boil it again.

Others

Others have built particular long Vaults under Ground, about three Yards deep, cover'd with Boards or with Roof of Pantiles The Mortar for it is prepared of three Parts Lime, flackened with Rain Water, which has fell with a North Wind, Sheeps Urin one Part, Sheeps Dung three Parts, all well beat together, and mix'd with common Salt, with this the Vault is built up two Bricks thick, then covered with old Stable Dung, every Fortnight, in the Increale of the Moon, it is water'd all over with North Wind Rain Water, and Sheeps Urin, and the Saltpetre has flooted out in the Vaults in Foffils

Another Method for the speedy Growth and Increase of Saltpetre is used, by building a Shed of Deal Boards, as large as one pleales or has Conveniency for, but if possible, in a Place where it may lay open to the four Winds, the Roof is either boarded or thatch'd, but the four Sides are left open Under this Shed a Lay of Earth is laid, about a Foot high, in four different Heaps, then is poured over it Brine of Salt, Lime mixt with the Urin of Men and Beasts, over this is laid another Lay of Earth, and proceeded as directed before, repeating it till the Shed is near full, and working each Heap gradually tapering up in the Form of a Roof, so that the Wind may the easier penetrate into each Heap, then laying a Coat of Earth over it, the Salt and other Liquids are pour'd over it again After these four Heaps have stood a Month, they are every third or fourth Day after the new Moon rak'd up with an Iron Rake, about a Foot deep, and moistened with Urin and Saltpetre Water, or Dung Lee, which is pour'd on out of a watering Pot. After these Heaps, thus prepared, have stood about four Months, they will be twice as rich of Saltpetre as common Saltpetre Earth, and may be boiled out every Quarter of a Year The boiled out Earth is laid up again under the Shed, work'd up as before, and whilst the last Heap is boiling out, the first is in its Bloom again, and encreales in Riches more and more, so that after a few Boilings, it may be boil'd out every Month The Conveniency, Dispatch, and Proftablenels of this Saltpetre-Work will require to have the Boiling-House in the Middle of the four or more Heaps, but then the Roof of the Shed should not be thatched, for Fear of an Accident· There may be (if the Shed is fill'd with large Heaps) four Coppers fix'd in the Boiling-House, and so contrived that one Fire may serve them all.

I shall

I shall here present the Reader with a Scheme for a Saltpeter Garden, which was form'd by *Cardil,* and use his own Direction, which is thus

Build a Vault about 60 or 80 Yards in Length, or according to what Room you have to spare, four Yards high, and
eight broad, on a firm Ground, let there be two Doors, the one
towards the North and the other towards the South, and dress
the Top of this Vault like a Garden; at one End whereof have
a little House for a Labourer to live in, who is to look after the
Saltpetre Work, and water the Garden every other or third
Day, when the Moon is encreasing, the Water he must save
beforehand of a South or North Wind Rain, which is best,
and mix it with Urin of Men, Horses, Oxen, Cows, Sheep,
&c flinging into it several Handful of common Salt, and stirring
it well together In the Winter Season, when there is hard
Frost and Snow, the Vault must be shelter'd with Boards, and
a little Charcoal Fire kept in it, leaving both Doors open,
but this is only to be observed in very hard Winters When
the Vault is thus finished and attended, the Owner thereof
will in six or nine Months time find the Saltpetre shoot out
in great Quantities, and the oftner the Fossils are broke off,
and the Garden nourish'd by watering, the more it will en
crease in Growth. It is not to be expressed of what Benefit
such a Work is, both for himself and his Generation or Suc
cessors

The Floor and Foundation of the Vault must be ram'd
down hard and close; the Side Walls, half an Ell thick, may
be built up with Pebble, Brick, or any other Stone, but the
Arch of the Vault must be done with Bricks, prepar'd in this
Manner Take the Earth for Bricks, work it up with North
or South Rain-Water, and Urin, of which you must have
a sufficient Quantity ready beforehand, with this, work and
form your Bricks, and burn them like other common Bricks
For Example Take 12 Barrels of Brick-Earth, four of Lime,
two of Salt, one of Saltpetre, all these well work'd together,
moulded and burn'd as usual

For the Mortar wherewith the Bricks of the Arch of the
Vault are joined together, you take four Barrels of Clay, four
of Lime, one of Salt, one half of Saltpetre, and half a Barrel
of Sheeps Dung, all well work'd together, and pour'd over
with the above Rain-Water and Urin, and temper'd to a proper Thickness for Mortar In the Middle of the Vault, let

an

an Opening be made, raifed like a Funnel, and fecured with Iron Bars at Top. After the Vault is thus built and inclofed, you raife a Ground over it about three Quarters of a Yard high, with common putrified Earth, but if it can be mix'd with Excrements or Stable Dung, it is better. This will be fufficient for the ingenious Adventurers to improve upon.

Another Method for furthering the Growth of Saltpetre, is the following.

FIRST erect Sheds, each of four Pofts, nine or ten Foot high, of a proportionable Thicknefs, fix Foot diftant from each other, faften'd with Joices, and thatch'd a top. When your Sheds are ready, lay fat black Earth, about a Foot high, upon a Level, then fling the following Mixture, about three Inches thick, upon it, which is thus: Take Salt 12 Pound, Saltpetre four Pound, Quick Lime 12 Pound; this well beaten and work'd together, is fit for Ufe.

After you have covered the firft Lay of Earth with this Mixture, then rake it well together with the Earth, and when done, pour over it Dung Lee and Urin, out of a Gardners Watering Pot, then rake and wet it again a fecond time.

After this, proceed thus with another Lay of a Foot high, fo as to go up tapering, one Lay after another, till it is about fix Foot high; then coat it all over with Sheeps Dung.

You muft obferve to begin this Work with the new Moon, and after your Heap has ftood three or four Nights, rake it all afunder, and proceed as you did at firft, this you muft do in the time of the Increafe three or four times, and repeat it for three Months together: In the Decreafe of the Moon you let it reft, and after the three Months are expired, you will have a very rich Saltpeter Earth.

Every Shed or Heap muft be at leaft eight Feet Diftance from one another, for the Benefit of the Air. After you have feveral of thofe Sheds brought to Perfection, you may boil Saltpetre fucceffively, for before you have done with three or four Heaps, the firft of them will be ready again to boil, before the fourth is done, and your Earth, the more and oftner it is boil'd, will grow the richer.

N B For Watering the Earth, you may, if it can be got, ufe the Pickle of Herrings, or other Salt-Liquors, Soap-

Lees

Lee after Cloaths are wash'd in, also Alum and other Liquors that are flung away by Dyers. You must also observe, to lay a Coat of Sheeps Dung over your Heaps every time you have railed them.

Glouser, in his Book, intitled *The Wellfare of Germany,* when he treats of the Growth of Saltpeter, and the Benefit it yields to many poor Families, expresses himself in this Manner.

' In the third Chapter of the first Part, about Concentring
' of Wood, the Pressing of Wood to boil Saltpeter, is only
' mention'd, but as Wood is not plenty every where, and
' as it cannot in many Places be spared, to cut it down for
' boiling Saltpetre out of it, it may be brought to bear that
' a large Quantity of Saltpetre may be produced out of the
' sided Leaves of Trees, as also out of wild Grass that
' grows under Trees, so as to have no occasion to cut
' Trees down on that Account. And in such Places where
' there is a Scarcity of Wood, but a Plenty of Corn, Salt
' peter may be prepared out of Straw and Stubble,
' and there is not a Place in the World which does not afford
' Matter for the Produce of Saltpetre. Wherefore I cannot
' neglect to communicate to all good and pious Husband
' men a valuable Art, by which they may provide and lay
' up a hidden Treasure (which Thieves cannot steal) for
' their Children, and for a Relief to themselves in time of
' Distress, thereby reflecting upon God's Providence, and
' remembring their Tutor. For as in the said Treatise
' I have taught three choice Secrets, both for rich and poor,
' great and mean, but they being useless to those who have
' neither Wine, Corn, nor Wood; I have thought it good,
' not to be forgetful of those who are destitute of either, and
' are yet willing to provide for their Wife and Children,
' with Honesty in the Fear of God, to teach them a benefi-
' cial Art, hoping it will attend to the Glory of God, and
' their own Advantage.

' First, then shall a young Beginner have God before
' his Eyes, and admonish his Wife and Children (if he has
' any) to fear God, keep his Commandments, and love their
' Neighbour. Then shall he determine within himself,
' to manage his Fortune left him by his Parents, or which
' he had with his Wife, with such Caution, Care and Fru
' gality, so as not to diminish, but to increase it every Year,

' that

' that when God fhould vifit him with Sicknefs, or a Charge
' of Children, he may have fomething laid by for a rainy
' Day Befides this, he ought not to lay his Hands in his
' Lap, but turn them early and late to labour, and look for
' the Blefling of God in his Endeavours And to fuch as
' have had but a flender Fortune of their Parents, I give
' them a Leffon, in what Manner they may lay up a
' Treafure for their Children, without much Trouble or
' Pains

' In the firft Place, let him build a Shed North Eaft of his
' Houfe or Habitation, if it can be done conveniently, elfe
' at any other Place, fo that the Sun and Air may come at
' it, but the Rain be kept out, in which Shed make a deep
' Pit, with the Earth which is flung up, wall it in to
' keep out the Rain-Water After this he fha'l begin to
' gather from Day to Day, from Year to Year the below
' fpecified Things, fo long and as much till one time or
' other, in Cafe of Neceffity, he is obliged to dig for them,
' and to fee what God has provided for him, and then reap
' the Benefit thereof

' The Things he is to fling in, are all Sorts of fharp and
' bitter Plants, which grow in uncultivated Places, Hedges,
' and Paths, and are no benefit to Cattle, fuch as are the
' Thiftles, Wormwood, the large Stalks of Tobacco, which
' (if they are planted) are flung away, alfo the hard Cab-
' bage Stalks and Leaves, and other Things unfit for Cattle to
' feed upon, Pine Apples, if they are to be had, and in
' Autumn the Leaves of Trees, alfo Pidgeons and Henns
' Dung, and the Dung of any other Creature If you can
' have Feathers of Poultry and wild Birds, fling them in;
' fling alfo in all the Afhes whereof Lee has been made,
' and fit for nothing but to be flung away, alfo the Chimney
' Soot, and from the Slaughters the Blood, if not ufed for
' any thing elfe, Hogs Hair, Horns and Shoes of Oxen
' and Cows, the Bones which the Dogs can't eat, fave
' them and fling them in the Pit, and not only the Out-
' caft and Scraps that are made in thy own Houfe, but alfo
' (to have the Pit the fooner full) thofe of thy Neighbours,
' if they have no ufe for it themfelves, and thus one may in
' one or two Years time fill a large Pit with fuch Things:
' In the mean while the Urin in the Houfe muft be faved,
' and flung into that Place, and if you can alfo have it from

' your

' your Neighbours for that Purpofe, it is good, for thofe
' Things in the Pit fhould be kept always moift, in order to
' caufe them the fooner to rot. If you can have no Urin,
' take common Water or Dung Lee, but if you can have
' Sea Water or any other Salt-Water, it is better · One may
' befpeak at the Fifhmongers the Pickle of Herrings, alfo
' the Brine of Salt Meat; for all the Brine wherein Meat
' has lain, turns to Saltpeter

' When you have fill'd the Pit full, and it is well putrified,
' wet it no more, but let it lay fo long till all is dry   Then
' if you have occafion for Money, look out for a Saltpetre
' Boiler, and bargain with him what you fhall give him to
' lee, boil, and fell your Saltpeter.   When he has done
' this, let the Saltpeter Earth that's boil'd out, be flung
' again into the Pit, with the Lee which did not fhoot to
' Saltpeter, and let it lay one or two Years, and pour fome-
' times fome Urin on it, or for Want of that, common Wa-
' ter; for that Earth will yield Saltpeter again, tho' not
' fo much as it did the firft time

' But if you have no need for Money, then let that Trea-
' fure lay, and as often as it is dry, moiften it, to make
' the Saltpeter grow and increafe more and more ; and thus
' you gather a hidden Treafure, and hardly know which
' way you come by it · If you do not want it, your Children
' will find it, Thieves will not rob you thereof, nor will
' the Plunderers in time of War carry it along with them
' When you have fill'd one Pit, you may make another next
' to it, to prevent the above fpecified Things from being
' flung away in Wafte, and if in every Village there were
' but one that would do this, the Produce in a fmall Country
' would amount to a furprifing Quantity in a Year, for the
' Service of the Publick, and there would never be Want of
' Saltpetre

' As foon as the Saltpeter is ready, your Money is ready,
' and Gold and Silver not far off   This mind, and be ad-
' vifed, you will furely grow once wife, and fee how blind
' you and your Equals have been But praife God firft, and
' be ferviceable to your Neighbour, for God has given it
' me, I give it you, give alfo fomething to your Neighbour,
' and we are all help d ".

How to cleanse Saltpeter.

PUT the Saltpeter into a Pot or Crucible, set it on a good Coal Fire, till it is diſſolv'd like Water. Then fling on one Pound, about the Bigneſs of a Nut, of coarſe pulveriz'd Sulpher, and it will flame, when this with the Smoak is vaniſh'd, then pour the Saltpetre into an Iron flat Pan, and let it congeal, which it ſoon will do, and looſes nothing, you may take an Earthen Diſh for this uſe, and pour the melted Saltpetre out of the Iron Pan into it by ſlow Degrees, letting it ſettle to the Diſh round about, for which end you may have one that keeps the Diſh in due motion to receive the Saltpeter, beginning in the middle, and ſo let it ſpread in a circular Form. The Settlings in the Iron Pan will be of a reddiſh Hue and impure, which boil and take from it what is ſerviceable.

A quick Cleanſing of Saltpeter.

IF one is in Haſte to have a quantity of Saltpetre cleanſed either for Aqua Fortis or any other Work, let him make a ſtrong Lee, and diſſolve the Saltpeter over a Fire in a Kettle, when all is diſſolv'd, pour the Solution through a coarſe Cloath into a Veſſel, , then rinſing the Kettle, boil it again ſo long till it is fit for ſhooting, then pour it into a Copper Pan, and the clear Saltpeter will ſhoot in Cryſtal, and the Salt remain in the Lee.

Another Way to cleanſe Saltpeter.

TAKE Saltpeter, as much as you will, pour freſh Water to it as much as is requiſite for its Solution, let it boil till all is diſſolv'd, and a great Scum raiſed. Then have a Tub at hand, which has a Hole at Bottom, under this let another Tub, at the Bottom of the firſt Tub put clean waſh'd Sand, about ſix Inches high, and over that a Linnen Cloath, upon this pour the warm Lee, and let it run off, and the Feces and common Salt will be kept back in the Cloath and Sand. When it has done running, pour it again into the Kettle, boil it, as much as is requiſite to coagulate it, pour it out in Troughs or Copper Pans as before, and the Cryſtal will ſhoot in two or three Days much finer and cleaner, theſe gather, the remaining Lee put again to boil; the oftner this is repeated, the cleaner will be the Saltpeter. A. other

Another Way to cleanse Saltpetre from all hurtful Matters

TAKE two Pound of Quick-Lime, one Pound of
Verdegreafe, one Pound of Roman Vitriol, one Pound
of Sal Armoniac, beat it all to Powder, and mix and put it
together, then put it into a wooden Veffel, pour on it as
much Vinegar as is fufficient to make a Solution, or for
want of Vinegar you may ufe clear Water, let it turn into Lee
and fettle for three Days, then put the Saltpetre into the
Copper, and as much of the forefaid Lee as will cover it,
boil it over a flow Fire, till it is half confum'd, what remains take out of the Copper, and put it in another Veffel,
the Fæces at the bottom fling away, let the Saltpetre Lee
cool, and proceed as has been directed before.

Another Method to purge Saltpetre after the firft Cleanfing,
by Thurnifer

PUT into a clean Tub fifted Beech Afhes, pour frefh
Water upon it, ftir it well with a ftirring Stick together, and let it fettle, then pour the firft Water off, and
pour frefh Water to the fettled Afhes, ftir this as before,
let it fettle, and repeat this fo long and often till the Lee
is fmooth and ftrong enough, which you may learn by pala-
ting a little of it on your Torgue.

Then take the once cleanfed Saltpetre, put it into a clean
Copper, pour on it the Afh Lee about a Hand high above the
Saltpetre, and meafure the Depth with any Stick or Rod to
the Bottom, then make a Fire underneath, and boil it, when
it boils, take the Scum off with a fcumming Ladle, but let the
Lee be well drain'd from it, to prevent Wafte, and when it
has boil'd fo much away as the Lee was above the Saltpetre, which you may infpect into by your Rod or Meafure,
then drop from your Ladle a few drops upon live Coals, and
if it gliftens and burns a blue Flame, it has boil'd enough,
but if you don't fee this, then it is not boil'd enough, and
you muft keep on boiling it till it gives a blue Fire. Then
take a clean Veffel, that's not too deep nor too fhallow,
place it where it may be cool, fpread over it a double or
treble Cloath that's clean, through this pour your boil'd
Saltpetre into the Veffel, then cut fome Splinters of Fir
about

about a Span long, lay them crofs one another in the Vef-
fel, and the Saltpetre will fhoot to them like Ificles, this
Saltpetre changes its Name, and is call'd Saliter, or refin'd
Saltpetre

To try Saltpetre whether it is good.

LAY a little Saltpetre upon an even clear Table, light
it with a Coal, if it crackles like common Salt when put
into the Fire, it is a Sign that it has much common Salt, if
it gives a fat and thick Scum, it fhews that it is full of Greafinefs, when the Saltpetre is burn'd, and there remain Fœces,
it is a Sign that it contains much Earth, but when it gives a
quick Flame, and many fparks, and the Table remains
without any Fœces, and burns like a clean Coal without Scum
or cracking, it is clear. Alfo, if after the fecond boiling
there is but four Pound out of a hundred diminifh'd, it is a
Sign the Saltpetre is good.

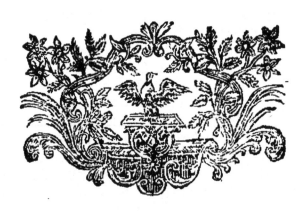

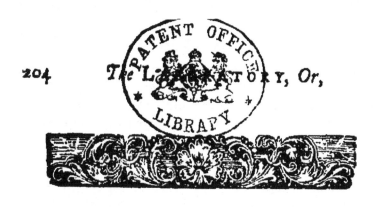

PART VIII.

Several Choice CURIOSITIES

I

Of the Regeneration of Plants

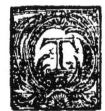

TAKE of any Plant the Seed, which has been gathered in a bright and clear Day, to the Quantity of four Pound. This beat in a Glass Mortar, and put it in a Phial, close it well up, and set it by in a warm Place. When this is done, choose a fine Evening in the Month of *May*, and prepare to catch the Dew you see is likely to fall that Night. Take the Seed out of the Phial, put it in a large earthen Dish, place that in a Garden or Field in the open Air, and in order to catch more Dew than what will fall into the Dish, you may hang some very clean Linnen Cloaths about the Gardens or Fields, and gather the Dew to the Quantity of two Gallons, by wringing it out of the Linnen, put all your Dew in a clean Glass, and the Seed which has been moistened therewith put, before the Sun rises, again into the Phial, close it well up, to keep it from evaporating, and put it to its former Place. You filter gathered Dew thro' a whited-brown Paper, and then distill it so often till you see it free from all earthly Particles; the Settling calcine, and you will have a fine Salt, which is presently dissolv'd in the distill'd Dew. Of this with Salt pregnated Dew, pour so much in the Phial upon the Grain, as will cover it three Fingers high a top. Then seal it with beaten Glass and Borax, put it into a warm damp Place, or in Horse-Dung for a Month, and after the Expiration thereof, you will, by examining the Phial, find the Seed change into a Jelly, and the Spirit thereof swim a top

like

like a Fleece of feveral Colours   Between the Fleece and the
clayifh Earth you will fee the Dew, which is pregnated by the
Seed, and is united to its Nature, refemble a green Grafs:
Thefe Phials well feal'd, hang throughout the whole Summer
in the Day-time in the Sun, and at Night in the Moon, but if
it fhould rain, then fet it in a warm and dry Place, till the
Heavens are clear again, and then put it again in the open Air.
It fometimes happens that this Work is accomplifh'd in two
Months time, and fometimes it will require a whole Year,
according to the Weather

The Marks or Signs by which one may know that it is come
to its Perfection, are thefe   The flimy Water at Bottom fwel-
leth up, the Spirit, together with the Fleece, daily diminifhes,
and altogether grows thick and troubled, then you fee in the
Glafs, when the Sun Beams reflect upon, innumerable delicate
Atoms arifing, yet very tender and without Colour, much like
Cobwebs, and like Shades of the growing Plant, but fall fud-
denly, as foon as the Sun withdraws its Beams from it   At
laft the flimy nafty Matter at Bottom changes into a whitifh
blue Afh, out of which by Degrees fhoot out Stalks, that
branch themfelves out in Plants and Bloffoms, in the Nature
of the Seed ufed for this Experiment, and this Phoenomen is
obferv'd only in warm Weather, but in cold Weather it is invi-
fible, fo long till it comes to be warm again   It will retain
this Quality as long as the Bottle is kept whole

A fine Curiofity to make Metals vifibly to grow.

CALCINE fine white and tranfparent Pebble-Stones, by
firft glowing them red hot, and quenching them in Water, this repeat till you have reduc'd them to a fine Powder. Of
this take one Part, and two Parts of Tartar, which has been
reduced by Saltpetre, put it in a clean Crucible in Fufion,
when cold beat it fine, ftrew it upon a Glafs Table or Marmor,
and let it in a moift Place flow to an Oil, or rather Liquid

Of this Liquid take about four, five, or fix Ounces, put it in
a white Phial, add to it a Dram and a half of metalline Calx,
which has been diffolv'd in Aqua Fortis, then let it to the Confiftence of the Calx evaporate, let this ftand, and when cold,
you will fee the Metal grow, and branch out in Twigs of
different Colours, according to the Calx you have put in.

N. *B.* It

N B. It is to be observ'd, that the Cause of this Growth is the volatile Acid meeting with a fix'd Alcali, we may conclude this from the following Experiment Take Quick Lime and common Salt, calcine this together to an Alcali, fling it on barren Ground, and it will make it fertile, and cause Vegetables to grow and thrive thereon, by contracting the Alcali, the Acid, the Air, and the volatile Salt.

You dissolve Iron in Spiritus Salis, and abstract the Spirit from it till it is dry, and there remains a fiery Red Mass, of this break about the Bigness of a Pea, put it into the before describ'd Liquid in a Phial, and in few Hours you will see a Tree in full Growth, of a dark brown Colour Gold for such Experiments is dissolv'd in Aqua Regis, the other Metals, as Silver, Copper, Tin and Lead, are reduc'd by Aqua Fortis. The Gold will produce a Growth of a yellow Colour, Silver a Blue, Copper a Green, Tin and Lead a white Colour

This affords a fine Speculation, particularly to those who delight in the Study of Mineral Productions

Cerescentia Lunæ, *or the Philosophical Lunar Tree*

THE Nature of the Growth and Increase of Silver Oar may visibly be demonstrated by the following Representation Take clean settled Aqua Fortis six Ounces, dissolve therein two or three Ounces of fine corned or beaten Silver, pour after this three times as much clean Rain-Water on; in this Solution you put to one Ounce of Silver, three or four Ounces of purified Mercury, let it stand undisturb'd in the cold, and you will plain and distinctly see, how by the Help of the Spirit of Tartar or Nitre in the Aqua Fortis, the Silver and Mercury work conjunctive, and form Varieties of pleasant Vegetables, Prospects of Hills, Rocks and Vallies This Manner is supposed to be the Beginning of the Growth of Metal Oar in the Mines.

Of Mines, *and how to discover them*

HUMAN Life would certainly have enjoy'd more Innocence and Satisfaction, were it not for the Riches and Lustre which Nature dazzles their Eyes with, and makes them indefatigable Searchers, into the innermost Recesses of the Earth, to her hidden Treasure.

Tho'e

Thofe fubterraneous Treafures, are difcovered feveral
Ways·

1. When after great Floods of Rain the Current in the
feveral Channels wafhes and difcovers the Veins of Oar
which Nature had concealed with Earth, as happen'd for-
merly at *Freyburg* in *Saxony*

2 Sometimes Metal Oars are difcovered after a great
Storm, when thereby Trees are tore up by the Roots, that
grew on the Surface of Gold or Silver Veins

3 *Juftinus* relates, that *Galicia* was very rich of Copper
and Lead, and *Baramaus* of Gold, and that it has often h ip-
pened that Husbandmen in plowing their Land, have plov ed
up Pieces of Gold Oar, and thereby difcovered the Mines
thereof   Nay, it frequently happens that Mines are difcovered by digging of Wells

4 *Diodorus Sicculus* mentions, that through the Fire the
Shepherds made in the Woods in *Spain*, the like Mines were
difcovered

5 It is reported for certain, that the Lead Mines at *Gof-
lar*, a City in Lower *Saxony*, were firft difcovered by a Horfe
beating his Hoof againft a Lead Oar, and the like has happen'd with Swine, in routing up the Ground, when they
fearch'd for Acorns.

But all thefe are Accidences   It is therefore better to have
certain Rules to direct one to the Difcovery of fuch Mines;
which indeed are beft learn'd by long Experience; however, thofe that have been obferv'd, are the following

1 When on the Surface of the Earth, Pieces of Oar of
ripe Metal are found, it is a certain Sign that Veins of Oar
are there.   By this was the rich Mine at *Kuttenburg* in *Bohemia* difcover'd, a Friar walking there for Pleafure in
a Wood, found a little Twig of Silver, which fprung
out of the Ground, he was fo careful as to cover the Place
with his Cloak, and carry the good News to his Convent

2 When a white Froft is all over the Country, there will
be none over the mineral Veins, becaufe they fend up fuch
Drought and warm Fumes as hinders the Froft, and for this
Reafon Snow fooner melts in thofe Places than in others.

3. It is a certain Sign that Minerals are found in fuch
Places where the Shrubs and Trees are obferv'd to fade by
the latter End of the Spring, become fpotty, and of a reddifh
Colour.

4 A

4 A Hill, the Foot whereof towards the North, and the Top towards the West, holds for the most part Silver Oar, the Silver inclining from West to North

5 By carefully examining into the Colour of the Earth, one may conjecture whether there are mineral Oars And the Colour of the mineral Earth will shew what Metal it carries, a Greenish Earth denotes Copper, Black gives good Hope to Gold and Silver, but the Gray and White for none but Iron or Lead

6 Dry, barren, and as it were, burn'd up Hills, contain all some Metal, because all the hurtful Vapours that fume out of the mineral Veins, dry up the Plants

7. When Stones or Earth are heavier then ordinary, it is a Sign of mineral Veins.

8. The Springs at the Bottom of Hills often discover Mines, either by their Colour, Smell or Taste, or by carrying some small metallick Substance, whereby one may perceive that there are mineral Veins

9. Some, but not many Plants and Trees which have a Sympathy with Metals, grow commonly over Oar Mines, and give thereby notice for the Discovery of them, as Juniper, wild Figs, and most Plants of a prickly Growth When Hills are always covered with Vapours and Smoak, it is a Sign that there are Metal Veins.

These are the Directions which are followed by such as are in Search after mineral Oar, as they are set down by *Agricola, Cardano, Glauber,* and *Kircher* This last Author proceeds thus " Lastly we must let it rest here that all the Knowledge " in Discovery of Mines here mentioned, are only founded on " weak Foundations, and that there is none of those supposed " Marks. whereby one can be sure and certain, after you have " discovered the Place that contains Oar, neither what Quan- " tity, nor what Kind it holds, for those Signs will direct as " well to Sulpher, Antimony, Salt, Mercury, Lead, Iron, " Copper, Tin, as to Silver and Gold But by Virtue of the " Winchel-Rod, one may with Confidence distinguish the one " from the other, and know what Kind of Oar the Mines con- " tain, for by holding in each Hand a Piece of Gold, the " Rod who thereby contracts the Atoms of the Gold, will " beat or move to no other Metal, with Silver it will be the " same. As those who profess themselves Possessors of that " Art, affirm "

How to search for, and to find Springs.

VITRUVIUS, in his Book of Architecture, takes Notice of the following Experiments, used in his Time to
discover Springs, *viz.* 1 If one will certainly know where
Water is to be found, he should a little before Sun-rising lie flat
upon his Belly, and rest his Chin upon the Ground, looking
round about him, and if he sees at any Place a rising Vapour
or Fog, in such Place he may be assur'd of Water. 2. In
looking for Springs, one ought well to examine the Condition
of the Earth, because in certain Places you have several Sorts:
The Water that's found in Chalky Grounds, is neither plenty,
nor of a good Taste, that which is discovered under a light
Sand, after you have bestow'd much Labour in digging deep
enough for it, will be very little, and thereby slimy and disagreeable, black Earth contains the best Water, because the
Rain, which falls in the Winter Season, soaks best into such
Earth, and (on account of its Closeness) preserves Water better than spungy Earth. Springs that are in dark Gravel, and
those not far from Rivers, are also very good, tho' they
afford no great Plenty, but those in coarse Gravel, Pebble, or
other Stone are more certain, and the Water very good. Springs
in red Sand are also good and strong, because the Water is not
suck'd up like in Stone Quarries. Those at the Bottom of
Hills, between Rocks and Stones, are the best, freshest, and
most wholesome. Springs in Vallies are black, heavy, faint,
and disagreeable, except they have their Source at some Distance under the Earth, or run through some shady Grove of
Trees whereby they are made agreeable and pleasant; as is
observ'd by such as spring out in the Vallies near Hills.

Besides the 'fore-mentioned Methods, there are others whereby one may conjecture the proper Place to dig for Springs;
namely, where-ever are seen (growing by themselves) small
Rushes, Willows, and such Plants which thrive no where else
than in watery Places, it is a Sign there is Water underneath
them, but this is only to be observ'd in Places that are free from
Pools, otherways Rain-Water may gather and occasion the
Growth of such Plants, without the help of any Springs. But
if one cannot come at these Trials, the following may be ventured
upon, *viz.* Dig a Hole, three Foot wide, and three or four Foot
deep, after Sun-set; then take a Copper or Leaden Bason, Dish,
Cup, or what you will, anoint the Inside with Oil, and let it on

P

the

the Bottom of the Hole, with the Infide downwards, then fill the Hole with Leaves of Trees, and over them Earth The next Day when you take up your Bafon, and you find Drops of Water hang the Infide thereof, it is a fure Sign, there is Water in that Place.

Or, put an earthen Pan that's not glaz'd in fuch a Hole, and in the 'forefaid Mannei , if there is Water in that Place, the Pan will be wet and damp Or, if you fling Wool in fuch a Hole, and you can the next Morning wring Water out of it, it is a fure Sign of a plentiful Spring

When a Lamp, light with a little Oil is put in fuch a Place, and neither the Wick nor the Oil confum'd the next Day, or the Lamp is damp, it is a Sign of a Spring, and that the Lamp has been fed with the Damps thereof

Another Tryal is, by making a Fire in fuch a Place, and when it is well heated, it will caufe a thick Vapour or Smoak, which is a Sign of Water

Caffiodorus will have it, that where fubtile Vapours or Mifts raife in perpendicular Pillars, in fuch Places one may be fure of Springs, which lay as deep under Ground as the Pillars are high. The fame Author recommends alfo for a fure Sign that which the Well Diggers have, who when after Sun-rife they fee a Swarm of Gnats as it were, in a Cloud, they conclude that underneath them the Earth contains Springs.

Pater *John François*, a Jefuit, is of Opinion, that Springs are beft difcovered by boreing, whereby the different Earths under the Surface may be brought up, and examined whether they have any Sign of Water, or not He adds, that fuch Gimlets might be made to bore through Quarries of Stone, and in cafe the Gimlet fhould not be long enough, to dig four or five Foot deep, and help it further that Way

Pater Kircher gives us another Method whereby to difcover Springs, or fubterraneous Water-Courfes, which he himfelf had tried with great Succefs, it being very eafy put in Practice Make a Ballance of Wood, in the Shape of the Needle of a Compafs, each Point thereof muft be made of different Sorts of Wood, one end too muft be of fuch a kind, that will eafily attract wet, as Elder, or the like. This Hand is ballanc'd between an Angle or Axis, or is hang'd on a Packthread, in a Place where Water is fuppofed to be If there really is Water, the Hand will foon loofe the Balance, and the Point of Elder

inclin.

incline towards the Ground. This Trial is (fays he) to be made in the Morning early, before the Sun has difperfed the Vapours of the Earth.

These are the beft of the common Methods, which I know, to difcover Water Springs, but how curious and ingenious however they are, the Searcher is often deceiv'd by them. *Pater Kircher*'s Method, indeed, is the eafieft, but his Project is not fo much for difcovering of Springs, as to determine whether there is any Water in that Place.

But the *Winchel-Rod*, is the moft wonderful Invention for that Purpofe, that has yet been difcovered and the Operation thereof is furprifing, for by Virtue of a Hafel-Rod or Stick, not only the Springs, but alfo the Depth to them is eafily difcovered to a great Nicety *Pater de Charles*, who made himfelf famous on Account of writing a Book intitled *Mundus Subterraneus*, after he has enumerated feveral Ways of difcovering Springs, concludes thus · " There is another Method to " fearch for Water, which is the moft wonderful of all, but " every one has not the Capacity of putting it in Practice. " The whole Myftery confifts in this; a fork'd Twig is cut off " a Hazel or Mulberry-Tree, and he who fearches carries it " loofe in his Hand, but as foon as he goes over a Spring, he " will obferve the Stick to turn in his Hand, and incline to the " Place where the Spring is" A large Account of this and the foregoing Matter, is given by the Author of the *Accurate Defcription of the Winchel Rod*, written in the *German* Language

A Camera Olfcura.

CHOOSE for the Trial of this an Apartment, out of which you may have a Profpect into five Garden-Walks or other Places of Refort, contrive a Hole, either through the Wall, or elfe in a Board fix'd in the Window, in which fix a round Glafs out of a pair of Spectacles, and fhut all the reft of the Light out of the Room, but what enters through that Glafs, then at a convenient diftance fix a Sheet of White Paper or a White Cloath, and you will with delight fee the Objects without, prefented thereon in their lively Colours, efpecially in a bright Sun-fhiny Day, you will fee the Birds in the Air flying, Ships (if you have fuch a Profpect) failing, People walking, Coaches riding, and every Thing elfe appear in fuch Beauty and Order, as will draw your Admira-

tion

tion to confider how the Colours are difplac'd in their proper Shades and Altitude, and how when two different Colours meet, the one is not changed by the conjunction of the
other, and what other Speculations it may afford you, both
ufeful and entertaining.

It is to be obferv'd, that all the Images which fall through
the Glafs upon the Paper, Cloath or white Wall, appear
upfide down, and to have them reprefented right, the fol
lowing Experiments have been approved of; the firft is, by
fixing another Glafs of a larger circumference at the outfide
of the Apartment, before t'other Glafs is fix'd in, this may
be done when the two Glaffes are fix'd in a proper Frame or
Tube made of Wood or Tin, for then they eafily may be
fix'd into a Hole made for that Purpofe in the Window Shut-
ter or Wall, but the Objects will not appear fo plain and
clear as through a fingle Glafs

We will here prefent the Curious with a Model and Defcription of a moveable *Camera obfcura*, whereby he may
draw Things, relating either to Orthography or Ichnography,
to the greateft Perfection. The Machine is prepared with
as little Trouble as Expence, in the following Manner.

Make a Cubical or an even-fided Frame, and clofe all the
Sides round with thick Pafte Board; on the oppofite Sides
make a little Hole, in each whereof fix a Glafs through which
the Images of the Profpect about may enter; fix a White
Paper oppofite the Glafs at a proper Diftance, and having
a little Hole made near the Glafs, you may through that
fee the Objects in a beautiful Manner on the Paper, which
enter through the Glafs.

To Illuminate an Apartment with various beautiful Colours

PUT three or four Pryfms, or Glaffes pinn'd in a Tri-
angular Form, together, of a Window, to make it
portable, as you fee in the Figure A, B, let the Pryfms
be fo fix'd Corner to Corner, that on one Side they
may make a Flat, and on the other a Trigonic Face, as
in the Figure, place this Frame thus finifhed before a
Window towards the Sun, fo that the flat Side be towards it,
and if there be any more Windows in the Apartment, let them
be clofed up As foon as the Beams of the Sun fhine
through thefe Trigonic Glaffes, your Apartment will appear
like

like a Paradife, in the greateft Beauty and of various Colours. If you catch thefe Beams in a concave Glafs, you fee the colours change quite different from what they were before; and if you look through thofe Glaffes into the Street, you fee every Thing in different Colours, fo that you will be in a Sort of Surprife and Admiration.

Diana, or the Philofophical Tree.

THIS Operation is a Mixture of Silver, Mercury, and Spirit of Nitre, cryftallized together in the Shape and Form of a Tree

Take one Ounce of Silver, and diffolve it in two or three Ounces of Spirit of Nitre, this Solution put into a Matrafs or Glafs Phial, into which you have put 18 or 20 Ounces of Water, and two Ounces of Quickfilver Let your Phial be fill'd up to the Neck, and place it in fome convenient Place where Nobody can meddle with it, for 40 Days together, in which Time you will fee a Tree fpread forth its Branches, with little Balls at the Ends thereof, reprefenting the Fruit

Another Manner to make a Tree of Diana.

DISSOLVE an Ounce of fine Silver in three Ounces of Aqua Fortis, in a Phial or fmall Matrafs, evaporate about half that Moifture in a warm Sand, by a gentle Fire; then add to it three Ounces of good diftill'd Vinegar, heat it a little, and ftir it about, then put your Matrafs in a fafe Place, where it may reft for a Month, and you will fee a Tree growing to the very Superficies of the Liquor, and refemble in its Branches a Fir-Tree.

Curious

✿✿✿✿✿✿✿✿✿✿✿✿✿✿✿✿✿✿✿✿

Curious Secrets for preserving Things from CORRUPTION.

To preserve Things from Corruption in Spirit of Wine

THIS is done with the most subtil rectified Spirit of Wine, camphariz'd, wherein many Sorts of Animals, Birds, Fish, Insects, Reptiles, &c may be kept many Years from Decay or Corruption *Porta* mentions to have seen a Fish at *Rome* thus preserv'd for above 20 Years, which was as fresh as if alive, likewise at *Florence*, where he saw one that had been preserv'd above 40 Years The Glasses, wherein they were kept, were Hermetically sealed, to keep the least Air from coming to it

The Preparation of the Spirit or Oil of Salt, whereby Things may be kept from Corruption, and is a great Restorer and Preserver of Health.

TAKE Sea Salt, as much as you will, put it in a Pan or Crucible cover'd, over a good Coal Fire, and when it has done crackling, take it off, put it in a damp Place, till it is dissolv'd, filter it often thro' a Paper, till it is thorough clear and fine Then let it digest in Horse-Dung, for about two Months, changing the Dung often for fresh, in order to keep it continually warm. Then distil it over some Sand, and you will have in your Receiver a Salt Oil, with a watery Phlegm, distil this gently in a *Balm* and the Oil will keep back, but the watery Substance be carried off, whatever is put into this Oil, will keep from Corruption without changing, for Hundreds of Years, This is the Salt Spirit which by *Paracelsus* is call'd *Croditas Salis*, and has incomparable Virtues, as well to restore Men to Health and Vigour, as also to preserve them from most Distempers, four or six drops taken in Wormwood Water, is good for the Dropsy, Convulsions, and the yellow Jaundice, three or four drops taken in Harts horn Water is good for all Sorts of Agues, for Worms, it is taken in Brandy, three Drops taken in *Carcit* or *Cordobenedictine* Water, is good for the Stoppage of Urin It is a fine Remedy for all Sorts of Sprains and Contractions of Nerves, it heals Bruises and Swellings, when mix'd with other Ointments, and the grieved Parts are anointed When mix'd therewith with Oil of Turpentine or Wax, or Camomile, it will asswage the Gout This Oil or Spirit of Salt, if it is well rectified, is a Solution for all Sorts of Metals and Stones, and a Key to many hidden Mysteries

But if this Preservative is too costly to keep things from Corruption, you may prepare a Sea-Water with a small Expence, which will keep Things for many Years, and this you do in the following Manner

After you have searced your Sea Salt, dissolve it in distill'd Rain Water, and make thereof a Lee which will bear an Egg

Or, when the Salt is searced, put it into a damp Place, and when it is dissolv'd, filter it through a Paper so long till it is clear and fine This you may use to preserve Things from Corruption, by stilling it, and pouring it over the Thing to be preserved.

A Regeneration of Coral.

TAKE Verdegrease three Pound, live Sulphur one Pound, clear Sand four Pound, pulverise and mix it, then still it in a Retort on Sand, first with a slow Fire, but augmenting it by degrees, and it will produce a Spirit, which has a sweetish sour Flavour.

If this Spirit is pour'd upon powdered Coral, or Harts-Horn Filings, and by a gentle Warmth is quite dry'd up, then put it into a Phial with some distill'd Rain-Water, and set it in a warm Place well closed up, the Coral or Harts-Horn will shoot and grow so natural that it will be delightful to behold it.

To prepare a Phosphorus.

TAKE Urin, as much as you please, put it into a Tub or Kettle, let it stand for three Weeks or a Month together and putrify, then boil away the humidity till the remainings become a black and tough Matter. Of this take

one

one Pound, Oil of Tartar Fœtid, or the ftinking Oil of
Harts-Horn, or for want of that, green Wax, mix it well with
the Matter, put it in a Retort, fet it on a ftrong Fire of a
Reverberatory Furnace, fit to it a large Receiver, lute the
Junctures, give firft a gentle, and laftly for four Hours the
moft fiercheft Heat you can; and you will find in the Receiver
in the firft Settlement the Volatile Salt, then fome Oil, and
after that the Phofphorus, who in the Receiver has fubli-
mated of a yellowifh Colour, let the firft fettlement ftay
over Night and grow cold, then take and wafh with the Li
quid that is at the bottom, all the Phofphorus and Oil, mix
it well together, put it into a Matrafs, ftill it out of a Sand
Coppel, and you will find in the firft Settlement Grains of
Phofphorus, which, whilft warm, prefs into little Sticks, and
preferve them in a little Phial as the former

Another fuch luminary Matter.

TAKE what by moft Apothecaries is known by the
Name of Land-Emerald, as much as you will, beat it
fine with Water on a Stone; temper it with Gum or Honey
Water, and write or paint therewith upon a polifh'd Copper
or Iron Plate, whatever you will, and let it dry, then lay it
upon a Charcoal Fire, or fet it before the fame, and in a
little while it will light, fo that when you bring it into a
dark Room, or put the Candles out, the Company who are
ignorant of what is done, will be furprized at fo fudden and
ftrange Appearance

To prepare a Room or Clofet in fuch a Manner that any one entering with a lighted Candle, will think himfelf furrounded with Fire.

TAKE a pretty large Quantity of Brandy, and put it in a
Bowl, fet it on a flow Coal Fire, to receive heat
enough to boil gently up, into the Brandy fling fome Camphir, cut in little Bits, which will foon diffolve, and when all
is diffolv'd, clofe both Windows and Door, and let the Brandy boil and evaporate; by this the whole Room will be
fill'd with fubtle Spirits, which, as foon as a Candle is
brought in, will be lighted, and feem as if all was a Fire   If
fome Perfume is diffolv'd in the Brandy, the Flame will be
attended with a fine Smell.   *To*

To prepare a Luminary Stone.

TAKE good rectified Spirit of Nitre, fling Quick-Lime and Chalk into it, till the said Spirit can t dissolve no more, and ceases to ebulate, filter the Solution, put it into a Retort, and still the Spirit of Nitre from it again; what remains in the Retort, place in the Air, and let it dissolve, then put it again in the Retort, draw off the Moisture till it is dry, set it again in the Air and let it dissolve, then pour it into Assay-Cups, put them into a Cucurbit, and distill all the Moisture from it, the Remains put under a Muffle to harden. Then hold it in the Light of Day, of the Moon, or the Light of a Candle, and it will contract that Light, so as to give it again when put into a dark Place.

The Preparation of a Phosphorus.

TAKE an earthen Plate or Dish, which is not glaz'd, about half an Inch thick, and make a Sort of Paste of Spirit of Nitre and pulverized Chalk, well stirred together; of this take the bigness of a Shilling, put it into the Plate, and set it in the Fire under a Muffle (where it will ebulate much) to dry, when dry, take it out, let it cool, and mix it up with Spirit of Nitre: This do six or eight Times, and it is ready: After it is cold, hold it a little while against a Candle, and shewing it in a dark Place, you will be surprised at the Light it gives.

How to prepare Thunder Powder.

THIS is done with three Ingredients, namely, three Parts Saltpeter, two Parts of Sal Tartar, and one Part of Sulpher, these are pounded and mixt together if you take about 60 Grains in a Spoon and warm it over a Candle or other Fire, it will give a Report, like a Cannon fired off, and thus the Flashing will beat downwards. If you make use of a Copper Spoon or Cup, you will after the Report find a Hole at Bottom, but when light it at Top, it will burn away like Lightning.

To reprefent a Philofophical Tree in a Glafs

TAKE of the fineft Silver one Ounce, Aqua Fortis and Mercury of each four Ounces; in this diffolve your Silver in a Phial, and after you have put over it a Pint of Water, clofe your Phial, and you will fee a fine Tree fpring forth in Branches, which will encreafe and grow thicker every Day.

To reprefent the four Elements in a Glafs Phial.

FIRST tincture in a Phial, good Spirit of Wine with *Terra Solis,* to reprefent the Air; then take well rectified Oil of Turpentine, this you tincture with Saffron, and red Ox-Tongue Root for Fire; Oil of Tartar, to which you add a little Ultramarine, to give it the Colour of the Sea or Water, and for to reprefent the Earth, take a little Smalt. This you may fhake together, and after it has ftood a little, every Thing will take its Place again, for the three Liquids will never keep or unite together.

Another

HAVE a Glafs made in the Shape of an Egg, fill the fourth Part thereof with clean Smalt, or common An timony, (*a*) to reprefent the Earth, for Water (*b*) take Spirit of Tartar; for the Air (*e*) Spirit of Wine three times rectified, and Oil of Benjamin, which in Colour and Bright- nefs may reprefent the Fire, (*d*) the Cover of the Glafs may be ornamented with a Flame, or what you pleafe

A Florence Flafk will anfwer the fame Purpofe, made with a Foot to it as you fee in the Figure.

An Elementary World in a Phial.

TAKE Black Glafs or Enamel, beat it to a midling Gravel Size, this, for reprefenting the Earth, will fettle at the Bottom, for the Water you may ufe calcin'd Tartar, or fandy Afhes, which you firft moiften, and what thereof diffolves, pour the cleareft into the Phial, and tincture it with a little Ultramarine, to give it the Sea Colour; for the Air ufe Aqua Vitæ, the beft you can get, which, when tinctured

with

with a little Turnfole, gives a Sky Colour, to reprefent the Fire, take Linfeed or Oil of Turpentine, and prepare the latter thus Diftil Turpentine in *Bain Mar.* the Water and Oil will raife tranfparently together, but the Oil will afterwards fwim a top, which take, after you have coloured it with Ox-Tongue and Saffron. All thefe Matters differ both in Weight and Quality, for if you fhike them together, you indeed obferve for a little while a Chaos full of Confufion and Diforder, but as foon you put the Phial down, every Matter takes its refpective Place in the fame Order as before.

To ornament a Room with a continual moving Picture.

PLACE a large Picture againft the Wainfcot, in a Summer-Houfe, or any other Room where the Wind may be convey'd to the Back of the Picture, bore little Holes through the Wainfcot, to correfpond with fome Paft-Board Wheels that are at the Back of the Picture; the Wind which blows on them through the little Holes, will put them in Motion, and having on the right Side of the Picture fuch Things painted and fix'd to the Paft-Board Wheel on one Spindle, they will have an equal Motion with them And there may be feveral Things reprefented in a Picture, and their Motion made agreeable, as for Example, a Man grinding of Knives, a Woman at her Spining Wheel, a Wind- or Water Mill, and feveral other Fancies, a Man's Curiofity will direct him to.

Of the Regeneration of ANIMALS.

Of Craw Fifh.

IT is to be obferved that if you will fucceed in this Experiment, you muft choofe the full Moon, and if poffible, when in a watery Sign, then take a parcel of live Craw-Fifh, which are catch'd in Rivulets and Brooks, divide them in two Parcels, one Parcel put into an Earthen

Pan

Pan that's not glaz'd, lute it well, and put it into a Furnace to calcine for feven or eight Hours, in a ftrong Fire After they are well calcined, beat them in a Marble Mortar to Powder, then take the other Parcel, and boil them in the fame Water they were catch'd in, pour off the Water in another Veffel, about half a Paleful, and fling into it about half a Handful of the calcined *Craw Fifh,* ftir it well together with a Stick, then let it fettle, and remain ftill, and in a few Days you will obferve in the Water a great Number of fmall Atoms in motion. When you fee them grow up to the bignefs of a fmall Button, you muft feed them with Beef Blood, flinging thereof by little and little into the Water, which will caufe them to thrive, and to grow to their natural bignefs ; but you muft obferve, that before you put them in the Veffel with Water, you lay Sand at the bottom about an Inch thick.

Petro Borello, in the 34th Paragraph of his Phyfical Hiftory, fays If one takes the Afhes of *Craw-Fifh,* and lays them in a damp Place or in an Earthen Pan, moiftened with a little Water, and lets it ftand, in lefs than 20 Days will be feen innumerable little Worms; and if after this you fprinkle Beef Blood upon it, they will by Degrees turn into Craw-Fifh.

The Sieur *Pegarius,* when he treats upon this Subject, fays " As to the Generation of Animals, a Friend of " mine did fee the Figures and Shapes of Craw-Fifh, in " a Lee he made of calcined ones, but what is more furprifing, out of fuch a Salt, not only the Refemblance of " fuch Creatures is produced, but alfo the very Animal " itfelf, alive and in its natural Form and Shape, as D *de* " *Chambulan* and others have experienced, by flinging the " Powder of calcined Craw-Fifh in ftanding Water, the " like may be done with the Afhes of Toads *Rochos,* in " his *Art of Nature* writes, that out of a rotten Duck have " grown feveral Toads, becaufe fhe had fed upon thefe " Creatures, and that the Carcafs of an Owl which has fed " upon Jacks, will bring forth great Numbers of that Fifh " after it is rotten, and if the faid Owl has fed upon Carps, " the rotten Carcafs will produce Carp And from hence it " is, that when a Fifh-Pond is quite dried up, and Water " is again let in, it will abound in a little Time with Fifh of " fuch Sort as never were in before".

Of

Of Eels.

KIRCHER in the first Part of his subterraneous World speaks thus of Eels.

Eels grow without a Sperm, or Seed, out of the Skin they throw off yearly, and corrupts, or of what sticks to the Stone against which they rub, the Truth of this may be easily experienced, by chopping an Eel in little Pieces, and flinging them in a muddy Pond, for in a Month's Time there will appear a Brood of small Eels.

Another Generation of Eels is perform'd thus; take two Spattles of Turff, let 'em lay that the Dew may fall upon 'em, then lay them Grass to Grass, and put them into a Pond or Ditch, so that the Water may play upon, and you will see first little Worms come from between, which in time will grow up to Eels.

According to *Aristotle*, there is neither Male nor Female among Eels, neither do they copulate, nor do they spawn, and there is never an Eel found with either a soft or hard Roe; from all which it may be conjectur'd, that when a slimy Water has been quite drain'd off, and the Slime been taken out, there has still been a Generation of Eels when fresh Water has been let in again; for in a dry Soil they don't generate, nor in the Sea that is always full of Water, because they have their Growth and Nourishment of the Rain.

They are also generated out of other corruptible Things, and we have seen, when a dead Horse has been flung into the Water, a vast Number of Eels have been perceived about the Carcase, and it is thought they come forth from other dead Carcases also. *Aristotle* says, they have their first Origin, in the inner Recesses of the Earth, where some of them break out into the Sea, and others in Rivers and Ponds.

That Vegetables produce all Sorts of Insects, and in particular Flies, we find in *Aldrovandro*'s Third Book of Reptiles, where Chap. 16. he says thus " As I will not deny " that out of the most putrified Matters, even out of " Carrion, grow Flies, I do believe that most of them have " their Origin from Vegetables, as we have Examples " of our own Experience, for a few Years ago, in a Win- " ter Season, when for Want of other green Plants I pounded

brown-

" brown Cabbage, and left them fome time in my Room, I
" found that Worms grew out of them, and that thefe Worms
" turn'd into Lady-Birds, I gathered them into a Box
" and opening the Box fome time after, a great Swarm of
" little Flies flew out of it, which before had been Lady
" Birds.

Something of the fame Kind did a good Friend and Cor
refpondent communicate to me in a Letter, *Dec* 28th 1671.
He writes thus " I once did read in an *Italian* Author,
" that out of *Cheledonia* a Tincture could be prepar'd, this
" did prompt me to make a ftricter Search into the Nature
" of that Herb, I took the whole Plant, chopt it fine, when
" it was in full Juice, and put it into a Matrais, then I luted
" a Head upon it, thinking to diftil it in *Baln Mar* but by fome
" accidental Hindrance, it remained almoft a whole Summer
" neglected in my Laboratory   Towards Autumn I found
" that the whole Mafs was liquified and full of Worms,
" hence I could eafily perceive what a fine Tincture I had
" to expect, however, I let it ftand the whole Winter, in the
" Beginning of the Spring I found that the Worms were all
" gone, and all was turned into a Black Powder, not long after
" out of this Powder grew Gnats, in fuch Abundance, that
" the whole Glafs was full of them, who made a buffing Noife
" and flew merrily about   I was in the Interim vifited by an
" Acquaintance, who fpied the Glafs with the Gnats as it
" ftood in the Window, we fell into a Difcourfe about them,
" when he maintained that thofe Gnats would not bear
" the open Air, but die as foon as it was convey'd to them
" I could hardly believe it, but to try the Experiment, I
" pull'd the Stopple out of the Retort, and perceiv'd all
" the Gnats dead in a Moment, after I open'd the Glafs,
" I found that moft of the Powder was turn'd into Gnats,
" except a little black Earth, which I tried, and found the
" Tafte very fiery, and produc'd, after it was light, a fix'd
" Salt, which without Doubt may have its particular Virtue

Scaliger fays, that every Tree and Herb has its particular
Worm or Infect, and almoft every fmall Vegetable its own
Fly. This a Virtuofo at *Rome* obferved in his Garden,
and had them painted together with the Plant in their natural Colours; but we need not go fo far as to *Rome*, we may
fatisfy our Curiofity by perufing Mr. *Albine*'s Natural Hiftory
of Englifh Infects

Peganus',

Peganus's Relation of what happen'd with his Experiment in the Generation of Serpents.

"WHEN *Anno* 1654, among other Authors I happen-
"ed to read *Theophrastus's* Book *de Vermibus,* where
"he in particular gives a surprising Account of our *Ger-*
"*man* Notters (Vipers) and having a Desire to try the Ex-
"periment of so great a Curiosity, order'd 25 Notters
"to be caught, I had them skinn'd, flung the Heads and
"Tails away, and saved the Heart and Liver for a particular
"Use, after I had made them into Powder, the Flesh and
"Bone I cut in little Pieces, put them into a glass Matrass,
"set over that another, and luted them close together.

"This I did in *July,* in my Laboratory at the Window,
"where the Sun only shined few Hours upon it; I let
"it stand for two Months, and observed every Day whe-
"ther there appeared any Change in the Glass, after a few
"Week I saw some oily or greasy Drops hang to the Upper
"Glass which were of a yellowish Colour, after I had
"look'd with great Attention upon these Drops for an Honr
"together, I observ'd issuing out of them snow white
"Worms very small, which crept downwards, and as these
"Worms encreased daily more and more, the first of them
"grew bigger, but the Matter at the Bottom of the Glass
"stood like a yellowish Oil with some watry Moisture,
"and the Settlement at Bottom appear'd of a black earthy
"Substance, after some Weeks the Number of Worms be-
"gan to decrease, the rest increased in Growth, at last they
"were all vanish'd to three or four, and they were about a
"Fingers Length, and had an uncommon Brightness. In a
"few Weeks they were all lost, save one, which was
"pretty long, and had the resemblance of a Serpent, but of a
"snow white Colour, smooth and shining, without Scales,
"although there were very subtil black Lineaments across,
"which in the Glass I could not well distinguish, the Head
"differed also something from that of a Serpent, the rest
"of the Mass grew dry, and resembled a black close Earth:
"I was in one Respect rejoic'd to have the Happiness of
"seeing this Curiosity of Nature, in Regenerating a
"Serpent, but on the other Hand I was cautious how to
"bring the Creature out of the Glass, and how to proceed
further

" further therewith, at laſt Fear got the Upperhand of
" Reaſon, and in a Sort of Horror I took the Glaſs and
" flung it into an Houſe of Office.

Of the Generation of Silk-Worms out of Veal.

TAKE about 10 or 12 Pound of Veal, all Meat without
Bone, warm, and as ſoon as 'tis kill'd, this chop with
a chopping Knife as fine as you can, afterwards put it in a
new earthen Pot, thus At the Bottom you make a Lay of
Mulberry Leaves, then a lay of Veal, and thus you proceed
till your Pot is full; then cover the Top with Mulberry
Leaves, and take an old Shirt, which has been well wore and
ſweated in by a labouring Man; this put at Top upon the
Leaves, and then tye the Pot cloſe with Leather. After
this is done, ſet the Pot into a Cellar, which is not too cool, but
ſomething warm and damp, let it ſtand for three or four
Weeks, till the Veal turns into Maggots, which happens
ſometimes ſooner, ſometimes later, according to the Nature
of the Place you put it in. Of theſe Maggots take as many
as you will, ſet them upon freſh Mulberry Leaves, which
they will eat; change their Form to Silk-Worms, will
ſoon content themſelves with that Nutriment, and ſpin and
generate like other Silk-Worms. I have produced them
twice, not without the Admiration of the late Mr. *Sperling,*
and yet I am of Opinion that this Generation is not of both,
but only of one Kind, the ſame Opinion I have of Toads
or Frogs, which are produced out of barren Earth.

The Time wherein Silk-Worms are to be raiſed, is in the
Beginning of *July,* to the eighth of that Month, when the
Proceſs is to begin *Vida* in his ſecond Book of Silk-Worms
teaches, when a young Ox is fed with Mulberry-Leaves,
that out of his Fleſh, after it is kill'd, will grow Silk-
Worms.

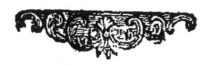

PART IX.

Several Curious and Useful Inſtructions in the Art of DISTILLING.

How to extraƈt the Quint-Eſſence of Roſes.

AKE freſh Roſes, which are gather'd before Sun Riſing, whilſt the Dew is upon them, bruiſe or ſtamp the Leaves thereof in a Stone Mortar, then put them into an earthen glaz'd Pan or Bowl, cover them cloſe, and let them ſtand till they putrify, which you may perceive when the Scent thereof is ſour, and turns ſo in about 12 or 14 Days, you may mix up with the Leaves a little Salt of Tartar, for this penetrates, cuts, and parts the contrary Particles, and will cauſe each the better to ſeparate.

After the Roſe-Leaves are thus putrified, take the fifth or ſeventh Part of them, put them into a Glaſs Cucurbit, and ſtill them in *Baln. Mar.* The diſtill'd Water pour upon the other Part of the Leaves, and after you have emptied the Cucurbit of the firſt Leaves, put in the ſecond Part, and ſtill them in *Baln. Mar.* as before, thus repeating it, you will draw a rectified Water, which contains the Spirit, and muſt be ſeparated in the following Manner. Put all the Water you have ſtill'd, into a Matraſs with a long Neck, and a Head belonging to it, lute to it a Receiver, then with a ſlow Aſh-Fire draw off the Spirit, and as there will go ſome of the Phlegm along with it, the Spirit muſt be, together with the Phlegm, put to another Diſtillation, with a ſlower Fire, and thus you will have a pure Spirit of Roſes, which will diffuſe its ſtrong Scent as ſoon as the Matraſs is open'd, over the whole Room.

Q   Save

Save this Spirit, well clos'd up in a Phial, as a precious and valuable Thing; for its Virtue is wonderful and admirable. Pour the greater Part of the distill'd Rose-Water over the already distill'd Rose-Leaves, in order to extract the Oil from the Water, which must be done by distilling it over a hotter Ash-Fire, than you did the Spirit The Oil will separate itself from the Phlegm, and swim on the Surface of the Water in a Gold-Colour, and although the Quantity is but small, the Virtue thereof is the greater and the more valuable

Separate this Oil from the Phlegm, and put it up apart by itself, and also the distill'd Rose-Water in a Glass by itself, after which take the distill'd Rose-Leaves, from which all the Spirit and Oil is extracted, burn them in a Crucible to Ashes, and in burning add a little Sulphur to them, give the Ashes a fierce Fire, and they will be as white as Snow.

These Ashes put into a Glass or Earthen Vessel, pour over them the above Phlegm or Rose-Water; boil it well, so long till the Water has extracted all the Salt from the Ashes, then filter it through a brown Paper into a Matrass, distill it, and carry off the Phlegm, and a clear Salt will settle at the Bottom of the Matrass· The Ashes you may calcine a-new in a strong reverberatory Fire, then boil them up again with the Phlegm, and draw out the Salt as before, this repeat till all the Salt is extracted, and there remains only a poor earthy Substance.

In this Manner are extracted from Roses the three pure Capital Parts, *viz.* Spirit, Oil, and Salt, from the three impure Parts Phlegm, Water, and *Cap. Mort.*

In case the Salt should not be clean enough, you must dissolve it again in the Phlegm, and repeat your Process by Distillation, as before, and you may make it as fine as you will

Each of these Substances has for itself great medicinal Virtues, but much more if all three are united together, which is done in the following Manner·

Put the clear Salt into a Glass Phial with a long Neck, and set it in a gentle Warmth, pour on it some of the Oil, and continue the Warmth till the Salt and Oil are united, then put another Part of Oil to it, and thus by uniting them by Degrees, your Boiling is finish'd Then add to it one Part of the Spirit, and augment the Quantity by slow Degrees, as you did with the Oil, and thus the three Substances will be united, that no Art is able to part them, and the medicinal Virtue thereof are inexpressible.

Anothe

Another Method to extract the Quint-Essence out of any Vegetables.

TAKE a Plant, Herb, or Flower, in the Month they flourish best, gather thereof before Sun-rising (with the Dew upon) what Quantity you please, chop it fine, and fill therewith a Glass Matrass, lute a Head over it, and place the Matrass in *Baln. Mar.* let it infuse over a very slow Fire for a Fortnight, after which time augment your Fire; when you find some of the Menstrum will go over into the Receiver, then take your Matrass out of the *Balneum*, and you will see the Herb infused in its own Juice, which pour off into a clean Glass. The Remains of the Herb take out of the Matrass, burn them to Ashes, and extract the Salt thereof with a Water distill'd from the same Herb.

How to abstract Oil of Herbs, Flowers or Seeds.

FILL a large Cucurbit with Herbs, Flowers, Seeds or what you chuse, infuse it in good *Spiritus Salis*, set it in Sand, and give it Fire enough to boil, and the Oil, as well as the Phlegm, will distil over into the Receiver; which you separate as has been directed; the Spirit you pour off, rectify it, and you may use it again for the like Process

A fine Secret to distil Herbs, so that the Water will retain both the Colour and Taste thereof.

TAKE the Leaves of the Herb you design to distil, infuse them for a Night and a Day in Rain-Water, then take a Still Head, pour into it some of the Water from off the Herbs, swing or rinse it about, and pour it through the Pipe on the Herbs again, fling more fresh Leaves upon it, put on the Head, lute it close, and distil it in *Bal Mar* with a slow Fire, and you will see the Drops, which have the Colour of the Herb or Flower When you have distill'd it all over into the Receiver, then burn the Leaves to Ashes, and extract the Salt from it in the Manner above directed; put half of it into the distill'd Water, let it dissolve in the Sun, and the Colour will be clear and fine.

To

To prepare a fixed Salt out of Vegetables.

TAKE Herbs, what Quantity you pleafe (thofe that fhoot up in long Stalks are the beft for this purpofe), burn them to Afhes in an open Place, or upon the Hearth, take of the Afhes and put as much as you will into a Kettle, pour Water upon it, and let it boil, then filter the Lee through a Linnen Rag, and pour frefh Water on the remaining Afhes, boil and filter it as before, and this conti nue to repeat till you can perceive no fharpnefs in the Afhes.

Then pour all the Lee into one Kettle, and boil it over a fierce Fire, till the Salt remains dry at the Bottom, of this take 12 Ounces, yellow Brimftone two Ounces, both well pulverifed, and mix'd together; put fome of this in the Iron Chaldron, which is made pretty hot, and in which you before boil'd your Salt; let the Brimftone burn gently away, taking care not to make the Cauldron too hot, left it fhould occafion the Salt to melt, which to prevent ftir the Matter continually, whilft the Sulphur is burning, with a Spatula When you find the Sulpher confumed, put the remainings upon a clean Paper, put more of the mixture into the Chaldron and proceed as before, till you have burn'd all the Sulpher, then put them with Sulpher Salt calcined all toge ther into the Cauldron, and make it red hot; fo that if there fhould be any Sulpher left, it may be confumed, and the Salt become a Whitifh Gray Colour, take it then off the Fire, pour, whilft it is hot, cold Water to it, and it will diffolve it immediately, then filter it through a brown Pafte board or Paper, if the Sulphur is all clear from it, the So lution will be of a Whitifh Yellow; if not, it will either be Green or of an Iron Grey.

This filtrated Solution pour again in the clean Cauldron, fet it upon a Wind Furnace, draw it off dry, and give it fo long Fire till the Salt is red hot, when fo, pour again quickly fome Water upon it, and it will diffolve, repeat this, till by taking a little of the Solution into a Spoon, and holding it in the Light, you fee not the leaft Film or Star on the Sur face thereof, but if you do, take it off the Fire, and filtrate it into a clean Cucurbit, fet it in warm Sand, and let it eva porate, without giving it the leaft motion, and in two or three Days, according to the Quantity of the Salt, it will shoot into fine Crystals, and when it has done Crystallising, there settles a Crystalline Crust upon the Surface; let it cool, take out the Crystal, and the remaining Liquor place again upon the warm Sand, to evaporate and shoot in Crystals.

You must observe not to be too sparing with your Water which you pour upon the red hot Salt, before you filter it, else the Salt would settle at the Bottom, and shoot no Crystals.

If it should happen, that in burning the Brimstone your Salt should dissolve, then take it off the Fire, let it cool, and beat it in a Mortar, and after you have dissolv'd and calcin'd it, burn it once again with the Sulphur, and then use it with the rest

The Ashes burn'd of green Herbs, or of such as are not too dry, yield more fix'd Salt than such as are dry'd up.

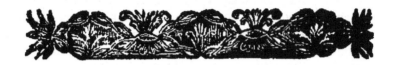

PART X.

Several Secrets relating to MARBLE.

How to stain Marble that's White, and paint upon it with various Colours ; which will penetrate into the Stone so as to bear polishing.

TAKE of Aqua Fortis two Ounces, Sal Armoniac one Ounce, of high rectified Spirit of Wine four Drams, then take some Gold, make of it an Amalgama with Mercury or Quickfilver, let the Mercury evaporate, and the Gold will remain at the Bottom of your Crucible like a brown Powder or Calx. Dissolve this in Aqua Regis, and evaporate it till it is of a yellow Colour, then pour on the Sal Armoniac and the Spirit of Wine, and when dissolv'd, evaporate the Spirit again, and there remains a bright Gold Colour

Calcine the Silver in a Phial, and then let the Aqua Fortis evaporate till you have a *Sky Colour,* which take off and preferve in a clean Phial, keeping the rest in a warm Sand to evaporate, and you will have a deep *Blue,* which you also preferve, the remains will, by more evaporating, turn into *Black*

By mixing these Colours you may produce several others, wherewith you may paint or stain what Figures you please; and the more you repeat laying on this Colour, the deeper they will penetrate into the Stone, and the stronger they will reprefent themfelves thereon After you have finifhed your Staining, you may polifh it like plain white Marble, and then you will have the Colours appear in their full Luftre.

Mar-

Marble may alfo be ftained with Colours which have been drawn from Vegetables, with *Spirit Sal Armoniac* or Urin, but, although they penetrate a good Way into the Marble, they will, on Account of their volatile Nature, be of no long Duration. The red Colour in this Procefs is made of Dragon's Blood, tempered with Urin of Horfes, Hogs, or Dogs; the Blue is treated in the fame Manner, for which they ufe blue Verditer· The Purple Colour is drawn from Cochineal, mix'd with any of the faid Urine; fome, inftead of Urin, ufe Spirit of Wine

To imitate Marble

TAKE Plaifter of Paris, Quick-Lime, Salt, Ox-Blood, Stones of different Colours, alfo Pieces of Glafs, all beat to Powder, and mixt up to the Confiftence of a Pafte, with Vinegar, Beer or four Milk, and then lay it into Tables, Pillars, or what you will, let it ftand fo long till it is thorough dry, then rub it firft with Pumice, and polifh it with Tripoli, giving it the finifhing Stroke with rubbing it over with Leather and Oil.

Another Method

WITH fine pulveriz'd Plaifter of Paris, and Size of Parchmens, make a Pafte, mix with it as many Colours as you pleafe, fpread it with a Trowel over a Board, and when dry, proceed as before.

To paint on Wood in Imitation of Marble.

FIRST lay a Ground (repeating it feven or eight times) with white, as you have been directed in the Method of gilding on Wood; then you marble it with what Colours you pleafe, after you have tempered them with the white of Eggs, and mix'd a little Saffron Water with it. If you are not ufed to marbling with a Pencil, you may pour one Sort of your Colour here and there a little, upon the white prepared Table, then holding and turning it fhelving, the Colour will difperfe all over the Ground in Varieties of Veins, then with another Colour proceed in the fame Manner, and fo with as many as you think proper, and it will anfwer your Purpofe: After it is dry, you may with a Pencil

　　　　　give

give it a Finishing by mending such Places as are faulty, then you may lay on a Varnish, and polish it in the best Manner you can.

To imitate a Jaspis.

TAKE Quick-Lime, mix it with the white of Eggs, and roll it up in Balls, this will serve for the White, for Red mix along with it Lake or Vermillion, for Blue add Indigo or Prussian Blue, for Green use Verdegrease, and so on

When you have made many different Sorts of colour'd Balls, to the Consistence of a Dough, then flat them with a Rolling-Pin, as you would Pye Crust, lay them one upon another, and with a thin Knife-Blade, cut it in long Pieces, and mix them confusedly in a Mortar together, then with a Trowel spread it over a Table, Pilasters, &c very smooth and even, when dry, pour boiling hot Oil upon it, and spreading it all over, it will soak in, then set it in a shady Place to dry

You may, if you will, mix your Quick Lime and your Colours with Oil at first, and then there will be no Occasion to oil it afterwards.

How to clean Alablaster or white Marble.

BEAT Pumice Stones to an impalpable Powder, and mix it up with Verjuice, let it stand thus for two Hours, then dip in it a Spunge and rub the Marble or Alablaster therewith, wash it with a Linnen Cloath and fresh Water, and dry it with clean Linnen Rags.

To imitate Marble in Brimstone

TO 'do this, you must provide your self with a flat and smooth Piece of Marble, on which you make a Border or Wall, to encompass either a Square or Oval Table, which you may do either with Wax or Clay When this is done, provide and have in readiness several Sorts of Colours, each separately reduced to a fine Powder, as for Example; White Lead, Vermillion, Lake, Orpiment, Masticot, Smalt, *Prussian* Blue, and such like Colours After you are provided with them then melt on a slow Fire in

several

several glaz'd Pannikins some Brimstone, put in each one particular Sort of Colour, and stir it well together, then having before oil'd the Marble all over within the Wall, drop with one Colour quickly spots upon, of large and less Sizes, then take another Colour and do as before, and so on, till the Stone is covered with Spots of all the Colours you design to use, then you must consult what Colour the Mass or the Ground of your Table is to be, if you will have it of a Grey Colour, then take fine sifted Ashes, and mix it up with melted Brimstone, or if red, with *English* red Oaker; if White, with white Lead, if Black, with Lampblack or Ivory Black   Your Brimstone for the Ground must be pretty hot, so that the Drops upon the Stone may unite and incorporate together, when you have pour'd your Ground even all over, then, if you will, put a thin Wainscot Board upon it; but this must be done whilst the Brimstone is hot, making also the Board, which must be thorough dry, as hot as it will bear, in order to cause the Brimstone to stick the better to it, and when it is cold, polish it with Oil and a Cloath, and it will look very beautiful.

To imitate a *Porphyr*

TAKE Red Oaker and Lake, grind it with Water of Gum Tragant, then, either on a Glass, Marble or a smooth Board (before anointed all over with Oil) you sprinkle out of a Brush or Feather, the Glass or Table, all over with that Colour, and having sprinkled it all over, mix Brown Red, or if that is too Red, add some Umber or Soot to it, mix it up with Gum Tragant to the Substance of a thick Paste, and roll it on the Glass, over the sprinkled Colours, as thick as you please, then let it dry, and when you are sure that it is thorough dry, you may polish it.

How to make Fret Work Cielings

TAKE Pebble, stamp them fine in an Iron Mortar, search it through a fine Hair Sieve, then take of powder'd Lime one Part, of the Pebble Powder two Parts, and mix it together with Water, then take the Mixture, and lay it all over the Cieling, very smooth, carve then on it what you please, or lay to it some Ornament with Moulds, which are cut

in

in fmooth Wood, or caft in Lead, fill the Form with the
Mixture, prefs it to the Cieling, and it will ftick and come
clean out of the Mould, let it dry, and when dry, and you
percei e that it is not every where of a good White, then
with a clean Pencil Brufh and clear Water ftrike it over, and
it whitens of itfelf. It will in Time grow as hard as Stone

PART XI.

Plain Inftructions for LIMNING and for Colouring COPPER-PLATE PRINTS, MAPPS, &c. with *Water-Colours.*

Of the Colours generally ufed in that A t

For White ufe
{
1. White Lead.
2. Flake White
3 Mufcle Silver

Yellow
{
1 Yellow Oaker
2 Mafticote.
3 Pale Mafticote
4. Dutch Pink
5 Gamboge.
6 Naples Yellow
7 Shell Gold

Blue
{
1 Indigo
2. Blue Lake
3 Blue Verditer
4. Smalt
5. Ultramarine
6 Latmus.
7. Blue.

Green
{
1. Sap Green
2 Verdegreafe
3 Terre Verde.

Red
{
1 Vermillion
2 Red Lead.
3 Red Oaker.
4. Lake.
5. Carmine.

Brown
{
1 Brown Oaker
2 Chimney Soot of a Wood Fire
3. Colln's Earth.
4 Umber.

Black.
{
1 Lamp-Black.
2 Ivory Black
3 Sea-Coal Black.
4 Indian Ink.

Out of thefe Colours you may temper all the reft which
your Work may require.

Some

Some Colours are to be washed and ground, as for Instance,
1. White Lead. 2. Brown Oaker 3. Dutch Pink   4 Umber 5 Colln's Earth 6 Ivory Black.

Some are only to be wash'd, and are, 1. Red-Lead.
2. Masticote 3. Blue Bise. 4 Smalt. 5. Ultramarine.
6 Vermillion.

Others are only steep'd in fair Water, as, 1. Gamboge.
2. French Yellow, to which you must add a little Allum.
3 Sap Green 4 Blue Lake. 5 Letmus.

And others again are only ground, *viz* 1 Flake White.
2. Indigo 3 Lake 4 Carmine 5 Distill'd Verdegreafe.

All your Colours you grind with fair Water on a hard
Stone, or on a Piece of Looking-Glass, which you fix with
white Pitch and Rosin upon a flat Board, having also a
Muller of that Kind.

Of the Colours (after you have ground them very fine) you
may take as much as will serve your present Occasion, and
temper 'em in a Gallipot or Shell with Gum Water, in which
you have also dissolv'd a small Matter of Sugar-Candy.
You must observe, that Colours which are very dry, require
a stronger Gum-Water, in others it must be used very sparingly

If your Colours won't stick, or the Paper or Print be
greasy, mix a very little Ear-Wax, or a little Drop of Fish
or Ox-Gall among your Colour, you may dry your Fish
or Ox-Gall and dilute it when you have Occasion for it,
with a little Brandy If your Paper or Print sinks, then
with clean Size and a spunge wipe it over, after you have
fastened the Edges round upon a Board, and let it dry

You must chuse Pencils of several Sizes, agreeable to
the Work you are to use them for, as for laying on a Ground
a Sky or Clouds, chuse a larger Size than those that you
use for Drapery, Trees, &c. wherein you must follow your
own Reason : Those Pencils of which the Hairs (after you
have wetted them between your Lips, and turn'd them upon
your Hand) keep close together, are the best

To paint or colour a clear Sky.

TAKE clear blue Verditer, mix'd with a little White,
with this begin at the Top of your Landskip or Picture,
and having laid on the Blue for some space, break it with a
little Lake or Purple, working it with a clean Pencil, one
Colour

it with a clean Pencil, one Colour imperceivably into another;
apply more White and Masticote, in order to make it
fainter and fainter towards the Horizon, working all the
while the Colours inperceptibly one into another, from the
Horizon to the Blue Sky; after which you may lay some
stronger Strokes of Purple over the Light, so as to make
them appear like Clouds at a Distance

For a fiery red Sky, you use Red Lead and a little White,
instead of the Purple Streaks or Clouds, working them
according to Art inperceptibly one into another

Clouds you lay on with White and Black, sometimes you
mix a little Purple along with, but the best and surest Di
rection you may enquire for of Nature herself

To lay a Ground for Walls of Chambers, Halls, &c

YOU must use for a common Wall, which is of a reddish
Hew, Brown, Red and White, and temper your
Colour according to the Newness or Decay thereof, shade it
with Brown Red, only mix'd with a little Bitre or Soot

Other Walls you lay on with Black and White, and shade
it with the same Colours; sometimes you mix a little Purple along with it, and then you shadow it with Black and
Lake.

For Wainscoting, that is embellish'd with carv'd Mouldings
and Figures, you must use one Colour, for both the Plain
and the Carve-Work, shading and heightning it with Judgment and Care

To paint a Fore Ground, in Imitation of Sand or Clay, lay
on the darker Parts with Brown Oaker, to what is in their
Distance, add a little White, and so on in Proportion, shading
it with Brown Oaker, and the strong Shades with Soot.

In a Carnation or Flesh Colour, use for young Women and
Children Flake-White, light Oaker, and a little Vermillion:
Some add a little Lake, but that must be but a very small
Matter, and having laid on the Colour for the Carnation,
you shade the Features about the Lips, Cheeks, Chin,
Knees, and Toes, with fine Lake and Vermillion, shadow-
ing the naked Part with Sea Coal and a little Lake, or
Brown Red, or with Brown Oaker and Lake, or else Indian-
Ink or Lake; for a brownish Complexion, you mix a little
Brown Oaker among the Carnation Colour

For

For ancient People, ufe Vermillion, Brown-Oaker and White, fhade it with Bitre and Lake.

A dead Corps of a young Perfon you paint with Flake-White, Brown-Oaker and a little Indigo, or Sea-Coal, and fhade it with Biftre or Sea Coal

For an old dead Corps, you leave out the Indigo, but fhade it as before.

For the Hair of young Women and Children you lay them on with light Oaker, fhade them with deep Oaker, and heighten them with Mafticot and White

Grey Hair you lay on with Black and White, fhade them with Black, and heighten them with White, and thus you proceed in painting any other colour'd Hair.

Trees, are laid on, fome with White, Black and Bitre, fhaded with brown Oaker, and heighten d with the fame Colour, with more White in it Thofe that ftand at a diftance, are laid on with Indigo Blue, Brown Oaker and White, and fhaded with Indigo and Brown Oaker Thofe that are further diftant you lay on faint, and fhadow them but flightly, which Order you muft obferve in colouring of Ships, Houfes, and other Buildings

In thatch'd Houfes you paint the Thatch or Straw, when new, with *Dutch* Pink, and fhade it with Brown Oaker, and to heighten the Straw, you ufe Mafticot and White Old Straw, you lay on with Brown Oaker, fometimes mix'd with Black and White, the Straw you heighten with Brown Oaker and White

In colouring Cities, Caftles or Ruins, you muft obferve Nature and cannot well be taught, but however to give a Beginner a little more light in that Affair, you muft obferve that thofe Houfes which lay neareft the Fore Ground muft be colour'd with Vermillion and White, adding to it a little Brown Oaker, fhading it with that and fome bitre; the heightenings are, upon occafion, done with Vermillion and more White

Houfes that lay further diftant, are laid on with Lake and a little Blue and White, fhaded with Blue and Lake, and heighten'd with adding more White.

Such Buildings as lay ftill further, are laid on with a faint Purple and a little Blue, fhaded foftly with Blue, and heighten'd with White, and the further they are off, the fainter and flighter muft be your Colour

In colouring of Rocks, Hills, &c that are at a great Distance, you obferve the fame Rule Such as lay nearer the Fore-Ground, you imitate according to Nature Trees that are upon the Fore-Ground, you paint with feveral Sorts of Greens, the better to diftinguifh one from the other, fuch as are on diftant Hills, muft be done with the fame Colour as the Hills

How to Paint or Colour Cattle.

HORSES of Chefnut Colour, you lay on with brown Red, fhaded with Brown Red and Black, and heighten it with Brown Red, White and Yellow; the Main and Tail of Horfes you may make White, as alfo the lower part of their Feet

One of an Afh-Colour you lay on with Black and White, fhade it with a bluifh Black, and heighten it with White.

A black Horfe, you lay on with all Black, fhade it with a deep Black, and heighten it with Black and White.

A white Horfe, you lay on with White-Lead, juft tainted or broke with a little Red, fhade it with black and white, and heighten it with pure White

Spotted Horfes muft be done according as Nature directs, and by thefe Directions you will govern yourfelf in painting or colouring any other Sort of Cattle.

Sheep you lay on with White, broke with a little Bitre, ufe in the Shadows a little Black.

Hogs or Pigs, you lay on with Brown-Oaker and Yellow Oaker, and fhade it with Bitre.

A Bear is laid on with Brown-Oaker, Black and Brown-Red, fhaded with Bitre and Black, and heightened with Brown Oaker and White.

A Leopard is laid on with Yellow Oaker, and fhaded with Bitre. The Spots are laid on with Bitre and Black, the Mouth with Black and White

An Afs is commonly of a Grizle, and laid on with Black and White, broke with a little Oaker

An Elephant is laid on with Black and White and a little Bitre.

A Monkey is laid on with Dutch Pink, Bitre and Black, the Hair is heightened with Mafticote, White and a little Bitre, the Paws muft be fhaded off with Black and Brown Red, with a little White

A Hart

A Hart is laid on with Brown-Oaker and English Red, and shaded on the Back and where it is requisite, with Bitre and Brown-Red; a Streak of White must be below the Neck, as must be the Belly and Breast of a white Colour.

A Hare is laid on with Brown Oaker, which loses itself by Degrees into White under the Belly; the Back is shaded with Bitre, and the Hair is heighten'd with Oaker and White.

A Rabbit is laid on with White, Black, and Bitre, the Belly is White. These Creatures are of various Colours, which may be imitated after Nature.

Of Birds.

A Falcon is laid on with Brown-Oaker, black and white, shaded with a pale black, the Feathers must be display'd and shadow'd with black, the Breast is white, the Legs are laid on with yellow, and shaded with Brown Oaker and Bitre.

A Turky Cock or Hen, is laid on with black and white, and shaded with black, working the Colours lighter and lighter towards the Belly, which must be all white, the Legs are laid on with Indigo and White, and shaded with Blue; when they are irritated, the Substance about their Bill must be laid on with Vermillion and Lake, deepening it with stronger Lake, otherwise when they are calm, that Part is a little upon the Purple.

A Swan is laid on with White, with a little Bitre, and heighten'd, where the Feathers seem to raise, with pure White. The Feet are blackish, and the Bill red, with a black Rising at the upper End.

Pidgeons, Drakes, Hens, are of so many various Colours, that there would be no End to give proper Lessons for every one, and thus it is with many other Birds, which an Artist ought to copy after Nature.

Of Fruit.

APPLES are laid on with fine Masticote mix'd with a little Verdegrease, or a little White, French Berry, Yellow and Verdegrease, shade it with Brown Oaker and Verdegrease, or Lake, heighten it with Masticote and White,

White, and the strongest Light with White alone; but you must regulate yourself to the Colour of the Apples as well as Pears.

Cherries are laid on with Vermillion and Lake, shaded with pure Lake, and heightened with Vermillion, or Vermillion and a little White

White-Heart Cherries, are laid on in the middle with Vermillion, Lake and White, working it to a Yellow towards the Stalk, and with Lake towards the Top.

Morello's are laid on with Lake and a little Black, shadow'd with Black, and heightened with Vermillion, Lake and Black, this must be so intermix'd that the Colours may seem all of one Piece

Mulberries are laid on with Lake and Bitre, shadow'd with Black, and heightened with Vermillion, on the highest Lights give little Dots with Lake and White

Strawberries are laid on with a yellowish White, then shaded with Lake and Vermillion, and heighten the Knobs with White and Vermillion

Grapes, the Black ones are laid on with Purple, shaded with blue Verditer and Indigo, and heightened with White

The white Grapes are laid on with pale Verdegrease, a little Masticote and White, the blue Bloom is very gently with a blunt Pencil just touch'd with the Blue Verditer dubb'd over them

Peaches and Apricocks are laid on with light Masticote, or French-Berry Yellow, and White, shaded with Red Oaker and Yellow, if there must be a Bloom upon them, you do it with Lake, and heighten it with White as you do the Grapes, some are of a more greener Colour than others, wherein you are to copy Nature as it lays before you

Radishes and Turnips, are laid on with White, shaded with Indian-Ink, and at the Top with Lake, working it down faint into White towards the Bottom   The Top is laid on with Verdegrease and Sap Green, shaded with Sap Green and Indigo, and heightened with Masticote.

Carrots, are laid on with Yellow Oaker, and if they are of a high Colour it is mix'd with Red Lead, they are shaded with Brown Oaker, Yellow Oaker and Bitre, and highten'd with Masticote. For the rest I direct the Practitioner to Nature.

Of Flowers

ROSES are laid on with a pale Carmine and White, Shadow'd with Carmine and lefs White, and the deepeft with Carmine by itfelf, the Heart you make always darker than the reft The Seed in open blown Rofes is Yellow

Tulips are of various Kinds, Colours, and Shapes, it is impoffible to give certain Rules for colouring of them

Some are done with Lake and Carmine on White, mix'd together, others with Purple, laid on with Ultramarine, Carmine and Lake, fometimes bluer, and fometimes redder, thefe Colours muft be ftreak'd according to Nature Thofe of one Colour, as Yellow, Red, &c are laid on with fuch Colours, and if there appear any Streaks you muft make your Colour either lighter or deeper, as Nature directs.

Emonies are of feveral Sorts, fome are laid on with Lake and White, and finifh'd with the fame Others with Vermillion and fhadow'd with that Colour, Carmine and Lake Yellow ones are laid on with Mafticote, and fhadow'd with that and Vermillion, fometimes with brown Lake

Red Lilies are laid on with Red Lead, fhaded with Vermillion and Carmine

The Piony is laid on with Lake and White, and fhaded with the fame Colour with lefs White.

Yellow Cowflips are laid on with Mafticot, and fhaded with Gumboge and Umber. Purple ones are laid on with Ultramarine, Carmine and White and fhadow'd with lefs White

Carnations and Pinks are managed like Emonies and Tulips. Some Pinks are of a pale Flefh-Colour Breaked with another that's a little higher; this is done with Vermillion, Lake and White, and ftreaked without White

The Blue Hyacinth, is laid on with Ultramarine and White, and fhaded with lefs White

The Red or Gridiline, is laid on with Lake and White, and a little Ultramarine, and finifh'd with lefs White.

The White Sort, is laid on with White, and fhadow'd with Black and White.

The Crocus are two Sorts, *viz* Yellow and Purple The Yellow is laid on with Mafticote, and fhaded with Gall-ftone or Gumboge, after which upon each Leaf on

R   the

the outside are made three separate Streaks with Bitre and Lake. The Purple ones are laid on with Carmine, Ultra marine and White, and finish'd with less White, the Streaks must be very dark on the outside of the Leaves. The Seed of both is Yellow.

Of Metals

GOLD is laid on with Red Lead, Saffron, and Yellow Oker, shadow'd with Lake and Bitre, in the deepest Places with Bitre, Lake and Black, then heighten'd with Shell-Gold

Silver is laid on with White, shadow'd with Black and Blue, and heighten'd with Shell-Silver

Tin or Pewter is done the same Way, only it is laid on with White, mixt with a little Indigo

Iron is done like Tin

Brass is done in the same Manner as Gold, only the Shades must not be so strong

Copper is laid on with Brown red and White, shadow'd with Brown red, Lake, and Bitre, and heighten'd with Brown, Red, and White.

These Directions will be sufficient to guide young Prac titioners to Nature, which is the best School they can go to, to their Live's

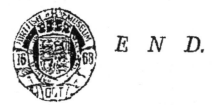 E N D.

AN
APPENDIX
TO THE
LABORATORY
OR
SCHOOL of ARTS:

CONTAINING,

I Plain Inſtructions in the Art of Dying SILKS, WORSTEDS, COTTONS, &c of various Colours

II Proper Leſſons for preparing and managing all Sorts of ROCKETS, CRACKERS, FIRE WHEELS, FIRE GLOBES, BALLS, STARS, SPARKS, &c. in the executing of artificial and recreative FIREWORKS.

Tranſlated from the HIGH DUTCH.

Illuſtrated with COPPER-PLATES

LONDON:

Printed for J HODGES, at the *Looking-glaſs* on *London-Bridge;* J JAMES, at *Horace's Head* under the *Royal Exchange,* and T. COOPER, at the *Globe* in *Pater-noſter Row* 1740

[Price One Shilling.]

APPENDIX

To the Second Edition of

LABORATORY

O R

SCHOOL of ARTS.

The Art of dying SILKS, WORSTEDS, COTTONS, &c. of various Colours.

HE art of dying in colours, is of great antiquity, as appears both from sacred and profane history, but who were the first inventers thereof, is uncertain, however, for the generality it is conjectured that like many others it had its first birth by accident. the juices of certain fruits, leaves, &c accidentally crushed, are supposed to have given the first hint. Purple, an animal juice, found in a mussel, was first discovered to be of a tinging quality, by a dog's catching one of the purple-fishes among the rocks, which in eating stained his mouth with that precious colour this colour was in so high esteem among the *Romans*, that none but their emperors were suffered to wear it I could give the curious a long historical and speculative account concerning this ingenious art, but

a

that

that being a fubject not fuitable to the intent of this work, I fhall only inform my readers in the practice thereof, in as concife and plain a manner as poffible My firft leffon is

How to dye Silk or Worfted of a fine Carnation Colour

FIRST take to each pound of filk, four handfuls of wheaten bran, put it in two pails of water, boil it, pour it into a tub, and let it ftand all night, then take half the quantity of that water, put into it ¼ a pound of allum, ¼ of a pound of red tartar, beaten to a fine powder, and ½ an ounce of fine powdered curcuma, boil them together, and ftir them well about with a flick, after they have boiled for a quarter of an hour, take the kettle off the fire, put in the filk, and cover the kettle clofe to prevent the fteam from flying out, leave it thus for three hours, then rince your filk in cold water, beat and wring it on a wooden pin, and hang it up to dry

Then take ¼ of a pound of gallnuts, beat them fine, and put the powder thereof into a pail of river water, boil it for one hour, then take off the kettle, and when you can bear your hand therein, put in your filk, and let it lay therein an hour, then take it out and hang it up to dry. When the filk is dry, and you would dye it of a crimfon colour, weigh to each pound of filk, ¾ of an ounce of cochineel, which beat to a fine powder, and fift it through a fine hair fieve, then put it in the pail with the remaining lee, and having mix'd it well, pour it into a kettle, and when it boils, cover it well to prevent any duft coming to it, after you have put in ⅔ of a pound, and two ounces and a half of tartar, both finely powdered, let it boil for a ¼ of an hour, then take it off the fire, let it cool a little, and put in the filk, ftir it well with a flick to prevent its being clouded, and when cold wring it out If the colour is not deep enough, hang the kettle again over the fire, and when it has boiled and is grown lukewarm again, repeat the ftirring of the filk therein, then hang it upon a wooden pin which is faftened in a poft, wring and beat it with a flick, after this, rince the dy'd filk in hot lee, wherein to one pound of filk, you have diffolved ½ an ounce of *Newcaftle* foap, afterwards rince it in cold water Hang the fkeins of raw-filk on a wooden pin, putting a little hand-ftick to the bottom part,

and

and thus having worked, wrung, and beat it round, you must hang it up to dry.

Another Method to dye Silk of a crimson Red.

TAKE of good *Roman* allum ½ an ounce, tartar one ounce, spirit of vitriol ¼ of an ounce, and put them pulverized into a pewter kettle, and pour as much water on them, as is sufficient for the quantity of ½ an ounce of the silk you propose to dye, when it is ready to boil, put in the silk, which before you must boil in bran, boil it for an hour or more, then wring it out, and put to the liquor ½ an ounce of cochineel finely powdered, and 60 drops of spirit of vitriol, when ready to boil, put in the silk again, and let it soak for four hours, then take clean water, drop into it a little spirit of vitriol, rince therein the silk, wring it out again, and dry it on sticks in the shade. This will be a high colour, but if you would have it of a deep crimson, you take instead of spirit of vitriol, spirit of sal ammoniac, to rince your silk in.

General Observations in dying Crimson, Scarlet, or Purple.

1 YOUR copper or kettle must be of good pewter, quite clean and free from any foul or grease.

2 The prepared tartar must be put in when the water is lukewarm.

3 If you intend to dye woolen or worsted yarn, you may put it in the first boiling, and let it boil for two hours.

4 When boil'd take it out, rince it, clean the kettle, and put in the water for the second boiling.

5 This second boiling is performed in the same manner as the first, then put in cochineel finely powdered, when it boils hard, and stir it well about.

6 Then the silk, which before has been washed and cleansed in the first lee, is put in on a winch, which is contin-

nually,

nually turned about, in order to prevent the colours from fixing in clouds.

7 When the colour is to your mind, take it out of the copper, rince it clean, and hang it up in a room or a shady place, where it may be free from dust

8 You must observe, that when the aqua fortis, is put into the second boiling, it causes a coarse froth to swim at top which you must carefully take off.

How to dissolve the Pewter for Dyer's Aqua Fortis

TAKE fine pewter, pour first a little clear water over it, then pour on the aqua fortis, which will dissolve it. The solution is of a whey or milk colour, temper it by adding more aqua fortis, till it is clear   The common proportion is, to one ounce of aqua fortis add a quarter of an ounce of pewter

To dye a Crimson with Orchal

PUT clean water into the copper, and to each pound of silk take 12 ounces of orchal· in this turn your silk and wring it out, then dissolve to each pound of silk $\frac{1}{4}$ of a pound of allum, and as much of white arsenic, in this liquor put the silk all night to soak, then wring it out, this done, take to each pound of silk, two ounces of cochineel, two ounces of galls, two ounces of gum, with a little curcuma· in this boil the silk for two hours, then put in a little zepsie, let it soak all night, and in the morning rince it out.

To dye a Violet Colour.

FIRST boil your silk in bran and allum, as has been shewn above, then clean your copper, and with clean water, put to each pound of silk, one pound of galls, one ounce and a half of cochineel finely powdered, and one ounce of gum arabick, boil it together like the crimson red, leave it all night, and the next morning take out your silk, and rince it in fair water.

To

To dye Worsted, Stuff, or Yarn of a Crimson Colour

TAKE to each pound of worsted, two ounces of allum, two ounces of white tartar, two ounces of aqua fortis, $\frac{1}{2}$ an ounce of pewter, $\frac{1}{4}$ of a pound of madder, and $\frac{1}{4}$ of a pound of logwood, put them together in fair water, boiling the worsted therein for a considerable time, then take it out of the copper, and when cool, rince it in clean water then boil it again, and put to each pound of worsted, $\frac{1}{4}$ of a pound of logwood

Another Method.

TAKE to eight pound of worsted, six gallons of water, and eight handfuls of wheaten bran, let them stand all night to settle, in the morning pour it clear off, and filtrate it, take thereof half the quantity, adding as much clear water to it, boil it up, and put into it one pound of allum, and half a pound of tartar, then put in the worsted, and let it boil for two hours, stirring it up and down all the while it is boiling with a stick Then boil the other half part of your bran-water, mixing it with the same quantity of fair water as before, when it boils put into it four ounces of cochineel, two ounces of fine powder'd tartar, stir it well about, and when it has boiled for a little while, put in your stuffs keep stirring it from one end of the copper to the other with a stick, or turn it on a winch, till you see the colour is to your mind, then take it out of the copper, let it cool, and rince it in fair water.

Another for Silk.

TAKE to each pound of silk, a quarter of a pound of fernambuca, boil it up, and strain it through a sieve into a tub, and pour water to it, till it is just lukewarm: in this turn your silk, which before has been prepared as has been directed, and when all the strength is drawn out, rince, wring and dry it.

A 3

Another for Carnation

TAKE to each pound of filk, after it is rinc'd and dry d, four pound of fafflower, put the fafflower in a bag, and wafh it in clean water, till the water comes clear from it, then take the fafflower out of the bag, prefs it between your hands, and rub it afunder in a clean tub, take to each pound of filk, four ounces of pot afhes, work it well together with the fafflower, divide it into two parts, pour one part thereof into a clofe fack, that will keep the pot-afhes from coming out, otherwife it will make the filk fpeck'ed, and pour clear water over it, to draw the ftrength out of the fafflower, then take to each pound of filk, a quarter of a pint of lemon juice, divide that alfo into two parts, and put each to the two quantities of fafflower hang your filk well dryed on clean fticks, and dip it in the firft part of the liquer continually for an hour; then wring it well out, and hang it again on fticks having prepared the other part of the fafflower as you did the firft, dip it therein as before for the fpace of an hour, then wring it well and hang it up to dry in the fhade, and you will have a fine colour

A Coction for Woolen

TAKE four ounces of ceruse, three ounces and a half of arfenic, one pound of burned tartar, one pound of illum, boil your ftuffs with thofe ingredients for two hours, then take it out, and hang it up the next morning make a dye of two pound of good madder, a quarter of a pound of orlean, two ounces of curcum, and three ounces of aqua fortis

To dye a Carnation on Silk or Cotton, with Fernambuca

TAKE three pound of allum, three ounces of arfenic, four ounces of ceruse, boil your filk or cotton therein for an hour, then take it out and rince it in fair water, after which make a lee of eight pound of madder, and two ounces of fal armoniac, foak the filk or cotton therein all night, then boil it a little in fair water, and put into it one ounce of pot afhes, then pour in fome of the lee, and every time you

pour,

pour, the colour will grow the deeper, so that you may bring it to what degree or shade you please.

Another Method.

TAKE to one pound of silk, cotton, or yarn, one ounce of tartar, and half an ounce of white starch, boil them together in fair water, then put in one quarter of an ounce of cochineel, a quarter of an ounce of starch, and a quarter of an ounce of pewter, dissolved in half an ounce of aqua fortis, and mixed with fair water, when the water with the starch and tartar has boiled for some time, supply it with the cochineel and the above aqua fortis, put in your silk or whatever you have a mind to dye, and you will have it of a fine colour.

Another Method.

TAKE one ounce of tartar, starch and lemon juice of each half an ounce, and cream of tartar a quarter of an ounce, boil them together in fair water, adding a quarter of an ounce of curcuma, put in half an ounce of cochineel, and a little while after one ounce of aqua fortis, in which you have dissolved a quarter of an ounce of pewter, and then put in your silk.

To dye Yarn or Linnen of a lasting Violet Colour.

TAKE one pound of tartar, half a pound of allum, two ounces of fernambuca, and half an ounce of saltpetre, boil them together, then let them cool a little, and put in your yarn, let it soak for four hours, keeping the dye hot but not boiling, after which rince and dry it.

How to prepare or set a blue Vat for dying.

HEAT soft water in a kettle or copper, fling four or five handfuls of wheaten bran, together with four pound of pot ashes into it, when that is dissolved boil it for an hour, and then add four pound of madder, with this boil it for an hour longer, then pour the water into the vat, fill it not full by the height of a foot, and then cover your vat, then set it with indigo and woad, of each six pound, and two

pound

pound of pot-aſhes, put this into a ſmall kettle in warm-water, ſet it on a ſlow fire, and let it boil gently for half an hour, ſtirring it all the while, then pour that to the other liquors already in the vat.

To ſet a vat with indigo only, you muſt boil the firſt lee with pot aſhes, four or five handfuls of bran, and half or three quarters of a pound of madder; this you boil a quarter of an hour, and when ſettled it will be fit for uſe. Then grind your indigo in a copper bowl, with an iron ſmooth ball very fine, pouring on ſome of the lee, and mixing it toge-ther, when ſettled, pour the clear into the blue vat, and on the ſediment of the indigo, pour again ſome of the lee, this you ſhould repeat till you ſee the blue tincture is extracted clearly from it

It is to be obſerved, that the madder muſt be but ſparingly uſed, for it only alters the colour, and makes it of a violet blue, which, if you deſign to have, cochineel is the fitter for. The mix'd colours in blue are the following dark blue, deep blue, high blue, ſky blue, pale blue, dead blue, and whitiſh blue

By mixing of blue and crimſon, is produced purple, columbine, amaranth, and violet colours, alſo from thoſe mixtures may be drawn the pearl, ſilver, gridelin, &c. colours

From a middling blue and crimſon are produced the following colours, *viz.* the panſy, brown gray, and deep brown

Care muſt be taken that in ſetting the blue vat, you do not overboil the lee, by which the colour becomes muddy and changeable, be alſo ſparing with the pot aſhes, for too much thereof gives the blue a greeniſh and falſe hue, but experience is the beſt inſtructer in this.

Another Direction how to ſet a Blue Vat, together with ſeveral Obſervations in the Management thereof, both for Silk or Worſted

TAKE half a buſhel of clean beech aſhes, well ſifted, of this make a lee with three pails of river or rain-water, pour it into a tub, and put in two handfuls of whea-ten bran, two ounces of madder, two ounces of white tartar

finely

finely powdered, one pound of pot-afhes, half a pound of indigo pounded, ftir it all well together, once every 12 hours for 14 days fucceffively, till the liquid appears green on your fingers, and then it is fit to dye, however when ready, ftir it every morning, and cover it when you have done

When you are going to dye filk, firft wafh the filk in a frefh warm lee, wring it out and dip it into the vat, you may dye it what fhade you pleafe, by holding it longer or fhorter in the dye.

When the colour is to your mind, wring the filk, and having another tub, ready at hand with a clear lee, rince therein your filk, then wafh and beat it in fair water and hang it up to dry

When the vat is wafted, fill it with the lee, but if it grows too weak fupply it with half a pound of pot-afhes half a pound of madder, one handful of wheat-bran, and half an handful of white tartar, let it ftand for eight days, ftirring it every 12 hours, and it will be again fit for ufe

Another Method for Woollen.

FILL a kettle or copper with water, boil it up, and put pot afhes into it, after it has boil'd with that a little, put in two or three handfuls of bran, let it boil for $\frac{1}{4}$ of an hour, then cover it, take it off the fire and let it fettle

Pound the indigo as fine as flower · then pour off the above lee to it, ftir it and let it fettle, and pour the clear lee into the vat; then pour more lee to the fediment, ftir it and when fettled pour that into the vat alfo, repeat this till the indigo is wafted *Or*,

Take to $\frac{1}{4}$ of a pound of indigo, $\frac{1}{2}$ a pound of pot-afhes, $\frac{1}{4}$ of a pound of madder, three handfuls of borax, let it boil for $\frac{1}{2}$ an hour, and then fettle, with this lee grind your indigo in a copper bowl, put this on an old vat of indigo, or on a new one of woad, and it will make it fit for ufe in 24 hours.

To dye Silk of a Straw Yellow

TAKE allum and rinfe your filk well, as has been di
rected before, then take and boil to each pound of
filk, one pound of fuftic or iocaw, and let them ftand for
¼ of an hour, then put into a tub, large enough for the
quantity of the filk, a fufficient quantity of that lee and fair
water, in this rince the filk, fill the kettle again with wa
ter, and let it boil for ¼ of an hour, and having wrung the
filk out of the firft liquor and hung it on fticks, prepare a
ftronger than the firft, in this you dip your filk fo long till
the colour is to your mind

Another Method

PUT into a clean copper or kettle to each pound of filk,
two pound of fuftic, let it boil for an hour, then put i.
fix ounces of gall, let it boil together ½ an hour longer, the
filk being allum'd and rinc'd, is turn'd about in this colour,
then take it out of the kettle, and wring it out, dip it in pot-
afh-lee, and wring it out again, then put it into the copper,
let it foak a whole night, and in the morning rince, beat
it out, and hang it up to dry.

Of dying Silk &c. of different Greens

THE middling colour of blue and yellow produces a
light green, grafs green, laurel green, fea-green, &c.
All olive-colours, from the deepeft to the lighteft are
nothing elfe but green colours, which by walnut tree root,
fuftic or foot of the chimneys, are chang d to what fhade
you pleafe.

A fine Green for dying Silk.

TAKE to one pound of filk ¼ of a pound of allum, two
ounces of white tartar, put them together in hot water
to diffolve, and when fo, put in your filk and let it foak
all night, take it out the next morning, and hang it up to
dry, then take one pound of fuftic, boil it in four gallons
of water, for an hour long, take out the fuftic, fling it away,
and put into the copper ½ an ounce of fine beaten verdigreafe,
ftir it about for ¼ of an hour, draw it off into a tub, and let

It

it cool, then put into that colour one ounce of pot aſhes, ſtir it together with a ſtick, dip into it your ſilk, ſo long till you think it yellow enough, then rince it in fair water and hang it up to dry, then dip it in the blue vat, till you think it enough, rince it again and beat it over the pin, and hang it up to dry, thus you may change the ſhades of your green by dipping either more or leſs, in the blue or yellow

For the green, take to one pound of ſilk three ounces of verdigreaſe, beaten to a fine powder, infuſe it in a pint of wine vinegar for a night, then put it before the fire, when hot ſtir it with a ſtick, and keep it from boiling, in this put your ſilk two or three hours, or it you would have it of a light colour, let it ſoak but for ½ an hour, then take ſcalding hot water, and in a trough, rub'd over with *New-caſtle* ſoap, beat and work it up to a clear lather, in this rince your ſilk, then hang it up to dry, rince it again in river water, beat it well, and when it is well clean'd, and dry'd, dreſs it

How to dye Linnen of a Green Colour

SOAK your linnen over night, in ſtrong allum water, then take it out to dry, take woad, boil it for an hour long, take out the woad, and put in one ounce of powder'd verdigreaſe, or according to the quantity you have to dye, more or leſs, ſtir it together with the linnen, briſkly about, then put in a piece of pot-aſh, the bigneſs of an hen's egg, and you will have your linnen of a yellow colour, which when dry'd a little, being put into a blue vat, will turn green

To dye Yarn of a Yellow Colour.

IN a copper of ſtrong lee put a bundle of woad, and let it boil, then pour off the lee and take one yard and a half of yarn, half an ounce of verdigreaſe, half an ounce of allum, put it into a quart of brown braſil-wood liquor, boil'd with lee, ſtir it well together and pour it in and mix it with the woad-lee, in this ſoak your yarn over night and it will be of a good yellow.

To dye Green Yarn or Linnen Black.

TAKE a sharp lee, put in three pound of brown brasil, and let it boil for some time, then pour off the colour from the chips, into a tub, add to it one ounce of gum arabick, one ounce of allum, one ounce of verdigrease, in this lay your yarn or linnen to soak over night, and it will be of a good black

To dye Silk an Orange Colour

AFTER you have clean'd your kettle well, fill it with clean rain-water, and take to each pound of silk four ounces of pot-ashes, and four ounces of orlean, sift it through a sieve into the kettle, when it is well melted, and you have taken care not to let any of those ingredients stick about the kettle, then put in your silk, which before you have prepared and allum'd as has been directed, turn it round on the winch and let it boil up, then take and wring it out, beat it and rince it, then prepare another kettle, and take to each pound of silk twelve ounces of gall-nuts, let the gall nuts boil for two hours, then cool for the same space of time, after which put in the silk for three or four hours, then wring it out, rince, beat and dry it

Another Orange Colour

SOAK the white silk in allum water like as you do in dying of yellow, then take two ounces of orleans yellow, put it over night in water together with one ounce of pot ashes boil it up, add to it, after it has boil'd half an hour, one ounce of powdered curcumi, stir it with a stick, and after a little while put your allum'd silk into it for two or three hours, according to what height you would have your colour, then rince it out in clear soap-suds, till it looks clear, afterwards clear it in fair water, and dress it according to art

A fine

A fine Brimstone Yellow for Worsted.

TAKE three pound of allum, one pound of tartar; three ounces of salt, boil the cloth with these materials for one hour, then pour off that water, and pour fresh into the kettle, make a lee of shart and pot ashes, let it boil well, and then turn the cloth twice or thrice quickly through upon the winch, and it will have a fine brimstone colour

A Lemon Colour.

TAKE three pound of allum, three ounces of ceruse, three ounces of arsenic, with these ingredients boil the cloth for an hour and a half, then pour off that water and make a lee of 16 pound of yellow flowers, three ounces of curcuma, then draw or winch your cloth through quickly, and you will have it of a fine lemon colour

To dye an Olive-Colour.

TO dye this colour observe the first directions for dying a brimstone colour, then make a lee of gall-nuts and vitriol, but not too strong, draw your stuff quickly thro', three or four times, according as you would have it, either deeper or lighter

To dye a Gold Colour

HAVING first dy'd your silk, worsted, cotton or linnen of a yellow colour, then take to each pound of the commodity, one ounce of filet-wood or yellow chips, and of pot ashes the quantity of a bean, boil this for half an hour, then put in your silk, and turn it so long, till the colour is to your liking.

The Dutch *Manner of dying Scarlet*

BOIL the cloth in allum, tartar, salgemma, aquafortis, and pea flowers, either in a pewter kettle or with aquafortis, in which pewter is dissolv'd, then put into the same kettle, starch, tartar and cochineel finely powdered, stirring or turning the cloth well about, and thus you may, by adding
more

more or lefs cochineel, raife the colour to what height you pleafe

General Obfervations for dying Cloth of a Red or Scarlet Colour.

1 THE cloth muft be well foak'd in a lee made of allum and tartar, this is commonly done with two parts of allum and one part of tartar.

2 For ftrengthening the red colour, you prepare a water of bran or ftarch, the bran water is thus prepared, take five or fix quarts of wheaten bran, boil it over a flow fire in rain-water for a quarter of an hour, and then put it with fome cold water into a fmall veffel, mixing it up with a handful of leaven, the fowerer it's made, the better it is, this caufes the water to be foft, and the cloth to become mellow, it is commonly ufed in the firft boiling, and mixt with the allum water

3 Arfenic, is an ingredient ufed in dying of reds, but few dyers can give any reafon for its virtue, but as it is of a dry fpungy nature, it may reafonably be fuppofed, that it contracts the greafinefs which might happen to be in the dye

4 The ufe of arfenic is not a very neceffary, but a very dangerous ingredient, aquafortis, or fpirit of falt will fupply its place as well.

5 To give a true defcription of fcarlet, it is nothing elfe but a fort of crimfon colour, the aqua fortis is the chief ingredient for the change thereof, this may be try'd in a wine glafs, wherein a deep crimfon colour may, by adding drops of aqua fortis to it, be changed into a fcarlet, or to a perfect yellow

6 Obferve that you always take one part of tartar to two part of allum, moft dyers prefer the white before the red tartar, but however, in crimfon colours and others that turn upon the brown, the red tartar is chofe by many as preferable to the white.

To

To dye Scarlet Cloth

FIRST take to one pound of cloth, one part of bran-water, and two parts of rain water, then put into it two ounces of allum and one ounce of tartar, when it boils and froths, fcum it, and put in the cloth, turn it therein for an hour, then take it out and rince it.

To dye Cloth of a common Red.

TAKE to twenty yards of cloth, three pound of allum, one pound and a half of tartar, and one third of a pound of chalk, put them in a copper with water and boil them, then take fix pound of good madder, and a wine-glafs full of vinegar, let it be warmed together, and put in the cloth, turn it round upon the winch, 'till you obferve it red enough, then rince it out, and it will be of a fine red.

Another Method.

TAKE four pound of allum, two pound of tartar, four ounces of white lead, and half a bufhel of wheat bran, put thefe ingredients, together with the cloth, into a copper; let it boil for an hour and half, and leave it therein to foak all night, then rince it, and take for the dye, one pound of good madder, two ounces of orlean, one ounce and a half of curcum, and two ounces of aqua fortis; boil them, turn the cloth with a winch for three quarters of an hour, and it will be of a good red

To dye Scarlet.

TAKE to two pound of goud, two ounces of tartar, and one ounce of fal armoniac, grind them fine, and boil them up in fair water, add to them two ounces of ftarch, half an ounce of gum cotta, and one ounce of cochineel, when thefe are boiling hot, put in an ounce and half of aqua fortis, and let it boil, then take it out, and when cool rince it

To dye Brown Colours

BROWN colours are produced from the root, bark and leaves of walnut-trees, as alfo of walnut fhells-china root might alfo be ufed for brown colours; but it being of a difagreeable fcent, it fhould only be ufed for hair colour in ftuffs, for which and the olive colours it is of more ufe The beft browns are dy'd with woad and walnut-tree root.

A Nutmeg Colour on Stuffs

TAKE three pound of allum, half a pound of tartar, put this into a copper of water, and boil your ftuff for an hour and a half; and take it out to cool Then take one pound and a half of fifet-wood or yellow flowers, three pound of madder, one pound of gall-nuts, put it together with the ftuff, into a copper, boil and turn it with a winch, till it is red enough, and take it out to cool, then take two pound of vitriol, which before is diffolv'd in warm water, put it in the copper, and turn the ftuff till the colour is to your mind; then rince it out.

Or,

Take half a bufhel of green walnut-fhells, or elfe walnut tree-root, infufe it in a kettle, and when it begins to boil put in the ftuff over a winch, turn it about three or four times, then take it out and let it cool; after it is cold, boil the liquor again, and put the ftuff in, turn it for half an hour, and take it out and let it cool, then put in one pound of gall-nuts, three pound of madder, together with the ftuffs into the kettle, let it boil for an hour, take it out and let it cool again, take one pound of vitriol, put it in, ftir it well about, then put in again the ftuffs over the winch, turn and boil it fo long till you perceive your colour deep enough, then take it out and rince it.

How to make Flax soft and mellow

MAKE a ftrong lee of wood or pot-afhes, and unflack'd lime, in which foak your flax for 24 hours, then put it together with the lee into a copper, and let it boil, and it will be as foft as filk. After this rince it in clean water, wring out the water, and put the flax again into a ftrong lee, repeat this thrice, then rince it out, dry it, and it will anfwer your purpofe. Some prefer cow-dung, with which the flax is daubed all over, or foak it in a lee of cow-dung for 24 hours, then rince and dry it.

An excellent Water for taking out Spots in Cloth, Stuff, &c.

TAKE two pound of fpring water, put in it a little pot-afhes, about the quantity of a walnut, and a lemon cut in fmall flices, mix this well together, and let it ftand for 24 hours in the fun, then ftrain it through a cloth, and put the clear liquid up for ufe, this water takes out all fpots, whether pitch, greafe or oil, as well in hats, as cloath, ftuffs, filk, cotton and linnen, immediately, but as foon as the fpot is taken off, wafh the place with water, and when dry you will fee nothing

To Dye Woolen Stuffs of a Black Colour

FINE cloaths and fuch ftuffs as will bear the price muft be firft dy'd of a deep blue in a frefh vat of pure indigo, after which you boil the ftuffs in allum and tartar, then you dye it in madder, and at laft with galls of *Aleppo*, vitriol and *Sumach Arab* * dye it black, to prevent the colour foiling when the cloaths are made up, they muft, before they are fent to the dye houfe, be well fcowered in a fcowring mill

Middling ftuffs, after they have been prepar'd by fcowring and drawn through a blue vat, are dy'd black with gall-nuts and vitriol

---

* Is a fhrub that grows in *Spain, Portugal* and *France*, from which coun tries it is carried in abundance to moft parts of *Europe* that which is good muft be dry and of a light green colour that of a brown hue is fpent and good for little It is ufed by black dyers, cordwainers &c The eaves boil'd in lee, dye hair black,

For ordinary wool or woolen ſtuffs take walnut tree branches and ſhells, a ſufficient quantity, with this boil your ſtuff to a brown colour, then draw it through the black dye made with the bark of elder, iron, or copper filings, and indian-wood.

To Dye Linnen of a Black Colour

TAKE filings of iron, waſh them, and add to them the bark of an elder tree, boil them up together, and dip your linnen therein.

To Dye Woolen of a good Black

1. TAKE two pound of gall-nuts, two pound of the bark of elder-tree, one pound and a half of yellow chips, boil them for three hours, then put in your ſtuff, turn it well with the winch, and when you perceive it black enough take it out and cool it

2 Take one ounce and a half of ſal armoniac, with this boil your ſtuff gently for an hour long, turning it all the while with the winch then take it out again and let it cool.

3. Take two pound and a half of vitriol, a quarter of a pound of *Sumach*, boil your ſtuff therein for an hour, then cool and rince it, and it will be of a good black

Another Black Colour for Woolen

FOR the firſt boiling take two pound of gall nuts, half a pound of braſil-wood, two pound and a half of madder, boil your cloth with theſe ingredients for three hours, then take it out to cool, for the ſecond boiling take one ounce and a half of ſal-armoniac, and for the third two ounces and a half of vitriol, three quarters of a pound of braſil, and a quarter of a pound of tallow.

Another

Another Black Colour for Plush.

PUT the following ingredients into a large veffel, *viz*
eight pound of elder bark, eight pound of *Sumach*,
twelve pound of oaken chips, nine pound of vitriol, two
pound of wild marjorum, fix pound of tile-duft, fome wafte
of a grind ftone, fix pound of walnut leaves, half a pound of
burnt tartar, two pound of falt, four pound of woad, on thefe
pour boiling water till your veffel is full, your plufh after it
is well boil'd and cleanfed muft be well galled, and this
you do by boiling it in one pound and a half of *Su-*
mach, eight ounces of madder, two ounces and a half of
burnt faltpetre, half an ounce of fal-armoniac, one ounce
and a half of vitriol, half an ounce of burnt tartar, then take
it out, and let it dry without rinceing it

Then you fill the copper with the above liquor, and boil
and dye your plufh in the manner as you do other ftuffs,
turning it round with the winch when the colour is to
your mind, take out the plufh, let it cool, and then rince
and hang it up to dry

To Dye Silk of a good Black.

IN a copper containing fix pails of water, put two pound of
beaten gall nuts, four pound of *Sumach*, a quarter of a
pound of madder, half a pound of antimony finely powdered,
four ox galls, four ounces of gum tragacant firft diffolv'd in
fair water, of fine beaten elder-bark of two ounces, and one
ounce and a half of iron file duft, put thefe ingredients into
the above water, and let them boil for two hours, then fill
it up with a pail full of barley water, and let it boil for an
hour longer, then put in your filk, and boil it for half an
hour flowly, then take it out and rince it in a tub with clean
water, and pour that again into the copper, the filk you rince
quite clean in a running water, then hang it up, and when
it is dry, put it in the copper again, boil it flowly for half
an hour as before, then rince it in a tub, and again in rain
water, when dry, take good lee, put into it two ounces
of pot afhes, and when they are diffolv'd, rince the filk therein

quickly,

quickly, then in running water, this done, hang it to dry and order it as you do other colour'd filks

This colour will alfo dye all forts of manufactur'd woollen ftuffs.

To give the black filk a fine glofs, you muft, before the laft dipping, put in for each pound one ounce of ifinglafs, firft diffolv d in water.

Another manner for dying Silk.

IN a copper of three pails of water put two ounces of borax, half a pound of *Agaricum*, a quarter of a pound of litharge of filver, four ounces of madder, one quartern of brandy, four ounces of verdigreafe, let them boil together for an hour, then cover the copper and let the liquid reft for 14 days· when you defign to ufe it, take two pound of *Sennes* leaves, two pound of *Gentian*, one pound of *Agarica*, two pound of granat fhells, let them boil together for two hours, and then put it to the other liquor fettled in the copper this colour will keep good for many years, and the longer you dye therein, the better it will grow, you muft be careful to keep it free from foap, which would fpoil it fo as not to be recover'd by any means; and in cafe by accident fome tallow fhould happen to drop from your candle into it, then forbear meddling with it 'till it is cold, when fo, take it off carefully, or heat your poker red hot and fweep it over the furface, this will take off all the greafinefs then take two or three little bags of canvas, fill'd with bran, hang them in the colour for two or three hours whilft the copper is heating, then clap whited brown paper on the furface of the colour, which will take off all the greafinefs that might remain, after that begin to dye.

Your filk that is to be dyed muft be firft boil'd in bran, then gall'd, to each pound of filk take twelve ounces of gall nuts, boil the gall nuts for two hours, before you put the filk into it, which muft foak therein for 30 hours

To Dye a Gray Colour.

GRAY is a middle colour, between black and white, which beginning with a white gray, approaches by degrees to a black gray it may be obferved, that if the black colour was to be prepared only of gall-nuts and vitriol, it would procure but an indifferent gray, but if to thefe ordinary ingredients for dying of ftuffs, you add fome indian-wood, you may procure white gray, pearl colour, lead colour, whitifh gray, iron gray, black gray, brown gray, &c. Some of thefe colours require a little tincture of the woad.

To Dye a Brown-red Colour either on Silk or Worfted.

FIRST, after you have prepar'd your filk or worfted in the manner directed for dying of red colours, boil it in madder, then flacken the fire under the copper, and add to the madder liquor fome black colour, prepared as has been fhewn, then ftir the fire, and when the dye is hot, work the commodities you have to dye therein, till you fee them dark enough

But the beft way to dye this colour is in a blue vat, therefore chufe one either lighter or darker, according as you would have your colour, then allum and rince your filk in fair water, this done, work it in the copper with madder, till you find it anfwer your purpofe

Another.

PUT into a kettle of hot water a handful of madder, ftir it together, and let it ftand a little then take the woolen ftuff, wet it firft, then let it run over the winch into the kettle, turning it conftantly, if you fee it does not make the colour high enough, add a handful more of madder, rincing the ftuff or filk fometimes to fee whether it is to your liking

Then put fome black colour into the kettle, mix it well together, ftir the fire, and when hot, turn your filks or ftuffs with the winch, and dye it either of a blacker hue by adding more black, or a redder by putting in lefs

*Of Madder and its Usefulness in Dying of Silk, Worsted,
Cotton,* &c

MADDER is a red colour, the best grows in *Holland*,
though the colour of that which grows in *Flanders* exceeds it, each sort of madder is mark'd with a particular
mark, to know what country it comes from The only
sign of the real goodness of madder, is the bright colour,
which when being ground to a fine powder, and put on a
blue or brown paper, sticks to it it must be kept close from
the air, otherwise it will loose the strength, and beauty of
its colour

The madder which comes from *Silesia*, under the name
of *Breslaw* red, resembles more a red earth than a root, it has
not so bright a colour as that which comes from *Holland* to
manure and cultivate the ground for the growth of madder, it must be observed, that it requires a good mould, which
is neither too damp nor dry, it must be plow'd pretty deep,
and be well dung'd before the winter season It is sown in
the month of *March* in the decrease of the moon, after the
land in which it is to be sown, is well clear'd of weeds,
least they should attract the strength and goodness thereof to
themselves, and their roots mix with the madder

About eight months after the madder is sown, they begin
to pull up the larger roots thereof, which is done to
hinder it from drawing the strength from the earth to themselves, which are to be a nourishment for the younger
sprouts, this is commonly done in the month of *September*,
when the feed is ripe for gathering The remaining roots
are then well covered with mould, till the next year, when
the larger roots are again gathered, thus it is managed 8 or
10 years together, after which the spot of ground may be
cultivated for the growth of corn, and a new plantation fix'd
upon in another place.

The roots of madder which grow in *Flanders* and *Zealand*,
when pull'd out are dry'd in the sun, but in hot countries
they are dry'd in shady places, in order to preserve their
colour and strength, after that they are ground in mills to a
powder, and pack'd up close in double bags.

The

The fresh madder yields a lively colour, that of a year old a more lively one, but after that time the older it is, the more it loses both its strength and beauty

Concerning the Dying with Madder.

IT has been a common rule to take to eight pound of madder, one pound of tartar; allum and tartar are used for preparing the commodities to be dy'd, for attracting and preserving the colour

Pot-ashes heightens the colour very much, as does bran-water, brandy is of peculiar use, it attracts the colour, makes it look clear and fine, and frees the subtilest particles from its dregs and impurities Some dyers, and indeed most, ascribe the same virtue to urine, but this is false, and although it may be of some use when fresh, it is highly pre-judicial to light colours when stale, for it expels its particles of salt too much, and causes the colour to be of a heavy and unpleasant hue this ought therefore to be a caution to such as would dye light and tender colours. The experiment may be tryed in a glass of clean water, in which litmus, being first dissolved and filtred, is poured in, if to this liquid, which is blue, you pour some spirit of salt, it will turn red, and mixing it with some dissolved salt of tartar it will resume its former colour, if you pour too much of the latter, the liquid will turn green, and thus you may change the colour by add-ing more or less of either the one or the other ingredient to it.

To dye Silk of a Madder Red

PREPARE it as has been directed under the article of dying silk of a crimson colour. This done put a pail full of river-water into a copper, together with half a pound of madder, boil it for an hour, and take care it boils not over, then let it run off clear into another vessel, stirring into it one ounce of curcuma, then put in your silk, let it lay therein till cold, then wring it out and beat it, this done take half a pound of good brasil-wood, boil it in bran-water for an hour, clear it off in another vessel, and put in your silk, rince

it

it out in soap-lee, and then in running water, after which dry and dress it.

Another Method.

AFTER you have prepared your silk for dying, hang it on sticks, and to each pound of silk, take eleven pound of madder, and four ounces of nut-galls, put these into a copper with clean rain-water, hang in your silk, and augment the heat of the copper till it is ready to boil, then turn your silk in it for half an hour, and prevent its boiling by lessening the fire; after this rince and beat it out, hang it again on sticks, in a tub with cold water, in which before you have put some pot-ashes, this gives it a beauty, then rince and dry it   How this madder is made use of for dying of worsteds or stuffs has been shewn already.

Of Cochineel and its Usefulness in Dying

COchineel, a costly fine red and purple-colour, are small dry'd up insects, in size of bed-bugs, which when brought into a powder and boiled, do yield a beautiful red juice or colour, and are used very much by scarlet dyers, for dying of silks, worsteds, cottons, &c   They are gathered in abundance in the *Spanish West Indies*, where they harbour on a certain tree, called the prickle-pear tree; the leaves are of a slimy nature, and the fruit of a blood red colour, full of seeds   the insect feeding on this fruit is ingendred with the tincture thereof   The *Indians* spreading a cloth under those trees, shake them, and by this means catch the insect, where they soon dye.   This is the manner of preparing cochineel.

Of Kermes, and its Use in Dying

THIS grain, by some called scarlet berry, on account of its containing that choice and noble colour, scarlet, grows in *Poland* and *Bohemia*, on small shrubs; they are about the bigness of a pepper-corn; the best comes from *Spain* it is also found in *France*, especially in *Languedoc*, and is gathered in the latter end of *May*, and the beginning of
June.

June. In *Germany* these berries are among the vulgar call'd
St *John's Blood,* because of their being found on the shrubs
about *Midsummer,* or the feast of St *John the Baptist*

The *Poles* call it purple-grains, they grow very plentifully in that country, and that people first discovered its
virtue for dying of crimson and purple, by a hen picking
those berries, and discharging her excrements of a crimson
colour The district about *Warsaw* affords great quantities.
In the *Ukrain* they are still in more plenty, and on the borders
of the sandy deserts of *Arabia,* they are gathered with great
pains by the poor people, whence, it is thought, they retain
the *Arabian* name of *Kermis* those berries or grains, when
ripe, contain an insect of a crimson red, which, if not timely
gathered, will disengage itself from the shell and fly away;
wherefore the people watch carefully the time for gathering,
when they roll them together in their hands into balls, dry
and sell them to the *European* and *Turkish* merchants, who
furnish therewith the colour dyers The *Dutch* mix it
among the cochineel, because it causes that colour to have a
higher and finer hue.

Of Indigo.

INDIGO is a dry and hard blue colour, which is brought
to us in lumps of different pieces or sizes, it is an
Indian shrub, which at certain times of the year, when in
blossom, is cut down and laid in heaps, so long till it is rotten; then the *Indians* carry it to the mills, which are
built in great numbers about that place, where it is ground,
boil'd and press'd, and when it is dry'd, they cut it in
pieces, pack it in chests, and send it abroad

There are several different sorts of indigo *viz* indigo
Guatimala and indigo *Lauro,* both which are exceeding
good and fine, their goodness is known when in breaking
it appears of a high blue, and not sandy, however that
with a deep gloss is not amiss These two sorts are followed by these, *Plato, Xerquies* and *Domingo,* which are
counted not so good as the former The *Indigo Plato* and
Xerquies, are of a high violet colour, and very light in
weight, so as to swim on the water, these are by some
reckoned better than that of *Guatimala,* because it is press'd
onl)

only from the leaves, and the other from the stalks and leaves together. *Indigo Domingo* is not of so lively a copper colour as the former, and is much mix'd with sand and earth, the merchants try this sort by lighting a piece, the good sort will burn like wax, and leave all the dross behind

Curcuma

IS a foreign root in the shape of ginger, of a saffron colour, it is brought to us from the *Indies*, where it is made use of both for dyers and spice.

It is also call'd the *Indian* crocus, the best is that which is heavy and in large pieces, without dust · there is no fitter ingredient to be found for heightening the scarlet to a yellow hue, and it is frequently used by colour dyers in tempering their reds, be they dy'd with kermes, cochineel, or madder, aqua fortis will do the same, but adds a greater life, especially to scarlet

Camphir or Brasil wood.

THIS comes from the country of *Brasil* in the *West-Indies*, it is cut out of a tree call'd by the inhabitants *Arbotan*, which, with its stem and branches is not much unlike an oak tree, only thicker, some will measure 24 foot round the stem, the leaves resemble those of boxtree. the finest brasil-wood is cut about *Fernambuca*, a town in the country of *Brasil*, this exceeds in colour all the other kinds of brasil wood, and is therefore sold at a dearer rate. this wood produces in dying of silks, &c. a fine colour, but it is very fading. It is best for black-dyers, who by using it with gall nuts, *Sumach, Rodoul, Fovic*, vitriol, and verdigrease, dye a good black or gray therewith.

Orchal.

ORCHAL is prepared from a small moss which grows on rocks and cliffs, the chief ingredients for its preparation are chalk and urine, and although the colour it produces

duces in dying of filks &c. is fading, yet whilft fiefh, I'is exceeding beautiful.

Orlean

COMES from the *Weft-Indies*, either in fquare pieces like *Newcaftle* foap, or in round lumps, or fmall cakes, the bignefs of a crown, which laft is reckoned to be the fineft fort, and has a fragrant fmell of violets; it is a tincture prefs'd from a feed, and when dry'd, of a dark red yellow colour. The druggifts fell two forts of orlean, the one is like a dough and is very cheap, the other is dry and very valuable. The dyers ufe it for dying of brown yellows, orange colours, &c.

Gall-nuts

IS a fruit of various forts, fome are fmall, others large, black and white, fmooth and knotty, they grow on high oak-trees, and by merchants are imported from *Smyrna*, *Tripoly*, *Turky*, and *Aleppo*; the heavieft is counted the beft, efpecially when black and knotty

PART

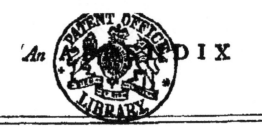

PART II.

Of Artificial FIRE-WORKS.

HAVING in the preceding seventh part of the *Laboratory*, already given a sufficient account not only concerning the nature and property, but also the management of saltpetre, in promoting of its growth, in cleansing and refining the same, &c. it would be needless here to enlarge upon that subject, except it were of such things that have there been omitted, and are of use in the management of artificial fire-works.

How to boil Saltpetre to a Powder.

TAKE a clean kettle or pan, put in as much saltpetre, as to lay at least two fingers thick, pour on it so much water as will just cover it; put it on a slow fire, and when the saltpetre is dissolved, take off the impurities with a skimmer, and let it boil gently till it begins to thicken, keep it stirring continually, till it is turned to a white fand or flower, then take off the kettle, and pour out the saltpetre on a table or board, spreading it thin, to cool.

How to melt Saltpetre.

PUT a crucible with saltpetre on charcoal, when melted, take off the scum carefully, then fling a little piece of brimstone upon it, and when that is burnt, pour the melted saltpetre on a clean metal plate or stone, and it will be of a fine white colour, transparent and like alabaster.

N B To one pound of saltpetre, take half an ounce of brimstone

Of

Of Sulphur or Brimstone.

SULPHUR is by nature the food of fire; it is the principal ingredient in gun-powder, and all forts of fireworks Among brimstone, that which is of a high yellow, and which when held in ones hand, crackles and bounces, is the beft.

How to ftrengthen Brimftone.

MELT as much of the cleareft brimftone as you will, in a kettle or other utenfil, and when the greateft heat is over, then put into it, for each pound of brimftone, half an ounce of quickfilver, ftir them well together, till the quickfilver and brimftone are united, then pour it out into brandy, inftead of quickfilver, you may ufe the fame quantity of zinnaber, and it will do as well.

How to break or granulate the Brimftone.

TAKE fome fpirits, put a handful of brimftone therein and let it diffolve; then take a broad ftick, and ftir it about till it grows mealy, and runs like fand. If you would have it ftrong and hard, fling a handful of faltpetre into it.

How to prepare the Oil of Saltpetre.

PUT fome good refined faltpetre upon a dry and well plained deal board, underneath which place a copper bafon, round about make a coal fire, and the heat thereof will draw the faltpetre, changed into an oil, through the board, and it will drop into the bafon this you may continue as long as you will, by recruiting the board with frefh faltpetre.

To prepare Oil of Sulphur.

FILL a matrass with fine pulverized brimstone about one third full, on this pour as much nut or elder oil as will fill the matrass half full, set it in warm ashes, and let it stand for 8 or 9 hours, and the oil will change the brimstone to a fiery red oil

To make Sal-armoniac Water.

TAKE three ounces of sal-armoniac, one dram of salt-petre, pulverize it fine, and mix it together, then put it into a matrass, pour on it strong vinegar, and distil it over a flow fire, then dry and refine it

To make Camphir and the Oil thereof

TAKE of pulveriz'd juniper-gum two pound, and of distill'd vinegar enough to cover it, put them together into a glass phial, set it for 20 days in warm horse dung, then take it out again, and pour it out into another glass, with a wide mouth to it, expose it to the sun for a month, and you will have a concreted camphir, like a crust of bread, which is in some measure like the natural camphir this, for use in fire works, is wrought to a powder by grinding it with sulphur in a mortar

The oil of camphir which answers the same end is produced by adding a little oil of sweet almonds, and working it together in a brass mortar and a pestle of the same metal, thus it will turn into a green oil

How to prepare Oil of Brimstone and Saltpetre at once together.

TAKE brimstone and saltpetre an equal quantity of each, mix them together, grind them to a fine powder, sift them through a fine sieve, then put it into a new earthen pot, pouring as much sharp vinegar or brandy to it as is sufficient to cover it, then lute up your pot close, so as to prevent any air entring into it, set it in a warm place, till the vinegar or brandy is quite digested, then take the remains, and extract it in a chymical manner.

To prepare Charcoal for Fire-works

COALS are a preservative, whereby the fire, which by the brimstone is brought into gun powder, may not suffocate the strong and windy exhalation of the saltpetre.

The charcoals are of several sorts, some prefer those burnt of hazle and willow wood, when you go to burn them, split the wood about one foot long, in four equal parts, scale off the bark, separate the pith and hard knots, dry them in the sun or in a baker's oven, then make in the earth a square hole, line it with bricks and lay the split wood therein, crossing one another, and set it on fire, when thoroughly lighted and in a flame, cover the hole with boards and fling earth over it close, to prevent the air from coming thereto, yet so as not to fall among the coals, having lain thus for 24 hours, take them out and lay them carefully up for use.

To make the Moulds for Rockets.

THE rockets bearing the pre-eminence, and being the principle things belonging to a fire-work, it is requisite to give some definition of every part of them, how they are made, finish'd and fired · in order to do this, I shall first endeavour to give the curious some idea concerning the moulds they are formed in, these are turn'd commonly of close and hard wood, as of white plumb tree, box, chesnut, cypress, juniper, *Indian* wood, &c

Some also are made of ivory, and for rockets of extraordinary large sizes, they are cast in brass or copper, and turn'd the inside in a nice manner, the foot or basis with its cylinder, wart or half bullet may in these as in others remain of solid wood   The whole is commonly turn'd in the size and form of a column in architecture, and embellish'd with ornaments, according as you fancy

The

The order to be obſerved in the ſize of the cylinder; it is agreed by the moſt famous artificers, that the moulds of all rockets from a half to ſix pound, ought to be ſix diameters, but the larger ſize of four, four and a half, or five diameters of their orifices high

Thoſe rockets which go under the denomination of ſmall ones, are thoſe whoſe inward diameter cannot receive a ball that exceeds one pound The middling ſort are thoſe whoſe diameter can admit balls of one, two or three pound ; and great ones are ſuch, whoſe bore will receive balls from three to a hundred pound.

Rocket moulds from ſome ounces to three pound, are ordinarily ſeven diameters of their bore long, the foot two or three diameters thick, the wart two thirds of the diameter, and the piercer one third of the bore, the roller two thirds, and always one or two diameters from the handle longer than the mould ; the rammer one diameter ſhorter than the mould, and ſomewhat thiner than the roller, to prevent the ſacking of the paper when the charge is ramm'd in, having always one ſtill ſhorter, that when the ſhell of the rocket is ramm'd half full, you may uſe that with more eaſe For the better illuſtration, ſee fig 1. repreſenting the mould with its baſes, cylinder, bore and piercer A B the interior diameter of the mould C D the height of the mould, ſeven diameters, from D to E, is the height of the breech at bottom, which ſtops the mould when the rocket is driving, and this is one and ⅓ diameter. Upon this bottom you have a ſolid cylinder, whoſe height is one diameter of the orifice A B, this cylinder is crowned with a wart or half bullet I, having a hole in the center, in which is fixed the iron or copper piercer F G an iron pin that keeps the bottom and cylinder together 2. The rowler. 3 The rammer 4 The ſhorter rammer

It is to be obſerved, that ſome of theſe moulds are made 9 diameters of their orifice long, the ſhell therefore with the wart will be 12 diameters. Theſe ſorts of rockets fly very high, becauſe of their length, they containing a greater charge than the ſhort, neverthelefs the piercer needs to be no longer than ſeven diameters, but ſubſtantial, ſo as to keep in its proper attitude, it will require the dimenſion of two thirds of the diameter at bottom, and from thence tapering to half the diameter

How

PLATE. I.

p 32

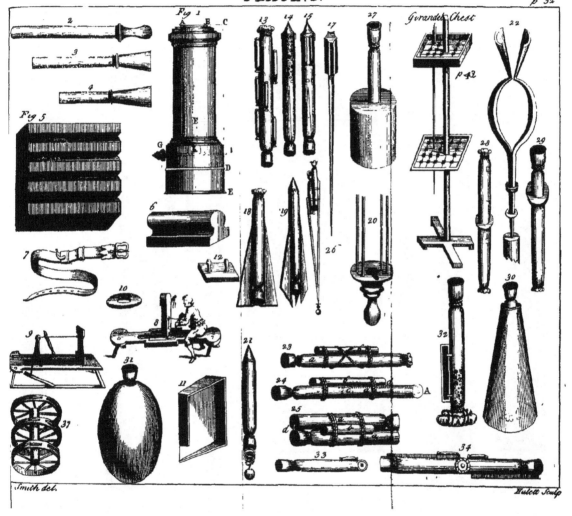

Girandole Chest

Smith del.

Hulett Sculp.

PLATE II

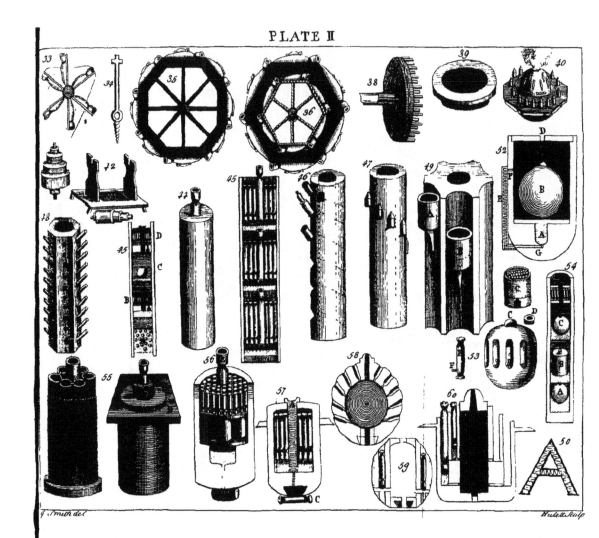

Charges for Water-cats.

MEAL powder two parts, faltpetre four parts, brimstone one part, coarfe coals two parts, faw duft two parts, and 'antimony three parts, moiften'd with linfeed oil.

Meal-powder two ounces and a half, faltpetre three ounces and a half, brimftone two ounces and a half, and antimony half an ounce.

Meal flower one pound, faltpetre two pound, brimftone one pound, and charcoal one pound

Saltpetre fifteen ounces, brimftone five ounces, faw-duft eight ounces, and antimony two ounces

Some general Remarks upon Rockets.

1. YOUR rockets muft have their proportionable height, according to the diameters of their orifices

2 Their necks muft be drawn or choak'd firm, and to prevent the cord giving way, they muft be glued over

3. Prepare your compofition juft before you want it.

4 Let it neither be too damp nor too dry, but fprinkle it over with a little oily fubftance, or a little brandy

5 When you drive your rockets, put always equal quantities of compofition in your cafes at a time

6 Carry with your mallet an even and perpendicular ftroke, when you charge your rockets

7. The cavity muft be bored upright and perpendicular, exactly in the middle of the compofition.

8 Bore your rockets juft before you ufe them; then handle them carefully, leaft their form fhould be fpoiled

9 Let the sticks and rods be well proportioned, strait and smooth.

10. Put your rockets, when compleated, in a place that is neither very damp nor dry.

11 Let most of your rockets have at top a conic figure, by that means they will the easier shoot through the air

12. Avoid, if possible, a damp, foggy, rainy or windy night, to play your rockets.

Defective Rockets are chiefly discovered by the following Observations

1 WHEN they are fired and in mounting two or three perches, they break and disperse without performing their proper effects.

2 When they remain suspended on the nail, and waste away slowly without rising at all.

3. When they form an arch in their ascent, or a semi circle, and return to the ground before their composition is burnt out.

4. When they mount in a winding posture, without an uniform motion.

5 When they move on slowly and heavy.

6. When the cases remain on the nails, and the composition rises and disperses in the air

More of these vexatious accidents will sometimes frustrate the hopes of a young practitioner, but as the above are the principal ones, he must endeavour to avoid them in his first beginning.

Of Rocket Flyers, and the manner of charging them.

THESE are of two forts, namely, the fingle and double, the latter are made after the following man ner.

Have a nave or button turn'd, the dimenfion of three inches, together with two knots upon it, perpendicular one againft the other, of an inch and an half long, and fo thick that both rocket cafes may fit over them, there muft alfo be a hole of the third of an inch in the centre of the nave, for the iron pin to go through, on which it is to fly, after this take two rocket cafes, of equal dimenfions, which are choak'd quite clofe at the neck, and glewed ram in the charge fo far as to leave only room to fix them on the two knobs upon the nave this done, bore into both rockets, near the clofed up necks, fmall touch holes, and one more near the pin, in that which is to burn firft, from this hole, carry a little pipe to the hole near the neck of the other rocket, having firft fill'd it with meal-powder, that when the rocket is almoft burnt out, the fecond may be lighted by the firft The three touch holes ftand in one row, and you may on the other fide fix a couple of reports, which will caufe a fwifter motion

The fingle flyers are made with more eafe, the neck in thefe muft not be tied clofe as in the former, but they muft be fired in that place, but thefe don't turn fo well as thofe that are made double, the figures hereof will give you a fuller idea to manage them See Fig 33 34.

Of Fire-Wheels.

OF thefe there are three forts, *viz* fingle, double, and triple, fome of their fills are of a circular form, others an hexagon, octogon or decagon form, fome like a ftar without fells, fome, and the moft of them, are made to run perpendicular to the earth, others horizontal, all may be ordered fo as to ferve either land or water.

The fire wheels that are to be used on land, turn upon an iron pin or bolt, drawn or screwed into a post. The nave is turn'd of close and firm wood, in which the joiners glew the spokes, according to the number of the fells, which must be carefully joined together, then have a groove hollowed round, so deep that the rocket or case may be about half lodg'd therein. See Fig. 35.

The double wheels must have their fells turn'd stronger and wider, with a groove for the rockets, not only at top, but also on one side thereof, plying the necks of the rockets at top to the right, and those of the sides to the left hand. Vid. Fig. 36.

A triple wheel has a groove at top, and one at each side, the matches are laid from one groove and rocket to another, with small pipes, fill'd with meal powder. you may also make a triple wheel on a long nave, and observe the placing of the rockets on each, contrary one to the other; and the communication you are to make with small pipes, which, after they are fix'd, you are to cover and glew over with paper. Vid. Fig. 37.

Your rockets being ready and cut behind a little shelving, bore them, the first three diameters of its orifice, the second two and three quarters, the third two and a quarter, the fourth two diameters, the fifth one and three quarters, the sixth one and a half, the seventh one and a quarter, the eighth one diameter, always the latter something shorter than the preceeding, after this they are prim'd with meal powder work'd up with brandy, and when dry, glew'd in the above describ'd grooves, you must bear the first fir'd rocket's neck up above the rest, underlaying it with a tin plate, or any thing else, the same you must observe in the head of the last fir'd one, where you put the charge of a report, you may also glew on every end of the rockets, a report of paper, with small pipes of copper, or goose quills, which are fix'd one end in the side of the rocket, and the other in the report. When all is dry, then you may cover your wheel on one or both sides, with linnen or paper, in what form you would have it.

The horizontal wheels, are made like the others with fells, or out of one entire piece, their grooves are furnished

wi'

with rockets, and their plane garnifhed with crackers. Vid.
Plate I. Fig. 38.

A fire wheel which is to whirl horizontally in the water
muft be thus ordered

Take a pretty large wooden difh or bowl, that has a broad
flat rim, See Fig 39 alfo a fmooth dry board, fomething
larger than the difh, and form'd into an octagon, in the
middle of this board make a round hole, that will hold
a water-ball, fo that one half be received in the difh, and
the other half rife above the furface of the board, nail
this board upon the rim of the difh, and fix the ball in the
middle, tying it faft with wire, then glew your rockets
in the grooves which are made round the edges of the
board, laying them clofe to one another, fo that fuc
ceffively taking fire from one another, they may keep
the wheel in an equal rotation You may add, if you pleafe,
on each fide of the wheel, a few boxes, fill'd with crac'ers
or cartouches, erected perpendicular, and alfo fix double and
fingle crackers, following in a range, one after another, for
two or three fires, or as many as the extent of the wheel
will admit

For your private fuzees, obferve that you conduct one
from the rocket, which is to be fix'd to the compofition
of the ball in a channel.

Fill thefe channels with meal powder, and cover them
clofe with paper alfo lay a train of fuzees of communication from the rockets to a cartouch, and from that to the reft.
See Fig 40.

Laftly, when all is ready and covered, dip the whole
machine into melted pitch, and fecure it from the injury of
the water, the ball is fired firft, and when lighted, you
place it gently on the furface of the water, and then fire
the rocket

To try a fire wheel, firft weigh one of the rockets, tie it
to a fell with cord, and according to that weight, fill little
long bags full of fand, tying them likewife on the reft of the
fells, then hang the wheel on an iron pin, fire the rocket,
and if it turns the wheel, then you may affure your felf it
will be compleat when finifh'd.

d 3

Wheels

Wheels form'd like stars, are to have their spokes fix'd upright in the nave, like other wheels, only with grooves on one of the sides of each, wherein you glew the rockets, at the bottom of each rocket is made a little hole, from whence the fire is convey'd through little pipes, fill'd with meal-powder up to the next, and so round, then cover it with linnen cloth or paper in the shape of a star, and place it on the iron axis

Observe that all the rockets used in fire-wheels, have their necks tied close, leaving only a small conveyance from one rocket to another, the last of all must be well secured below, where you may place a strong report of corn-powder See Fig 40

Charges for Fire flyers and Wheels, of four, five, and six Ounce Rockets

MEAL powder three pound, saltpetre two pound, charcoal five ounces, and sea coal three ounces.

Meal powder fourteen ounces, saltpetre six ounces, charcoal three ounces and a half, brimstone three ounces, and sea coal three ounces

Meal powder fifteen ounces, saltpetre six ounces, brimstone three ounces, and charcoal three ounces

Saltpetre five pound, brimstone three quarters of a pound, charcoal one pound four ounces.

These charges are bored a little with a round bodkin.

Meal powder two pound, sea coal eight ounces, and charcoal ten ounces

Meal powder three pound, brimstone eight ounces, and charcoal ten ounces.

These charges may be used for triple wheels, and must be bored one third with a bodkin.

For Wheels of one Pound Rockets.

MEAL powder six pound, saltpetre three pound, brimstone one pound seven ounces, charcoal two pound nine ounces, and tanners dust one ounce

The bore must be an inch and an half.

For Wheels of one and a half, and two Pound Rockets.

MEAL powder fix pound, faltpetre three pound and a half, brimftone one pound and a half, charcoal two pound three quarters, and faw duft one ounce and a half.

The firft rocket in the wheel is in length two diameters and a half of its orifice.

For Wheels of three and four Pound Rockets

MEAL powder nine pound, faltpetre one pound and a half, brimftone one pound two ounces, and charcoal three pound four ounces

The firft rocket is bored but one and a half of its diameter.

To make fingle and double CARTOUCHES or BOXES, TUBES, STARS, SPARKS, *&c.*

WHEN fome hundred boxes or cartouches, are adjufted and fixed in machines of great fire-works, they afford among the towring rockets great delight to the fpectators. Thefe boxes are made either of wood, pafte board, or copper, and are charged and proportioned according to their ftrength, with the charge and compofition that is defigned for them. If made of wood they muft fit exactly, and receive each other, fo as to feem but one continual piece; and if pafte board, you muft glue on a foot at bottom, of a hand high, to each of them. the infide of thefe machines muft exactly fit and correfpond with the outfide of the cartouches themfelves, and be fo contrived as to flip into one another.

The engine, Fig 42. is very proper for the conftruction of thofe boxes, the latter reprefents the bench, and B the cylinders, upon which, (having greafed them firft over with foap,) you fafhion your boxes, juft as you think proper, by pafting one thicknefs of paper upon another, and fixing a handle to the end of the cylinder.

Hav-

Having formed them, put them to dry in a moderate heat, too great a heat will shrivel them up; when dry, take one after another off the cylinder, and immediately clap round wooden bottoms, the edges being first done over with glue, into them, and sprig them on the outside to make them secure.

The single boxes are to be charged in the following manner:

1 Put in some corn powder

2. Upon that charge fix a round paste-board, well fitted to the concave side of the box, which has five or six small holes, and is on both sides laid over with meal-powder tempered with brandy

3 Put upon the paste-board a little meal powder, and upon that well pierced crackers, so as to stand with their necks downwards the principal rocket is put in the middle, with the neck downwards open at both ends, so that being lighted above and burning down it may fire the rest of the crackers, which are blown up in the air by the corn powder.

4. The empty spaces between the large fire case and the crackers are carefully filled up, and the cartouch is stuffed at top with tow, or else boiled in saltpetre lee, with saw-dust.

5 The cartouch is covered with a cap, which is glewed very closely thereon, and for the great case reaching out of the cartouch, make in the middle of the cap a hole, through which it is put, and close the opening by glewing some slips of paper round it The fire-case is loose, covered with a paste-board cap

Double Boxes or Cartouches

IN Fig 43 is exhibited the construction of a case, called a double one, to enlarge on the description thereof seems

to

to be needlefs, only obferve, that the bottoms of the upper boxes, ferve for the covers of the lower, a hole being made, through which the compofition of the lower box is fired, after the upper rocket has forced away the empty box, which already has difcharged its load. The upper box you cover as has been fhewn above If there are more than two cartouches upon one another, they are called Burning Tubes, which when fired fhorten by degrees, the cartouches following one another till all are fired, fome are intermixed with artificial globes, and feveral other fancies, which afford great pleafure to the fpectators

Thefe boxes or cartouches are placed in long cafes made for that purpofe. The vacancies about the cartouches may be filled up with fand See Fig 44.

Another Sort of Fire Tubes

ARE made of folid, hard and dry wood, of what height and thicknefs you think proper, bore the middle of the wood one third or a quarter of its diameter, after which divide the whole height into equal parts, each exactly correfponding with the sky rockets you defign to fix upon them, but rather a fmall matter fhorter, all thefe divifions are cut floping downwards, except the uppermoft, which muft run out in a cylinder On the rims of each of thefe divifions make a groove all round, of about a fingers breadth, in thefe grooves bore fmall holes, by which the fire may be conveyed through pipes from the cavity of the tube, to light the rockets that ftand behind the paper cartouches, which muft be made fecure to the wood, leaft they fhould fly up along with the rockets

The conftruction of the hollow tube in this and other fuch like tubes is expreffed in Fig 45 A the fire ftars and fparks, interfperfed with corn powder B a box filled with paper or crackers. C a fire-ball or water-globe, which of them you pleafe. D another box filled with crackers. The hollows between thefe fires are filled up with corn powder, to blow up the globes and boxes one after another.

The ftars and fparks made ufe of on this occafion are prepared in the following manner.

Take

Take of beaten faltpetre five pound and a half, meal powder two pound four ounces, and brimftone one pound twelve ounces

Meal powder three pound, faltpetre fix pound, brimftone one pound, camphir half an ounce, tanners bark two ounces, or elfe faw duft; all finely fifted and moiften'd with linfeed oil.

Meal powder one pound, faltpetre four pound, brimftone half a pound, and pounded glafs fix ounces, moiftened with linfeed oil

Saltpetre half a pound, brimftone two ounces, antimony one ounce, and meal powder three ounces.

Saltpetre half a pound, brimftone three ounces, antimony one ounce, and iron file duft half an ounce

Saltpetre two pound, meal powder ten pound, and brimftone one pound.

Saltpetre one pound, brimftone half a pound, meal powder three ounces, and antimony one ounce

Saltpetre one pound, fulphur two ounces, powder of yellow amber one ounce, crude antimony one ounce, meal-powder three ounces.

Sulphur two ounces and a half, faltpetre fix ounces, fine meal-powder five ounces, frankincenfe in drops, maftick, mercury fublimate, of each four ounces; white amber and camphir of each one ounce, antimony and orpiment of each half an ounce

Thefe ingredients being well beaten, and fearced thro' a fearcer, muft be fprinkled over with a little glew or gum water, and form'd into little balls, of the bignefs of a fmall nut, then dry'd in the fun, or near a fire, and lay'd up in a dry place, to be ready, on occafion, for playing off with fire-works. When you ufe them, wrap them up in tow.

The following Stars are of a more yellowifh Caft, inclining to White

TAKE four ounces of gum tragacant, or gum-arabick pounded and fifted through a fine fieve, camphir dif-folv'd in brandy two ounces, faltpetre one pound, fulphur half

half a pound, coarfe powder of glafs four ounces, white amber one ounce and a half, orpiment two ounces, incorporate them, and make balls of them, as directed before

Sparks are prepared thus.

TAKE faltpetre one ounce, ditto melted half an ounce, meal-powder half an ounce, and camphir two ounces; having melted thefe things by themfelves, (when you ufe them) put them together in an earthen pot, pour on them water of gum tragacant, or brandy that has had gumarabick, or gum tragacant diffolv'd in it, that the whole may have the confiftence of a pretty thick liquid, this done take one ounce of lint, which before has been boil'd in brandy, vinegar, or faltpetre, when dry, throw it into the compofition, mix and ftir it about, till it has foak'd it up; then roll them up in pills about the bignefs of great pins-heads, and fet them to dry, having firft fprinkled them with meal-powder.

Some of thefe pyramidical tubes and fire-works, are now and then fired in large rooms, upon grand entertainments in miniature, wherein are employ'd odoriferous pills, and other ingredients, that have a fragant fmell, thefe pills are commonly compofed of *Storax Calamita*, benjamin, gum juniper, of each two ounces, *Olibanum*, maftick, frankincenfe, whiteamber, yellow amber, and camphir, of each one ounce, faltpetre three ounces, lime-tree-coal four ounces, beat thefe ingredients very fine, pulverize and incorporate them together, and moiften it with rofe water, wherein before you have diffolv'd fome gum-arabick or gum-tragacant, you may form them into pills, and dry them in the fun or before a fire.

Single Tubes or Cafes

ARE only filled with compofitions, and to the outfide are faftened fome crackers, ferpents, or cartouches; thefe cafes being generally round and uniform, like a cylinder, you are to trace out a winding line from the top to the bottom, on which cut holes to the depth of two or three inches, See Fig 46 B and C Into thefe holes contrive to fix paper

cafes

cafes with wooden bottoms, wherein you may put any for^t of rockets you pleafe, as you fee in A and E, but take care you provide little holes, to lead from the great tube to the corn powder under your rockets

Another fire-tube is delineated Fig. 47. This is furrounded with cartouches, difpofed in a ferpentine order, like the firft, which are glewed and nailed as fecure as poffible; out of thefe are difperfed great numbers of fquibs, as for the reft, they have nothing but what is common in others

Another Fire Tube

THE circumference of this cylinder is by a cord divided into a certain number of equal parts, and being brought into a poligonal figure, by cutting away the convex parts it is brought into angles

Then bore the plain fides with a number of holes perpendicular, fo as to penetrate obliquely to the great boring in the middle. into thefe holes thruft crackers, fquibs, or ferpents. See Fig 48

Fig 49 exhibits a tube, whofe length is fix diameters of its thicknefs The cylinder being divided round the rim into fix parts, then fubdividing each of thofe into feven parts, referve one of them for the lift, between each of which make channels, which being fix in number, place little mortars of the fame dimenfions therein

The mortars muft be turned of wood, bore the bottoms and add a chamber to them, as you fee at E, each chamber muft be one third or one half of the depth of the fluting, and the breadth one fixth only. Thefe chambers are defigned to hold corn powder

Secure thofe mortars on the outfide with ftrong paper cafes, and nail them faft in the hollow channels, whofe cavity they are to fit exactly, their length may be doubled to their breadth, each mortar muft contain a globe made of paper, with a wooden bottom, and their chambers muft be charged with corn powder

Thefe mortars fix in a fpiral line, one only in each fluting, with iron ftays, and bind the middle with an iron plate, faftened

tened on each side of the interstices; but before you fix the mortars, you must not forget to pierce little holes in the tube, and to fix the touch holes of your mortars exactly upon them, priming both with meal powder. Every thing relating to this may be plainly conceived in the figure, where A and B describes the mortars, and C the globe or cartouch.

Of Salvo's

THESE, in fire-works, are a great number of strong iron reports fixed either in a post or plank, and with a fire discharged at once.

Charges for Cartouches or Boxes.

MEAL powder six ounces, saltpetre one pound eight ounces, brimstone four ounces, and charcoal four ounces and a half

Meal powder fourteen ounces, saltpetre five ounces, brimstone two ounces, and charcoal three ounces

Meal powder one pound, saltpetre three quarters of a pound, brimstone four ounces and a half, tanners bark or saw dust two ounces, and charcoal four ounces

Charges for Fire Tubes

MEAL powder six pound, saltpetre four pound, charcoal two pound, rosin half a pound, tanners bark five ounces, moistened with a little linseed oil

Meal powder three quarters of a pound, saltpetre four pound, brimstone ten ounces, and saw dust four ounces. This charge may be used dry

Meal powder five pound, saltpetre three pound, charcoal one pound six ounces, rosin three quarters of a pound; not moistened

A Preservative for Wood against Fire.

THIS being a necessary article in the execution of fire-works, it will not be improper to set it down in this place.

Take

Take brick duft, afhes, and iron filings, of each an equal quantity, put them together in a pot, pour glew water or fize upon it, then put it near the fire, and when warm ftir it together. With this fize wafh over your wood-work, and when dry repeat it, and it will be proof againft fire.

The Manner of preparing and making Letters and Names in Fire-Works

BURNING letters may be reprefented after feveral methods

Order a joiner to cut capital letters, of what length and breadth you pleafe, or about two foot long and three or four inches wide, and an inch and a half thick, hollow out of the body of the letters, a groove, a quarter of an inch deep, referving for the edges of the letters a quarter or half an inch of wood   If you defign to have the letters burn of a blue fire, then make wicks of cotton or flax, according to the bignefs and depth of the grooves in the letters, and draw them leifurely through melted brimftone, and place them in the grooves, brufh them over with brandy, ftrew meal pow-der thereon, and again with brandy and thin diffolved gum tragacant, and on that ftrew meal powder again ; when dry drive fmall tacks all round the edges of the grooves, and twift fmall wire to thofe tacks, that it may crofs the letters and keep the cotton or flax clofe therein, then lay over it brandy pafte ; ftrew over that meal-powder, and at laft glue over it a fingle paper

If you would have the letters burn white, diffolve fix pound of faltpetre, and add to it a little corn powder, in that dip your wicks of cotton or flax   You may inftead thereof ufe dry touch wood, which cut into pieces of an inch thick, put them in melted faltpetre over a fire, let them lay therein till the faltpetre is quite foaked thro' the wood, after which mix powdered faltpetre with good ftrong brandy, take fome cotton, and with a fpatula or your hands, work that, the faltpetre and brandy, together, then fqueeze it out, ftrew the cotton over with powder'd faltpetre, and thereof make wicks, having placed firft the touch wood in the

the grooves, lay the wicks over that and the vacancies about it, and then proceed to make it tight and secure, as has been directed above See Fig. 40

There is another method for burning letters without grooves, and this is done by boreing small holes in the letters, of about an inch distance, one from the other, the diameter of those holes must not be above the eighth of an inch, into them put and glew cases, ram'd with burning charges, but these letters do not burn so long as the others, except the charges are very long.

Another method for burning of letters is us'd, when they are form'd by a smith of coarse wire, about a quarter of an inch thick; when this is done get some cotton spun into match-thread, but not much twifted, to two yards of this take one pound of brimstone, six ounces of saltpetre, and two ounces of antimony; melt these ingredients in a kettle, first the brimstone by itself, and then the rest all together, when melted, put in the match thread, and stir it about, till it has drawn in all the matter, then take it out, and strew it over with meal powder, let it dry, and wind it about the white letters, fasten these upon a board, that has been well laid over with a preservative to keep it from firing When you have lighted one letter, all the rest will take fire immediately.

Letters cut in a smooth board, which is made to slide in grooves of a chest are ordered thus: The lid of the box is made full of holes for difperfing the smoak of the lamps, or wax-tapers, which are set behind, to illuminate the letters, behind the cut out letters is pasted oil paper of various colours, which, when the lamps are lighted, has a fine effect. By these means, various changes may be made, in reprefenting devices, names, coats of arms, &c. But this way is more practifed on the stage in plays than in fire-works.

Charges for Burning Letters with Cafes.

MEAL-powder six ounces, saltpetre one pound, mix'd with *Potrolio* oil

Meal-powder three quarters of a pound, saltpetre nine ounces, and brimstone three ounces, mix'd up dry.

Meal

Meal-powder five ounces, faltpetre feven ounces, brimftone three ounces, and file-duft half an ounce, moiftened
with linfeed oil.

*To order and preferve Leading-fires, Trains, and Quick-
matches.*

FIRE works being of various kinds and inventions, it is
impoffible to affign certain rules for their feveral performances. But to fay fomething of what concerns a mafter's
praife, it is to be obferved, that great fire works are not to be
fired above once or twice at moft, for it would not be
deemed an artful performance, to fire one cartouch after
another; likewife the match pipes, the moft preferable of
which are either iron, lead, or wood, and fhould be
ftrengthened or clofely twifted round with the finews of
beafts, fteeped in diffolved *Feather-white* and filled with
flow charges, which ought to be well tried. Or elfe fur-
nifhed with match-thread of *Stupinen*, dry and well prepared, and afterwards either joined to the grooves made in
the boards, or only laid free from one work to another
The joinings of the pipes muft be well clofed and luted with
potter's clay, fo as to prevent the fire from breaking out,
thefe pipes muft alfo have little vent holes to give the fire
air, or elfe it would be ftifled, or burft the pipes; but thefe
holes muft be fo contrived, that the flame may vent itfelf
in the open air, and at fome diftance from the works, fo as to
prevent touching them

All burning matches are to be as diftant from the machines as poffible, to prevent accidents.

A particular direction for conducting your trains and fuzees, cannot be given, becaufe of the variety of poftures, fi-
tuations and contrivances of machinery; thofe rules already
given will be fufficient for the ingenious, add to this the advantage a novice in this art, may gather from the fufficient
direction in this matter from the figures, which, with much
care and induftry, have been traced out for their information
and benefit.

Charges

Charges for Fuzees or Leading-matches.

MEAL powder three ounces and a half, faltpetre four ounces, brimſtone one ounce and three quarters, and charcoal one ounce and three quarters.

Meal-powder three ounces, faltpetre nine ounces, brimſtone four ounces and a half, and charcoal half an ounce.

Meal powder four ounces, charcoal half an ounce, and coarſe coal half an ounce.

Meal-powder half a part, faltpetre three parts, brimſtone two parts, and charcoal one part. this laſt is very flow.

Of Water-balls

BALLS, in fire works, are made of different faſhions, ſome are globular, ſome oval, ſome conical, ſome cylindrical, and others in the form of a pendant or drop

The water-balls are commonly made of knitted cord-bags, or of wood, thoſe made of bags are ſhaped like oſtriches eggs, and are

1. Fill'd with their proper charge

2. The outſide is dip'd in glew, and wound about with hemp or flax, till it is a quarter of an inch thick thereon

3 This ball is then coated over with cloth, and about the touch-hole is glewed over with a piece of leather.

4 The touch-hole is bored with a gimlet, and ſtop'd with a wooden peg.

5. At the bottom of the globe pierce a ſmall hole thro' to the compoſition, in which faſten a ſmall copper pipe, furniſhed with a paper report, together with a leaden balance, glew the report faſt to the ball, then dip the ball in melted pitch, open the touch-hole, and prime it with a quick burning charge

Theſe balls keep a long time under water, before they riſe, and if a true balance is not obſerved in the lead, or the ball is overcharg'd, they will ſink to the bottom and burn out, therefore you muſt well obſerve, that when a water-ball without the ballance is two pound weight, you muſt give it four or four ounces and a half of lead, but if it weighs one

c pound

pound and a half, balance it with three or three ounces and a half.

Water balls or globes made of wood, which swim and burn upon the water without any further effect, are of two forts, *viz* single and double, the single ones are made thus have a hollow globe turn'd somewhat oblong, with a vent-hole, fill that with a good and approv'd charge, but not too close, prime the end with some meal-powder, then glew a stopple in the hole, which must be thrice as thick, as the shell of the globe, in which beforehand the counterpoise is cast of lead, when dry, make a hole at top, large enough for a two ounce cracker to enter, through this ram down the charge in the globe, and fill it quite full with the same composition, then glew it over with a paste-board. and lastly fix a small copper-pipe through the stopple, having bored a hole through it for that purpose; to the pipe fasten a paper report; when this is done dip the whole in pitch these are call'd single water-globes. Both forts of globes are, for the better security, twisted and tied round with several rows of strong packthread.

Double water-globes are such which after one is fired, discharges another. These have chambers at bottom which are fill'd with gun powder; on these put a cover of thick leather, which has several holes in the middle, and goes close to the sides, on this strew meal-powder, and place thereon a fire-globe, which is charged Fig. 52 will demonstrate the construction with more ease than a long lesson; observe,

1. That the little chamber at bottom ought to be the fifth of the breadth of the whole globe, and that its height be one and a half thereof

2. That the water-ball B, should be encompass'd with a water ball composition, as you see by H

3 The partition C is for this purpose, that when the powder in it shall have the fire conveyed to it through the pipes E F G, it may with more force blow up the ball, in the body of the first; this taking fire at the hole D, will burn upon the water for some time, and then, to the astonishment of the spectators, on a sudden, it will blow up the ball that was in it.

4. You

4 You muft be very careful to fecure the piece of leather or board that covers the little chamber, leaft it fhould
be blown up by the compofition of the greater globe, before
it is all burn'd out.

How to charge a Water-globe with many Crackers.

TAKE, for this purpofe, a fingle water globe, which
may be round or of an oval form, fill the fame with
the compofition hereafter mentioned. Hollow the outfide
thereof in feveral places, to the fize of your reports or crackers,
which are to be fix'd in them, to each of the crackers be-
longs a fmall copper tube, fill'd with meal powder, which
are to be fitted to the fmall holes in the flutings, in the
manner as expreffed in the print, where Fig. 53 A are the
flutings, B the little holes for the fuzees, C the upper orifice
for priming, D the hollow ftopple, through which the
ball is primed, E the form of the crackers, which are to
be fix'd in the flutings, F little fuzees belonging to them.

How to prepare a Water-mortar, or Water pump with feveral Tubes

TAKE feven wooden tubes, wrap them about with
cloth that is either pitch'd or dipp'd in glue, twift-
ing them round very tight with packthread Their height,
thicknefs and diameter you may order as you think proper,
only allowing the middlemoft a greater height than the reft;
bind them together in one cylindrical body, to the bottom
fix a round board with nails, and then with ftrong glew ftop
up all the crevices to prevent the air getting to the compofition ⁘ this done fill the tubes according to the order reprefented in Fig. 54. Firft pour into each tube, a little corn-
powder, about half an inch high; upon that put a water-ball
A, upon that a flow compofition, then again corn powder;
upon which put a water-globe fill'd with fquibs, as you fee
in B, on that again a flow compofition, then corn powder,
and then a light ball, as may be feen in C, over this put a
third time a flow compofition on corn-powder, as before,
which you muft cover with a wooden cap on this fix running rockets, not too clofe, but to leave room enough
C 2   between

between for a wooden cafe fill'd with a water compofition; the remainder of the tube fill with a flow charge, and clofe it up. Your tubes being all fill'd in this manner, get a fquare or round piece of plank, with a round hole in the middle, large enough to receive the ends of all the tubes, which cover clofe, to preferve the powder and compofition from being wet, this float-board is mark'd with the letter D, Fig 55. Thus prepared, dip it in a quantity of tar, or melted pitch, then put the rocket E, or a fmall wooden tube fill'd with a ftrong compofition that will burn on the water into the orifice of the middle tube, the compofition of which fhould be more flow than of the reft

If you would have the tubes take fire all round at once, you muft pierce the fides of the great one with fmall holes, correfponding with thofe in each of the other tubes, by this means the fire may be convey'd to all of them at once, and confume them equally and at the fame time, but if you would have them burn one after another, you muft clofe them well up with pafteboard, and to each tube fix a fuzee of communication, fill'd with meal powder or a flow compofition, thro' which the fire may be convey'd from the bottom of that which is confumed, to the orifice of that next to it, and fo on fuccefively to fuch as have not been fired.

How to Charge a large Water-globe, with feveral little ones, and with Crackers

HAVE a wooden cylinder made, let the orifice thereof be at leaft one foot diameter, and its height one and a half, let there be a lodge or chamber at bottom to hold the powder, which muft be confin'd therein, by a tampion or ftopple joined to a round board, fitted exactly to the infide of the globe, through the middle of the ftopple muft pafs an iron tube fill'd with meal-powder, then prepare fix water-balls, or more if you think fit, fo that when all are fet together in the circumference of the globe, they may fill up that circle, each of thefe balls muft be provided with an iron-fuzee in its orifice, fill'd with meal powder. Having charged the chamber of the globe with corn-powder, let down the forementioned board with the ftopple upon it, then range the fix water-balls, cover them with another round board,

board that has fix little round holes, correfponding with the fix iron fuzees of the balls, and which muft a little furmount it. This laft board fpread over with meal and corn powder mix'd together, and upon it you place as many rockets as the globe can hold in the midft of thefe you fix a large rocket, into whofe orifice the iron tube may enter, which is the fame you fee in E, Fig. 56

This tube muft have holes drill'd all round the plane of the 'forefaid partition or board, to the end that the fire having a communication through them, it may reach the running rockets, and at the fame time fire the water-balls, whofe tubes rife out of the board, and from thence, after having penetrated down to the chamber below, it may blow up the whole into the air, and make a great noife See the figure, where A points out the fix water balls, B the great rocket in the middle of the running ones, C the chamber for the powder, D a communication, or the iron pipe, to convey the fire to the paper cracker, F the globe, which having adjufted after the manner directed, cover it clofe round, dip it in tar, to preferve it from the water.

To prepare the Water Bee-hive or Bee fwarm, both fingle and double.

THE fingle bee-fwarm is thus prepared Have an oblong globe turn'd, whofe length is two diameters of its breadth, or proportioned to the height of your rounding rockets, which place round the wooden tube marked with A; this muft be of an equal height with the globe, and be fill'd with a compofition of three parts of powder, two of faltpetre and one of brimftone, at the lower end of the globe fix a paper cracker C; the letter D is a counterpoife of lead, through which you convey a little pipe or fuzee, to communicate with the charge in the wooden tube, at top fix a round board for a balance, F two little holes which convey the fire to the charge for blowing up the rockets See Fig 57.

How

How to prepare a Water-globe on the outside with Running-Rockets

GET a wooden globe perfectly round and hollow, bore on the outside several cavities, sufficient to receive running rockets, leaving a quarter of an inch between the extremities of them, and the composition within the ball, then bore the wood, left between each, with a small gimlet, fill them with meal powder, then put in your rockets, close the top of the globe with a wooden cylinder, that has a hollow top, with a touch-hole to receive the priming, the bottom stop with a stopple, which likewise has a conveyance to the cracker that is commonly fix'd beneath it, between which and the stopple fix also a leaden counterpoise, to keep the whole upright in the water. See Fig. 58.

To prepare Water-globes with single or double ascending Rockets.

FOR the first sort have a globe turn'd with a tube in the middle, half its diameter wide, leaving two inches for the placing of solid wood at bottom, round this tube bore holes for small rockets thereon, after which you burn, with a red hot wire or small iron, touch-holes, out of the large tubes, into the little ones, then fill the globe with the following composition, *viz*

Two pound of saltpetre, eight ounces of brimstone, eight ounces of meal powder, twelve ounces of saw dust, this done close the top with a stopple, which has a touch-hole in the middle, then put a good deal of meal powder in the small tubes, up to the touch-holes, and after you have plac'd your rockets upon that, fill the vacancy round with a little corn powder, glew over them paper caps, then dip the globe into pitch, but not over the paper covering, fix a counterpoise at bottom, and when the fire has burn'd half way or further, in the large tube, it will communicate through the touch holes, and discharge all the rockets at once

The second sort is done after the same manner, only the middle tube is not bored so wide, because of giving more

room

room for two rows of small tubes round it, the first row next to the tube is bored a little below the middle, the second almost near to the end thereof, the touch holes for the former are burnt from the inside of the great tube, and those of the latter from the outside hole are closed again with a wooden pin in the large tube you may lodge a strong report of iron, charg'd with corn-powder, having a touch-hole left at top. See Fig. 59, 60.

Charges for single Water-globes

CORN-powder half a pound, saltpetre sixteen pound, brimstone four pound, ivory shavings four ounces, saw-dust boil'd in saltpetre lee four pound

Meal-powder one pound, saltpetre six pound, brimstone three pound, iron-filings two pound, and rosin half a pound.

Meal powder four pound, saltpetre twenty-four pound, brimstone twelve pound, saw-dust eight pound, powdered glass half a pound, and camphir half a pound.

Corn powder one ounce, saltpetre twelve ounces, brimstone four ounces, and saw dust three ounces

Saltpetre twelve ounces, brimstone four ounces, saw-dust two ounces, melted stuff three quarters, this must be ram'd in tight.

Meal powder one pound four ounces, saltpetre one pound eight ounces, brimstone nine ounces, saw-dust five ounces, pounded glass one ounce, melted stuff four ounces, mix them together with a little linseed oil.

Meal powder eight ounces, saltpetre five pound, brimstone two pound, copper filings eight ounces and a half, and coarse coal dust eight ounces and a half

Saltpetre eight ounces, brimstone three ounces, saw-dust one ounce, and tanners bark two ounces

Saltpetre six pound twelve ounces, brimstone two pound fourteen ounces, melted stuff half a pound, saw-dust one pound, coarse coal dust one pound, and pounded glass one pound, mix'd up and moisten'd with vinegar

Saltpetre two pound twelve ounces, brimstone two pound six ounces, melted stuff four ounces, saw-dust eight ounces, charcoal one ounce and a half, and pounded glass three

quarters

quarters of an ounce, moiften'd with linfeed oil, and mix'd up with a little corn-powder.

Charges for double Water-globes.

SAltpetre four pound fix ounces, brimftone one pound four ounces, faw duft half a pound, and coarfe-coal duft fix ounces, moiftened with a little vinegar or linfeed oil.

Meal-powder one pound four ounces, brimftone four ounces, and charcoal two ounces, moiftened with *Petrolium* oil

Saltpetre three pound, brimftone a quarters of a pound, and faw-duft boiled in faltpetre ten ounces, moiftened a little.

Charges for Bee fwurms.

MEAL-powder thirteen ounces and a half, faltpetre fix ounces, brimftone two ounres and a half, fine charcoal three ounces, coarfe charcoal one ounce, and fine faw duft three ounces

Meal-powder three quarters of a pound, faltpetre fix ounces, brimftone three ounces and a half, fine charcoal four ounces, and coarfe charcoal two ounces and a half.

Meal-powder four parts, faltpetre eight parts, brimftone two parts, coarfe charcoal two parts, and fine charcoal one part

Odoriferous or perfumed Water-balls.

HAVE balls turned about the fize of large walnuts, fill them with any of the compofitions fpecified below; after they are filled and ready, light and put them into water This is generally done in a large room or hall, at grand entertainments.

The Compofitions for them are as follows ·

SAltpetre four ounces, *Storax Calamita*, one ounce, frankincenfe one ounce, maftic one ounce, amber half an ounce, civet half an ounce, faw-duft of juniper two ounces, faw-duft of cyprels two ounces, and oil of fpike one ounce.

Salt-

Saltpetre two ounces, flower of fulphur one ounce, camphir half an ounce, rafpings of yellow amber half an ounce, coal of lime-tree wood one ounce, flower of benjamin, or *Affa odorata* half an ounce; let thofe which are to be powdered, be done very fine; then mix them together as ufual.

Saltpetre two ounces, myrrh four ounces, frankincenfe three ounces, amber three ounces, maftic one ounce, camphir half an ounce, rofin one ounce, boiled faw-duft one ounce, lime-tree coals half an ounce, bees wax half an ounce, mix them up with a little oil of juniper

Saltpetre one ounce, myrrh four ounces, frankincenfe two ounces and a half, amber two ounces, mother of pearl four ounces, melted ftuff half an ounce, and rofin half an ounce; mix them up with oil of rofes.

Meal-powder three ounces faltpetre twelve ounces, frankincenfe one ounce, myrrh half an ounce, and charcoal three ounces, mix'd with oil of fpike

The Manner of preparing the Melted Stuff.

MELT twenty four pound of fulphur in a fhallow earthen pan, over a clear fire, and as it melts fling in fixteen pound of faltpetre, ftir them well together with an iron fpatula; as foon as they are melted take it off the fire, and add to it eight pound of corn-powder, mix it well together, and being cooled, pour out this compofition upon a polifhed marble, or metal plates, and then divide it into pieces about the fize of a walnut This compofition is chiefly ufed in military fire-works, and not for thofe I am treating of, but for thofe fire-works which are only for pleafure it is diftinguifh'd by warm and cold melted ftuff, and is prepared in the following manner.

Take for the firft fort half a pound of faltpetre, grind among it three quarters of an ounce of antimony, till one cannot be diftinguifhed from the other; then melt one pound and a half of brimftone, put the mix'd faltpetre and antimony to it, and mix them well together, this done put it warm into a wooden mould of two pieces, which fhould be well greafed on the infide this ftuff you break afterwards in bigger or leffer pieces, it is, on account of its clear fire, ufed to imitate ftars.

The

The Manner of preparing the cold melted Stuff

GRIND the above ingredients, or eight ounces of meal pou
der, four ounces of saltpetre, three ounces of brimstone
and one ounce of coal dust, together, till all is of one colour
this done, moisten that stuff with the white of eggs, gum
water, or size, and make thereof a stiff dough, then
strew on a smooth board some meal powder, roll the dough
upon that a quarter of an inch thick, strew again meal
powder upon it, then cut it in square pieces, and let them
dry, or else form small balls of it, of the size of a small
nut or larger; then roll them in meal powder and put them
up to dry.

*To prepare a Globe which burns like a Star, and leap
about both on Land and Water.*

CAUSE a globe to be turned of dry wood, whose dia
meter is the length of a half pound or a pound rocket
divide this globe into two equal parts, in the middle of one
of the half globes, on the inside, make a cavity, deep, long
and wide enough to hold three or four rockets or crackers
so that the other half of the globe may be easily and closely
fitted upon them, after this take three crackers, one with
strong reports and two without any, place them so into the hol
low, that the head of the one may lay to the others neck, and
be so ordered that as soon as the one is spent, the other may
take fire and force the globe back, and thus alternately from
one to the other till it comes to the report, which finishes
Care must be taken that the fire passes not from the first
to the next cracker, before it has quite consumed the first,
but as I have given a caution in the article about rockets that
run on a cord, the same may be observed here

Having taken care to fix the rockets, cover them with the
other half globe, and join them firmly with strong pasted
paper

*To charge Globes, which leap on Land, with Iron and
Paper Crackers*

TAKE a hollow wooden globe, which has a touch-hole
at the top, in the form of a small cylinder, fill it
with an aquatic composition quite full, then bore into the
charge

charge five or fix holes about half an inch wide, in which put iron petards or crackers, which run tapering, provide them at the lower end with a fmall touch-hole, and cover the top with a tin-plate, in which there is four holes, which you muft clofe up with wads of paper or tow, after you have filled them with the beft corn-powder, and when you fire them on even ground, you will fee them leap as often as a cracker goes off. See fig. 61.

The other fort is not much unlike the firft, except that to this you add a certain number of crackers, which are difpofed as you may obferve in Fig. 62. A the crackers, B the touch-hole.

How the Globes difcharg'd out of a Mortar, are made and ordered.

FIRST find the mouth of the mortar, and divide it in twelve parts, then have a globe turn'd of wood, which is two diameters of the mouth high, divide the diameter in fix equal parts, and let the height between A and C be the diameter of the globe, the radius of the femi circle C I, fhall be one fixth, or half the height of the globe, the thicknefs of the wood H I, fhall be $\frac{1}{12}$ of the above diameter, and the thicknefs of the cover of the diameter of the globe; the diameter of the cavity of the globe five fixths of its whole diameter, the height of the priming chamber B F fhall be one fixth and a half of the diameter, but its breadth only one fixth, the diameter of the touch hole is one fourth or one fixth of that of the chamber. for the better underftanding thefe directions, fee Fig 63.

The manner of filling thefe globes is thus.

Take hollow canes or common reeds, cut them into lengths to fit the cavity of the globe, and fill them with a weak compofition made of three parts of meal powder, two of coal, and one of brimftone, moiften'd with a little linfeed oil; excepting the lower ends of them which reft upon the bottom of the globe, which muft have meal-powder only, moiften'd likewife with the fame oil, or fprinkled over with brandy and dry'd the bottom of the globe cover with meal-powder mix'd with an equal quantity of corn-powder, the reed

being

being fill'd in this manner, fet as many of them upright in
the cavity of the globe, as it will contain, then cover it well
at top; and wrap it up with a cloth dip'd in glue, the priming muſt be of the ſame compoſition with the reeds

The globes repreſented, N° 97 and 98 are contrived like
the above, only the firſt of theſe is fill'd with running rock
ets, and the laſt with crackers, ſtars, and ſparks, interſperſed
with meal-powder, and put promiſcuouſly over the crackers,
the figures are ſo plain, that I need not give any further ex
planation.

N° 99 is the repreſentation of a globe, which plainly
ſhews its conſtruction the great globe which contains the
leſſer is the ſame as deſcribed above, for it is charged with
running rockets; as that of 97. However with this difference, that this is lined but with ſingle rockets, and the other
is fill'd up with them. In the midſt of theſe rockets fix a
globe in a cylindrical form, with a flat bottom, and a chamber and touch-hole at A, the cavity of this inner globe is
fill'd with iron crackers, and cover'd with a flat covering
the priming chamber fill with the ſame compoſition as has
been directed for the above globes, the fuzees muſt be
fill'd with good meal-powder

N° 100 ſhews another ſort of globe, which is prepared
thus Firſt get a wooden globe, in the middle whereof fix
a mortar with a little chamber for powder, round which form
a lodge, for ranging paper tubes, this lodge muſt have a
groove or channel, fill'd with meal powder, to convey the
fire all round, this done, put a globe into the mortar, fill'd
with running rockets, crackers, reeds, or ſtars and ſparks,
and having placed your paper tubes fill'd with running rock
ets round the groove, cover them about with ſtrong paſted
paper and cloth, dipp'd in glue, as has been directed. The
figure of this globe will illuſtrate the deſcription, A ſhews
the mortar, B the touch-hole, C the priming chamber, D
the priming of the mortar, E in the other figure repreſents
the order in which the paper tubes are placed upon the
groove.

To form Letters, and all Sorts of Figures which may be represented in the open Air in a dark Night.

PROVIDE a wooden globe of the same form, height, breadth and thickness, as those already describ'd, only the priming chamber must be the height and breadth of one sixth of the diameter of the whole globe. Besides this chamber there must be another B, for corn-powder, the height and breadth must be equal $\frac{1}{6}$ of the diameter of the globe, the vent-hole must be a quarter of the powder or priming chamber, you must also have another globe in a cylindrical form, the bottom of which must be rounded on the outside, as may be observed in the same figure by F, the cover must be let a little into the inner surface of the cover of the great globe, to keep it firm, placing this lesser globe perpendicularly over the chamber, which is fill'd with corn powder.

Fill the cavity of the little globe with running rockets, stars and sparks, as may be seen in the figure at the bottom of the large globe, having furnished the vent-hole with meal and the chamber with corn powder, put about the small globe the same composition, mix'd promiscuously together, and on this fit a flat wooden ring, very tight to the globe, in which bore holes, as you see in Fig. 101. Your globe being thus prepared, take two long thin slips of whale-bone, which bend easily without breaking, join them together parallel, so as to have their bendings opposite to each other, and make a straight piece, take two of these long pieces and join them as is seen in A by two shorter pieces at both ends, so as to make a right-angled paralellogram, R S T U, within this frame form your letters either of wire or whale-bone, placing each about a hands breadth from the other, and having fix'd your letters, wrap them neatly round in quick tow from one end to the other, taking care that none of it entangle about the frame, least when the letters burn, their flame should be confounded in one another, then steep your letters in brandy, wherein before you have dissolv'd some gum-arabick, and in drying strew them over with meal-powder, if you would have your letters descend perpendicular to the horizon, you must fasten

two

two small weights to your frame, at T and U, but if parallel to the plane of the horizon, you must have a weight at
each corner, having order'd it thus, bend it round to go in
the inner circumference of the great globe, and let it rest
perpendicular on the wooden ring, and fill the empty places
about the letters with meal powder, then cover it up, and
prepare the globe fit for the mortar, as usual, it will have
a delightful effect.

To prepare the *Quick Tow*

TAKE either flax, hemp or cotton, of two or three strands,
twist them slightly, and put them into a clean glaz'd earthen pan, pour on them good white wine-vinegar four parts,
urine two parts, brandy one part, purified saltpetre one part,
meal-powder one part, boil it all together over a quick fire,
and till all the moisture is evaporated, then strew meal-powder on an even board, and roll your match therein, then let it
dry either in the sun or shade This sort of match burns and
consumes very quick, but if you would have it burn slower,
make the liquor weaker, boiling the match in saltpetre and
vinegar only, and strewing meal-powder in it, let it dry

Another sort of match is made by some which is not
twisted at all, but only dip'd in brandy for some hours,
then powdered over with meal-powder and dry'd, some
dissolve a little gum-arabic or tragacant in the brandy, this
will make it stick the better to any thing

To prepare the light *Balls*, proper to be used at Bon-fires.

TAKE two pound of crude-antimony, four pound of
brimstone, four pound of rosin, and four pound of
coal, and half a pound of pitch, having powdered all these
ingredients, put them into a kettle or glaz'd earthen
pan, over a coal fire, and let it melt; then throw as much
hemp or flax into it as may be sufficient to soak it up,
then take it off the fire, and whilst it is cooling, form
it into balls.

You may wrap them up in tow, and put them either into
rockets or globes.

To

To prepare the Paste for Stars and Sparks

TAKE five ounces and a half of meal powder, one pound twelve ounces of brimstone. *Or,*

Take three pound of meal powder, six pound of saltpetre, one pound of brimstone, two pound of camphir, and two ounces of tanner's bark or saw-dust. Moisten all these ingredients with linseed oil.

Take meal-powder one pound, saltpetre four pound, brimstone half a pound, and powder'd glass six ounces; moistened with a little linseed oil.

Saltpetre half a pound, brimstone two ounces, antimony one ounce, and meal-powder three ounces.

Saltpetre half a pound, brimstone three ounces, antimony one ounce, and iron file-dust half an ounce.

Saltpetre two pound, meal-powder ten pound, and brimstone one pound.

Saltpetre one pound, brimstone half a pound, meal-powder three ounces, and antimony one ounce.

Having mixed and prepared your ingredients, boil some flax in saltpetre lee and camphir, then cut it small and mix it up with any of the above compositions which must be moistened with either the white of eggs, gum, or size form this into little balls of the size of a hazel-nut, strew them over with meal powder and let them dry.

To cause the stars to burn very bright, make your composition of one ounce and three quarters of saltpetre, three quarters of an ounce of brimstone, and a quarter of an ounce of powder.

Saltpetre two pound, brimstone fourteen pound and a half, and meal-powder six ounces.

The paste or melted stuff above mentioned, is also made use of for the same purpose, wrapt in tow.

To project Globes from a Mortar, and the Quantity of Powder required for that Purpose

THE globes being of wood, it is requisite that the charges for them should be agreeable to their substance, for which end they are first weighed, allowing for each pound of its weight a quarter of an ounce of gun-powder. For example, if your globe weighs forty pound, you must, to difcharge it, allow ten ounces of powder

The charge is thus performed: put the powder into the chamber of the mortar, and cover it with ftraw, hay, hemp or flax, fo as to fill it quite full, or if the chamber of the mortar be too big, get one turned of wood equal in height and breadth to the chamber of the mortar, that contains the charge of powder required, pierce this with a red hot wire, from the bottom of the wood to the centre of the bottom of the chamber in it, not perpendicular but flanting, as from *c* to *b* in Fig. A. The place, where the touch-hole begins, muft be mark'd, fo that you may turn it to correfpond with the touch-hole of the mortar. When you would load your mortar, cover the bottom of the chamber with a little meal and corn powder, mix'd together, and upon that put the wooden chamber, in which is the powder requir'd to difcharge the globe, then fix the touch-hole of the globe exactly upon the chamber, wrapping it in hemp, &c to make it ftand upright

The mortars contrived on purpofe for globes are more commodious, and one is more certain in projecting them: thefe are caft as follows: the length of the mortar with the chamber, without the bottom, is two diameters of the mouth, the bottom is one fifth thick, the chamber is half the diameter of the mouth long, and a quarter wide, oval at bottom; the fides are an eighth of the diameter of the mouth thick, which is increafed at bottom to a third, the thicknefs about the chamber is a fourth part.

Some prepare thefe balls with faltpetre four pound, brimftone one pound and a half, powder half a pound, antimony fix ounces, and charcoal half an ounce.

Saltpetre four pound, brimftone three pound, camphir a quarter of a pound, and powder half a pound.

FINIS.

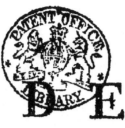

INDEX.

Illumi-

An INDEX.

An INDEX.

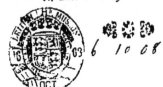

Lightning Source UK Ltd.
Milton Keynes UK
UKOW05f0246140716

278363UK00010B/449/P